WOMEN in HEALTH & ILLNESS

LIFE EXPERIENCES AND CRISES

Diane K. Kjervik, R.N., M.S., J.D.

Associate Professor, School of Nursing, Adjunct Faculty, Women's Studies,
University of Minnesota, Minneapolis, Minnesota

Ida M. Martinson, R.N., Ph.D.

Professor and Chair, Department of Family Health Care Nursing, School of Nursing,
University of California, San Francisco, San Francisco, California

1986   W.B. SAUNDERS COMPANY

Philadelphia ○ London ○ Toronto ○ Mexico City ○ Rio de Janeiro ○ Sydney ○ Tokyo ○ Hong Kong

W. B. Saunders Company: West Washington Square
Philadelphia, PA 19105

Library of Congress Cataloging-in-Publication Data

Women in health and illness: life experiences and crises.

1. Women—Mental Health. 2. Stress (Psychology). 3. Women—
Psychology. 4. Life change events.   I. Kjervik, Diane K.,
1945–   II. Martinson, Ida Marie, 1936– . [DNLM: 1.
Life Change Events. 2. Stress, Psychological. 3. Women—
psychology. WM 172 W872]

RC451.4.W6W656 1986   155.6′33   86-6576

ISBN 0–7216–2086–8

Editor: Dudley Kay
Designer: Bill Donnelly
Production Manager: Bill Preston
Manuscript Editor: W. B. Saunders Staff
Illustration Coordinator: Walt Verbitski
Indexer: David Harvey

Women in Health and Illness: Life Experiences and Crises   ISBN 0–7216–2086–8

Last digit is the print number: 9   8   7   6   5   4   3   2   1

CONTRIBUTORS

Marie Albrecht-Sundt, R.N., M.S.
Assistant Professor (Retired), University of Minnesota School of Nursing
Forsyth, Montana
The Experience of Widowhood

Holly Branch, R.N., M.S., C.S.
Health Counseling Services
St. Louis Park, Minnesota
Women in Pain

Kathleen Dineen, M.S.N., C.N.M.
Assistant Professor and Director, Nurse-Midwifery Program, University of Minnesota School of Nursing
Minneapolis, Minnesota
The Stress of Infertility

Ruth Dyer, R.N., M.S.
Menopause: A Closer Look for Nurses

Karen Storlie Finck, R.N., M.S.
Health Counseling Services
St. Louis Park, Minnesota
The Potential Health Care Crisis of Hysterectomy

Verona C. Gordon, R.N., Ph.D.
Professor, University of Minnesota School of Nursing
Minneapolis, Minnesota
Divorce and Depression in Women

Rosemary Huerter, R.N., M.S.
Deceased
Female Sexuality

Marjorie Jamieson, R.N., M.S.
Chair, Board of Directors, St. Anthony Block Nurse Program
St. Paul, Minnesota
Women and Chemicals

La Vohn E. Josten, R.N., Ph.D., F.A.A.N.
Director of Public Health Nursing, Minnesota Department of Health
Minneapolis, Minnesota
Child Abuse

Thomas Kiresuk, Ph.D.
Chief and Clinical Psychologist, Hennepin County Medical Center; Director, Program Evaluation Resource Center
Minneapolis, Minnesota
Impact of Rape on Victims and Families: Treatment and Research Considerations

Diane K. Kjervik, R.N., M.S., J.D.
Associate Professor, School of Nursing; Adjunct Faculty, Women's Studies, University of Minnesota
Minneapolis, Minnesota
A Conceptualization of Women's Stress; Dependency in Women; Sexism and Its Resulting Effect on the Mental Health of Women

Marcea E. Kjervik, R.N., M.S., C.S.
Clinical Nurse Specialist, Hennepin County Mental Health Center
Crystal, Minnesota
Eating Disorders and Women

Linda Ledray, R.N., Ph.D., F.A.A.N.
Director, Sexual Assault Research Service
Minneapolis, Minnesota
Impact of Rape on Victims and Families: Treatment and Research Considerations

Sandra G. Lindell, M.S., C.N.M.
Instructor, University of Minnesota School of Nursing
Minneapolis, Minnesota
The Stress of Infertility

Sander Lund, A.B.
Associate Director, Program Evaluation Research Center, Hennepin County Medical Center
Minneapolis, Minnesota
Impact of Rape on Victims and Families: Treatment and Research Considerations

Ida M. Martinson, R.N., Ph.D., F.A.A.N.
Professor and Chair, Department of Family Health Care Nursing, School of Nursing, University of California, San Francisco
San Francisco, California
Older Women's Health Care; Loss of the Child: Two Case Studies

Beverly LaBelle McElmurry, Ed.D., F.A.A.N.
Professor, College of Nursing, University of Illinois
Chicago, Illinois
Health Appraisal of Low-Income Women

Linda Crockett McKeever, R.N., M.S.N.
Santa Ana, California
Older Women's Health Care; Menopause: A Closer Look for Nurses

Marie Menikheim, R.N., M.S.
Interim Executive Director, Minnesota Nurses Association
St. Paul, Minnesota
Communication Patterns of Women and Nurses

Miriam Watkins Meyers
Professor of Communications, Metropolitan State University
St. Paul, Minnesota
Communication Patterns of Women and Nurses

Georgia K. Millor, M.S., R.N., D.N.S.
Assistant Professor, School of Nursing, University of Rochester
Rochester, New York
Child Abuse

Elizabeth G. Morrison, D.N.S., R.N., C.S.
Professor, School of Nursing, University of Alabama
Birmingham, Alabama
Lesbians

Elizabeth A. Peterson, R.N., M.S.
Assistant Professor of Nursing, Bethel College
St. Paul, Minnesota
Dependency in Women

Sharon L. Rising, R.N., C.N.M.
Cheshire, Connecticut
Childbearing: Its Dilemmas

Catherine Schabot, R.N., B.S.N.
Assistant Director of Nursing Services, St. Mary's Rehabilitation Center
Minneapolis, Minnesota
Women and Chemicals

Kathleen Sodergren, R.N., M.S.N.
Assistant Professor, University of Minnesota School of Nursing
Minneapolis, Minnesota
Health Assessment

Carol Valenti, R.N., B.S.N., M.S.W., A.C.S.W.
Psychotherapist, West Hennepin Community Mental Health Center
Minnetonka, Minnesota
Working with the Physically Abused Woman

Mary G. Weisensee, R.N., Ph.D.
Assistant Professor, University of Minnesota School of Nursing
Minneapolis, Minnesota
Women's Health Perceptions in a Male-Dominated Medical World

PREFACE

This book, *Women in Health and Illness: Life Experiences and Crises,* by Diane Kjervik and Ida Martinson, is an outgrowth of our first book on issues related to women, *Women in Stress: A Nursing Perspective,* which appeared in press several years ago. The personal encouragement by various leading women theorists, especially Angela McBride, who encouraged us on numerous occasions to continue to develop material on women's studies, was extremely important.

Stress was a popular concept then, but as time passed, the book needed to have major revisions, for stress had been heavily examined and the complexity of the stress reaction was more fully appreciated. "Illness" in the title does not reflect merely physical illness; for example, we do not discuss diabetes or stroke. The illness talked about in this book is the broader social illness of tragedy for both children and women.

All contributors from the first book were encouraged to bring their material up to date, and numerous new authors were added, so this is a new book with materials that may be used both inside and outside the nursing profession. Students and teachers of nursing courses focusing on women's health and illness may consider this book as a text, because a framework for understanding the nature of a woman's health status throughout her life cycle and methods to assist her when crises develop are addressed. Women's studies faculty will find the book useful in presenting the myriad life experiences and crises facing women in the context of the changing societal roles of women and men.

Students and faculty of nursing and women's studies will benefit from this material, and ultimately the clients of nurses and recipients of the evolving philosophies of women's studies will also be served. Our contributors have been patient, our publisher has been brave, and we hope you will learn as we have from unique authors who shared much with us for you.

D. KJERVIK

I. MARTINSON

CONTENTS

I

WOMEN'S STRESS AND HEALTH

II

BIOPSYCHOSOCIAL FACTORS IN HEALTH AND ILLNESS

III

WOMEN'S LIFE EXPERIENCES AND
THEIR RESOLUTIONS

IV

LOSS

WOMEN'S STRESS AND HEALTH

This first section begins with a chapter on women's stress, continues with information regarding health assessment and the perceptions of women in dealing with a male-dominated medical profession, and then concludes with a chapter regarding older women and their special health concerns.

1

A CONCEPTUAL-
IZATION OF
WOMEN'S STRESS

DIANE KJERVIK

In this chapter Diane Kjervik conceptualizes women's stress. She states her assumptions underlying the concepts and provides a description of the relationship between stress and self-esteem, adaptability, motivations, and power. She closes with suggestions for nursing interventions and the role of women helping women.

Stress, as it affects a woman's life, can be understood as existing within a woman or as coming from outside a woman. She may experience the stress subjectively, in which case her feeling of stress is in response to external or internal stressor events; or stress may be seen as impinging upon her, leading to her efforts to adapt or cope with the stress. In either view of stress, energy is necessary to cope with the situation. Some authors define stress as encompassing both the internal reaction and the external stressor events.[1] The conceptualization of stress here presented adopts the former view of stress as a subjective experience of the woman.

Stress that is experienced by the woman is either positive in nature when it helps her grow or negative in nature when it thwarts or diminishes growth. Stress becomes positive when the woman's positive internal adaptors to stress outweigh the negative stress factors (Fig. 1.1). Negative stress occurs when negative stress factors inside the woman outweigh the positive adaptors. Numerous variables such as age, economic status, number of children, race, religion or cultural heritage become negative stress factors or positive adaptors, depending on the type of stress experienced by the woman. For instance, a large number of children could be a negative stress factor when a woman gives birth to an additional child but a positive adaptor when one child dies and the other children form a supportive network for their mother. The cultural variable places a special burden on women because of the underevaluation of women in society. Reinforced every day in the media are images of helpless women, women sex objects, or "absent" women (for example, in movies with few if any women present). Women must endure insults from men who are sexual harassers or abusers. The devaluation of women by society usually becomes a negative stress factor inside a woman. Only rarely has she creatively found a way to use devaluation to her advantage (for example, by seeing a verbally abusive remark about women as an opportunity to learn how to deal with such aggression). This advantage quickly becomes a disadvantage as the woman's energy is overly drained.

Certain assumptions underlie this conceptualization of women's stress. First, life contains intrinsic paradoxes, ironies, and stressful circumstances (stressors) that exist within a woman and in the world external to her. Concurrently, alleviators of stress exist both within a woman and external to her. A woman will be aware of some of these stressors and alleviators but probably not all of them, unless she has undergone extensive self-analysis. Sec-

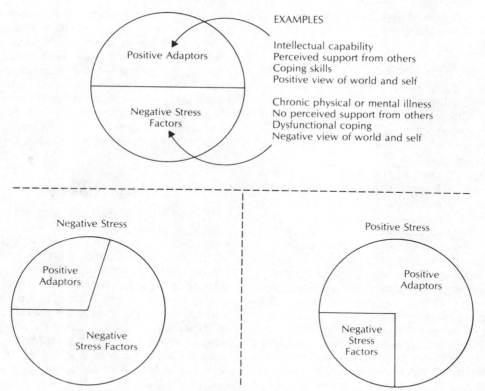

Figure 1.1. Female adaptation to stress.

ond, a woman may move toward positive or negative adaptation to stress. She will have no control over some events, (for instance, the death of a friend). But in response to such an event, she may draw on her internal positive adaptors. Third, when negative stress factors outweigh positive adaptors (negative stress), the woman will experience the effect of this stress in subjective reactions, such as pain, fear, anxiety, or illness. Positive stress is experienced as stimulation, creativity, or euphoria. Finally, stress is an innate part of health that is experienced in different ways at different times. Health may be viewed as a complex phenomenon, within which exist states of passive balance to states of dynamic change, and striving for wellness.[2] Health may also be viewed as a life process to be experienced.[3] Stress as a subjective life experience is part of either view of health.

STRESS AND SELF-ESTEEM

Whenever a woman can look within herself and identify stressors and alleviators of stress, she steps closer to improved self-esteem. Her self-awareness means she experiences her state of health. When she moves beyond identifica-

tion to action, she further improves her self-esteem. Her first step is learning what stresses her; that is, what happens inside and outside herself that precedes her subjective experience of stress. Next, she can become aware of resources outside and inside herself that she can use to cope with the stress she feels. Because women have learned to be dependent on others economically and for a sense of self-identity, they will often try to seek outside help before they can appreciate their inner resources.

When a woman learns how to reach out for a resource that does, in fact, help her, and when she learns to draw on her inner resources for help in diminishing negative stress, she learns to appreciate, like, and value herself.

Women must learn to deal positively with stressors that are common to both males and females (such as the loss of a parent) and stressors that are common only to females, (such as pregnancy, hysterectomy, and the cultural denigration of women). If she is able to experience these stressors as positive stress, she will develop self-esteem. The self-esteem will give her energy that will be available for work and play, increased competence in work and interactions with others, and self-growth.

She will feel steadily more satisfied with her own femininity and her humanness.

STRESS AND ADAPTABILITY

Successful resolution of negative stress requires adaptability on the woman's part. She must be able to shift from one behavior, feeling, or thought to another. This is where women's ability to compromise becomes useful. Women have learned that to be accepted in a male-oriented world, they must sacrifice their own perceptions, values, and beliefs. They must somehow incorporate negative images of the female. Some women incorporate these images so thoroughly that they display promasculine values and beliefs openly (for example, by espousing the inferiority of females, fighting against equal rights for women, or developing arguments supportive of female masochism). Other women who have incorporated negative views of the female allow masculine domination and degradation of women to go on without comment. Believing they are inferior, they allow the perceived superiors to influence and dominate them.

Whereas this form of compromise has been detrimental to women, the ability to compromise as a skill is valuable in adapting to negative stress. The woman is able to change a pattern of behavior or a belief that has been detrimental to her self-esteem. Her ability to change can then be considered the striving for wellness. She can use her ability to compromise to benefit herself, rather than to cater to others. This moves her from a negative caretaking role to a positive caring role. Instead of caretaking through supporting negative behaviors of others by excusing them from the effects of their irresponsibility or giving unsolicited help, she will care by allowing them to feel the effects of their failure and giving what she has the genuine capacity and willingness to give. Caring for others in a way that facilitates their growth rather than their dependence will reward the woman. Her self-esteem will improve and be added to her list of positive adaptors.

STRESS AS A POSITIVE FORCE

As is true with beauty, stress exists in the eye of the beholder. With stress, the important beholder is the woman herself. When she feels stress, she is in stress. If an outsider does not find an obvious reason for the stress, for instance, no situational or developmental stressor events, the woman's feeling of stress is no less real. In order to respond to the stress, she must generate energy, so in a sense, stress becomes an energy impetus.

Once energy is generated, it becomes available for use by the woman in developing new coping skills, changing old detrimental attitudes, and making more fulfilling interpersonal connections. Stress, therefore, can be a positive force in moving the woman toward growth, self-fulfillment, and the health state of wellness.

STRESS AND POWER

Women have been kept from positions of power outside a very narrow sphere of influence. Women have exerted power within the home as household managers or within the organizations of certain occupations such as nursing or clerical work. But women have, until recently, exerted little group influence over public policy or over their own economic or social status. There is evidence that persons who are powerless have higher levels of stress than those who are powerful.[2] Women must learn to reclaim or acquire power in order to reduce their stress.

The acquisition of power by women can be made without apology or deference to others. As one takes more responsibility for oneself and learns to depend less on others economically and psychologically, one is empowered. One's negative stress is lessened by the actions of oneself. A positive sign of growth is the ability to care for oneself without expecting or needing others to reduce one's stress. (This is not to say that other persons play no role in the reduction of stress.) The woman's relationship to others is different; the woman directs her own life such that she determines what kind of help is needed and who can be of help. This is a far cry from helplessly waiting for the solution to her problem to appear magically.

The negative stress that a woman feels when she is in a position of relative powerlessness can serve as a cue to the need to reclaim or acquire power over her life circumstances. In this sense, negative stress serves as a tool of empowerment. It signals the woman's need to act on her own behalf.

NURSING INTERVENTION

Helping a woman to confront situations that produce stress for her involves a thorough assessment of external or internal stressor events and both positive adaptors and negative stress factors within the woman. The stressor event might be rape, incest, death, pregnancy, marriage, or any other situational or developmental change that results in stress to the woman. Negative stress itself is reported as pain, anxiety, illness, grief, anger, or other internal responses that indicate that the woman feels a sense of imbalance as opposed to her steady internal state of equilibrium.

Intervention is focused on moving the woman away from negative stress factors such as low self-esteem to positive adaptors (that is, those elements that aid her growth). Garland and Bush have classified coping behaviors as either adaptive or maladaptive and subdivided each category into conscious or unconscious types of coping.[5] The notion of unconscious coping skills implies the need of nursing assessment that goes beyond the woman's self-report. Her methods of coping may be beyond her awareness, and therefore, the nurse must examine the woman's actions and the meaning implied from her words. An example of an unconscious coping skill is projection, in which the woman allows other persons in the environment to carry her own emotional load for her. The allowing, however, occurs on an unconscious level, and as she becomes more self-aware, she reowns these lost emotional aspects of herself.

In addition to increasing the woman's self-awareness, nursing intervention strives to increase the woman's knowledge of her power in stressful situations and her willingness to exercise that power. Anne Wilson Schaef correctly points out the caveat that if a woman is told that she has power too early in therapeutic process, her belief in her own inferiority and stupidity will be reinforced rather than alleviated.[6] She will feel stupid, because she did not know she had this power. Schaef suggests that a woman's perceptions of the world must first be acknowledged, even if they are self-denigrating perceptions.[7] Acknowledgment by the caregivers does not mean approval; acknowledgment means recognition of the woman's view of the world and herself in a society where her perceptions have been and continue to be undervalued or overlooked entirely.

In a support group for female rape victims that I conducted, the victims talked in the early sessions about the rapists, not in angry tones, but with concern for how ashamed and miserable the rapists must now feel about what they had done. As the expression of these feelings was accepted through acknowledgment by the leaders of the group, the victims moved to the subject of their own grief and anger over what had happened to them.

Once the woman recognizes her power of choice to act in one of several possible ways in response to her negative stress, she will exercise her choice timidly at first, and later more boldly. She begins choicemaking very carefully, because she does not know how others around will respond to her choice. As she presents her own limits to others, she discovers that one or two friends disappear because they had counted on her adaptation to their needs and wants. She discovers that she can survive the loss of one or two friends and that other friends can be found who appreciate her openness and her ability to take care of herself (that is, to not enter into a dependent relationship with them). Her perception of a supportive person will change from the expectation that a supportive person is one who solves her problems for her to one who listens carefully to her, gives some suggestions, but encourages the woman to exercise her own power of choice. With the redefinition of support, the woman will discover, or perceive, more support from those around her. As her ability to solve her own problems increases, so too will her self-esteem. Thus, her view of herself and her support system will become positive adaptors.

One clarification is needed concerning the positive view of the world mentioned as a positive adaptor in Diagram 1. To perceive our society as sexist is a negative view of society. However, within the sexist society are forces that resist the sexism, which are also capable of being perceived. When a woman has a positive view of herself and the world, she focuses primarily on those elements of society that nurture the feminine spirit rather than on those that seek to subvert or destroy it.

Nursing intervention should also focus on negative stress prevention with clients who are at risk; that is, those in whom negative stress factors exist but who have not yet experienced the stressful event. Working with women to increase their self-esteem and teach them healthy coping behaviors prepares them for the stressful event. For instance, childbirth preparation is useful, because the woman learns how to cope with the pain and how to use a support person throughout labor and delivery. Similar preparation is used to get people ready for retirement. More difficult is preparation for the emotional pain accompanying loss of a spouse or dear friend, or for the disruption of self-esteem after the loss of

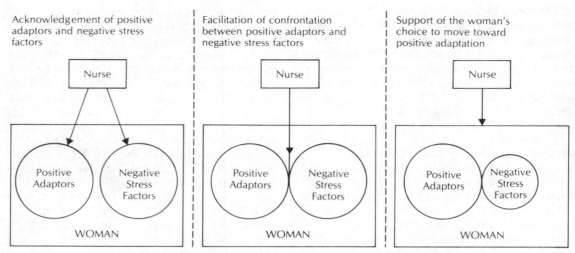

Acknowledgement of positive adaptors and negative stress factors

Facilitation of confrontation between positive adaptors and negative stress factors

Support of the woman's choice to move toward positive adaptation

Figure 1.2. The nurse's role as negotiator in situations that produce stress.

bodily function following an accident or accompanying the aging process.

Whether the nurse intervenes before the negative stress is felt by the woman or afterward, the principle of enhancing positive adaptors and diminishing negative stress factors remains. The nurse acts as an agent of negotiation in helping the woman to confront these aspects of herself (Fig. 1.2). When the negative stress factors within the woman predominate, the nurse encourages the woman's positive adaptors to be expressed. When her positive adaptors predominate but she is not making needed changes for growth, the nurse acquaints her with the remnants of negative stress factors still within her that are blocking her growth and change. Psychodrama can be used to assist the negotiation between the competing facets within the woman. The resulting self-awareness and self-confrontation demonstrate graphically to the woman that she can choose which aspect of herself to believe in, to use, and to display to others. She can nourish either a strong, kind, competent image of herself, or a weak, mean, useless image. She can focus on the cruel, unjust, and harsh forces within the world or on the spirited, enlightened, and humane forces.

WOMEN HELPING WOMEN

Female nurses are in a position to offer special help to women experiencing negative stress. Because female nurses experience being women in a society that undervalues their contributions, they can sympathize with female clients' pain from being overlooked and unappreciated. Because they are women, female nurses can also perceive and value the growing female consciousness in society and can rec-

ognize the attempts by their female clients to connect with the efforts of many women to assert their newly appreciated perceptions of the world and themselves.

This is not to imply that male nurses have nothing to offer female clients, for example, regarding changing male-female roles. Male nurses have an opportunity to demonstrate what a sensitive, nurturing male can give to a self-respecting female. What is implied here is that female nurses have something special to offer by virtue of their experience as women in a sexist society, and our purpose is to spell out the nature of this special skill. Although it cannot be overlooked that recent studies have shown that male attitudes toward women have not been adapting to the changing roles of women,[8-11] the opportunity is there for male nurses to break the male norm of resistance to the change.

Self-aware female nurses understand firsthand the nature of self-deprecation. They know about women denigrating other women, because they have observed it. They know about women not valuing other women and not valuing themselves, because they have read about it in respectable research journals.[12-15] They know about self-denigration after self-analysis, in which they discover their own harsh self-criticism and perfectionism. They learn that they have incorporated into their own self-images society's negative images of women; and after they learn this, they act to overcome the self-deprecation.

Through the struggle with self-deprecation, female nurses learn how this negative stress factor can be confronted. In fact, they learn that there must be a grappling with the internal self-hatred if the female client is to know herself thoroughly. Also, overcoming internalized attitudes of female self-deprecation in the student is necessary to supervising female student family therapists, because if the female supervisor is to be accepted as a positive role model, the student's negative opinion of women must be addressed and overcome.[16] Likewise, if the role modeling of a female nurse is to be accepted by a female client, the denigration of women must be addressed directly. If the role modeling of the nurse can be accepted, the female client will observe a female nurse functioning competently in a patriarchal system and working to redefine that sytem. The client, therefore, is more likely to value and appreciate advice given by the nurse.

CONCLUSION

Women's stress can be conceptualized as a subjective experience in response to stressor events originating either outside or inside the woman. Awareness of this subjective experience can be considered an important part of health, because the woman is then in touch with her own life process and state of wellness. The woman's ability to use the stress as a positive impetus for growth depends on her adjustment of her inner balance toward positive adaptors and away from negative stress factors. The nurse acts as a negotiator between the competing internal forces within the woman and uses her own self-awareness of the growth process as a guidepost in helping her female client to choose positive adaptation to stress.

References

1. Garland, L. M., and Bush, C.T. *Coping Behaviors and Nursing*. Reston, VA: Reston Publishing Company, 1982, p. 24.

2. Dunn, H. L. High level wellness for man and society. *American Journal of Public Health*, Vol. 49, no. 6, 1959, pp. 786–792.

3. Newman, M. Newman's health theory. *In* Clements, I., and Roberts, F. *Family Health: A Theoretical Approach to Nursing Care.* New York, NY: John Wiley and Sons, 1983, p. 168.

4. Horwitz, A. Sex-Role Expectations, Power, and Psychological Distress. *Sex Roles: A Journal of Research*, Vol. 8, no. 6, June 1982, p. 619.

5. Garland and Bush, p. 115.

6. Schaef, Anne Wilson. *Women's Reality*. Minneapolis, MN: Winston Press, Inc., 1981, p. 96.

7. Ibid., p. 91.

8. Stolk, Y. and Brotherton, P. Attitudes towards single women. *Sex Roles: A Journal of Research*, Vol. 7, no. 1, Jan. 1981, p. 77.

9. Benson, R., and Jerdee, T. H. Perceived sex differences in managerially relevant characteristics. *Sex Roles: A Journal of Research*, Vol. 4, no. 6, Dec. 1978, pp. 837–843.

10. Brooks-Gunn, J., and Fisch, M. Psychological androgyny and college students' judgments of mental health for women. *Sex Roles: A Journal of Research*, Vol. 6, no. 4, August 1980, p. 575.

11. Aslin, A. L. Feminist and community mental health center psychotherapists' expectations of mental health for women. *Sex Roles: A Journal of Research*, Vol. 3, no. 6, Dec. 1977, p. 537.

12. Woodward, C., et al. Client, treatment and therapist variables related to outcomes in brief systems-oriented family therapy. *Family Process*, Vol. 20, no. 2, June 1981, p. 196.

13. Deaux, K. Self-evaluations of male and female managers. *Sex Roles: A Journal of Research*, Vol. 5, no. 5, Oct. 1979, p. 571.

14. Kutner, N. G., and Brogan, D. R. Problems of colleagueship for women entering the medical profession. *Sex roles: A Journal of Research*, Vol. 7, no. 7, July 1981, p. 739.

15. Gruber, K., and Gaebelein, J. Sex differences in listening comprehension. *Sex Roles: A Journal of Research*, Vol. 5, no. 3, June 1979, p. 299.

16. Caust, B. L., Libow, J. A., and Raskin, P. A. Challenges and promises of training women as family systems therapists. *Family Process*, Vol. 20, no. 4, Dec. 1981, p. 443.

2

HEALTH ASSESSMENT

KATHLEEN SODERGREN

This chapter by Kathleen Sodergren addresses the values concept of health as a disease-free state, as a social role, and as the ability to contribute to the economic system; and then describes the health history and physical examination, including skin, hair, nails, mucosa, and the gynecologic examination. The chapter closes with an assessment of the social and economic roles of women.

The health of women has been a major concern throughout history. Although in America women live longer than men, have lower mortality rates for most illnesses, appear to have a genetic advantage over men, particularly regarding recessive traits carried on the X chromosome, women have been shown to report more illness than men. Many reasons for these differences have been suggested, including (1) that what constitutes illness has been defined by physicians (that is, men) and therefore reflects a sex bias, as demonstrated by the fact that female reproductive functions and feminine traits in general are tinged with illness attributions; (2) that women report more illness than men do, because it is culturally more acceptable for them to do so; and (3) women have more illness than men, because their roles are more stressful.[1]

In determining the health status of women, the persons interested in fostering the health status of women must consider these hypotheses, determine for themselves an acceptable definition as to what constitutes health, and determine indices of health with which to make judgments about the health status of the individual woman. It is for this reason that we begin this discussion of assessment of women's health with reference to these hypotheses and a brief discussion of several views of health.

HEALTH AS AN IDEA

Health is an evaluative concept based on a set of values a person has about the state of affairs that should exist in some realm of one's being. What constitutes health for the fundamentalist Christian, the militant feminist, the traditional physician, and the barefoot doctor is very similar in some respects and differs greatly in others.

Health as a Disease-Free State

In its simplest form, health is defined as the absence of disease. Using this definition places one in the difficult position of first demonstrating that no disease indicators are present before reaching a judgment about the presence of health. Given this definition, there probably is no independent entity one can call health. Although it is somewhat negative, this is the idea of health to which most persons refer when asked about the state of their health. This is the definition of health on which the traditional medical history and physical examination are based. Its usefulness in providing a basis for practice in the health disciplines is difficult to deny.

Tillich[2] elaborates on this view of health in a philosophically consistent manner by clarifying the realm of the person's being that sets the boundaries for a discussion of health. The life processes, in Tillich's view, consist of a dialectic between self-alteration and self-identity; that is, between "going out from" oneself and "turning into" oneself within every dimension of one's being, from the level of the individual cell, to the social level, to the spiritual level. The dialectic of the life process contains two dangers: one danger consists of a wrong kind of growth where one goes so far out from oneself that one cannot return, losing self-identity; the other is in preserving self-identity such that one is unable to change, or go out from oneself into self-alteration. Disease consists of a distortion or alteration in these processes, an "interruption in the flow," which is produced by the ambiguities of life.[3] The greatest ambiguity is that one must risk disease to avoid disease. Health, in Tillich's view, can only be seen as the absence of disease and can only be assessed by measurements that indicate distortion in the processes of self-alteration and self-identity.

Traditionally, indicators of health, given its definition as a disease-free state, have been determined from several sources. Morbidity and mortality statistics have led to analyses of the likelihood of illness and to a focus on risk factors for illness. These risk factors have produced the basis for selection of many health indicators, especially those associated with life stress and lifestyle. This definition has also led to the measurement of disease-free individuals by various parameters, such as blood values, organ size, height-weight ratios, and to the establishment of the "normal range."[4] By comparing a specific individual with the normal range, one could make a judgment about his or her health status.

Tillich's analysis might incorporate some of these same indicators, but the direction his analysis would offer the caregiver also offers some indicators or assessment variables, or both, that are very untraditional. For example, in the chemical dimension of being, health would be measured by determining the balance among various body chemicals and comparing them with the normal range. In the biologic dimension, one would determine health by looking at the total organism and its relation to the environment through rest, awakening of interest, initiation of movement, and engagement in acts designed to change nutritional intake and respond to changes in climate.[5] Tillich believes that balance between self-alteration and self-identity in this dimension can

be seen in the recreative activity of the being; that the presence of recreation indicates that the "created vitality was stopped in the process of going out beyond itself or in its power to return to itself."[6]

Health as a Social Role

A second view of health is that it is a socially defined state;[7] that is, society establishes standards for adequate performance regarding social roles and role tasks. Deviations from adequate performance are given meaning, and it is the meaning attached to these deviations that determines the attribution of health and illness. Social health arises as a consequence of the individual's interaction with persons and objects in the environment. This interaction is commonly evaluated within the context of the normal developmental process. Illness is the inability to carry out one's expected level of performance as a consequence of a disturbance in interaction or of a physical inability. An alteration in the ability to carry out one's roles and role tasks and the meaning others attach to this alteration in ability, then, is the primary indicator of alteration in health status. Such indicators are measures of task performance, relationships with others, assumptions of expected roles, and performance at an expected level of growth and development.

This social definition of health is useful for consideration of mental health, for describing the implications of physical inabilities on health, and for examining the social causes of disease. It is also useful for suggesting social and interactive modes of cure, extending even to the creation of new social norms and status structures, as is done in the therapeutic communities.

Health as the Ability to Contribute to the Economic System

A third conception of health is that it is defined by the economic system of the society.[8] In a capitalist society, the economic system is one in which the means of production and distribution are privately owned and operated for profit and in which the individual and the social institution are viewed as subordinate to the economic process. Individuals in such a system are objectified; that is, they are considered as material objects and valued for what they can contribute to the system as consumers or producers. When individuals ultimately cannot control the system affecting them, they experience alienation or separation. Kelman[9] states that health in such a system is defined as "the organismic condition of the population most consistent with, or least disruptive of, the process of capital accumulation." He equates this with the capacity to do productive work. Lovell[10] expands this view by recognizing that health and disease are defined primarily by those who control profits, traditionally men, and that as a consequence, nonmale functions (menstruation, childbirth, pregnancy, menopause) are defined as pathologic and are exploited for profit. In this system, the female is defined as unfit for the economic system because of her pathologic functions and their accompaniments: nervous susceptibility and emotional instability.

An economic definition of health creates a dilemma, in that the maintenance of the productive capacity of the worker interferes with the accumulation of capital. Production, in a system where the worker is alienated, tends to be bolstered by the introduction of a competitive goal structure, so that while production increases, anxiety and stress in the worker also increase, creating forces that ultimately reduce production (such as absenteeism and psychologic and somatic illness). In addition, although environmental conditions present in the workplace or resulting from production may interfere with the productivity of the worker, their elimination would interfere with profits. The worker is thus reduced to an expendable resource of the system of production. Kelman indicates that the individual, in contrast to the system, has a concept of how health should be experienced. This concept, coupled with the individual's absence of control over the economic system of which he or she is a part, produces alienation. In this condition, persons often act against their view of their own self-interest as regarding exposure to environmental carcinogens and occupational illnesses. They will often cope with alienating circumstances in unhealthy ways, such as with alcohol and mind-altering drugs. This concept of health is useful for considering how much control an individual has over the conditions that influence his or her health, for examining the economic causes of disease, and for suggesting modes of cure involving changes in philosophic systems.

It is my view that all of these conceptions of health help guide this consideration of the assessment of women's health status. It must be recognized that in the scope of one chapter, a thorough consideration of relevant health indices cannot be outlined. The views of health discussed here are not theoretically developed adequately enough to give complete direction to the assessment process or to permit the evaluation of their consistency. It is hoped that these views will be an eclectic compilation useful to the reader, who will develop a complete and conceptually coherent view of health that will suggest indicators to guide the assessment process.

HEALTH HISTORY AND PHYSICAL EXAMINATION

The health history and physical examination, as they are traditionally conceived—with their emphases on immunizations, medical-surgical events, family and genetic disease patterns, and review of systems, coupled with basic laboratory tests—continue to be the best tool available for health assessment, given the absence-of-illness definition of health. This kind of assessment requires sufficient knowledge of anatomic structure and physiologic determinants of function and their "normal" variations to permit associations among findings and to allow for the formulation of conclusions about health status. Considerable skill is also required in gathering data through interview, observation, palpation, percussion, and auscultation. Discussions of these skills and of the tools that give direction as to the nature of the data to collect are so readily available that another discussion of them would be superfluous. Emphasis here will be on some indicators of health in areas that are judged to be particularly useful in the health assessment of women and that are often neglected in other contexts.

The setting in which health assessment takes place, whether in an institution or in the woman's home, must be conducive to the comfortable exchange of information. It is well documented that most useful information in health assessment comes from the use of effective interview techniques. The interviewer's role is to bring about the conditions that facilitate the provision of information by the woman being assessed; this will often require that the direction be set by this woman and not the interviewer.

Optimal conditions for the sharing of information include demonstrations of empathic understanding and of genuineness.[11] Communication of positive regard, or unconditional acceptance, is conveyed by nonverbal attending, by verbal messages that are nonjudgmental, and by a minimum of verbal responses. Empathic understanding, or understanding from the point of view of the other rather than from one's own point of view, can best be demonstrated by offering responses that are interchangeable with those of the other or that state what the other leaves unstated, and by withholding advice and empty reassurance.[12] Genuineness or being oneself can best be demonstrated by communicating actions and words that match one's feelings, especially when those feelings are negative and interfere with the communication of positive regard. This includes abstaining from playing false roles, such as assuming the role of expert when this role is unjustified.

Environmental conditions require that the assessor ensure privacy from intrusion and observation by others. During physical observation, the environment and objects used for observation should be of a comfortable temperature. The surroundings should help the woman relax and feel physically at ease. Lighting sources, both direct and indirect, should be available and easily manipulated.

Measurement of the absence of disease can be accomplished through indirect means; that is, health is reflected in the general appearance of the woman, in the condition of her skin and hair, and in the condition of the mucous membranes, all of which are accessible to the observer even under conditions not optimal for carrying out a complete physical examination.

GENERAL OBSERVATIONS

The assessor might elicit the woman's own perception of her health status initially and determine the factors that she uses to make her judgment. This approach will give the interviewer knowledge about the woman's own beliefs about the nature of health, the specificity of her self-knowledge, her sensitivity to inner states, and her knowledge of factors that determine health status. When the woman identifies symptoms of concern, the assessor must determine what these symptoms mean to the woman. For example, the premenopausal woman often has little information about normal accompaniments of the early stages of menopause and frequently interprets irregularity in menstruation, increase in dysmenorrhea, and other common disruptions as indications of disease, most frequently cancer. The assessor should explore any identified problems and symptoms pertaining to history, duration, character or quality, relationships to activities

and to environmental factors, and relationships to other symptoms. Questions such as "When is the last time you felt completely well?" or "When did you first suspect your health condition was not normal? are particularly useful when beginning to elicit such data.

Although the health professional may view some of the relationships identified by a patient as trivial, attention to the details surrounding her explanation of the connection may provide valuable insights concerning the nature of the problem or the patient's interpretation of it. Exploration of past medical history and the traditional review of systems provides a framework for the assessor's questions and serves to alert the assessor to problems or symptoms the patient may have dismissed or forgotten to mention. Family medical history assists in the exploration of hereditary tendencies to illness and the identification of risk factors, such as familial history of breast cancer or of drug abuse. For further assistance in eliciting a health history, the reader is referred to any of the excellent nursing textbooks focusing on health assessment.

The absence-of-disease view of health, especially as advanced by Tillich, would require some assessment of energy balance. Energy can be perceived as the capability for vigorous action or the capability to overcome resistance. When we speak of energy, we often incorporate an idea of velocity. The body must move fast enough to overcome resistance but not so fast that it "burns up." When the energy of the body is not in balance, one experiences fatigue. In order to maintain energy balance, the resources and expenditures of the body must remain equal. Someone who expends a great deal of energy must maintain a higher input.

The easiest way to measure the balance between input and output is by noting constancy of weight. If body weight is going down, there is more output than input. If body weight is increasing, there is more input than output. Constancy in weight, however, is not a sufficient index of energy balance. The quality of the input and output are necessary factors in energy balance. Assessment of energy balance, then, would require an assessment of nutritional quality. Nutritional records can be assessed for quality by comparing the nutritive value of the foods eaten with the quantity or caloric value of the foods eaten. The ideal is a diet that is high in nutrients and that supplies sufficient calories to meet the requirements of the body for energy output. Intake of nutrients is necessary for energy expenditure, but the body must also have the capability to nourish itself with these nutrients. An indirect index of this capability is the condition of the hair, skin, and mucous membranes.

Energy expenditure must be sufficient to meet the requirements of the individual. If the individual experiences fatigue in carrying out the tasks of daily living, including those associated with carrying out her roles, it is an indication of some problem with her health. Indicators of fatigue are subjective accounts by the woman concerning insufficient energy to carry out tasks, depression, and an inability to overcome resistance offered by organisms, chemicals, and other environmental stressors.

PHYSICAL ASSESSMENT

Observation of the woman affords some indication of her health status. Listlessness, apathy, and dullness of the eyes characterize the low energy state and contrast markedly with the alert, bright-eyed appearance usually associated with high energy and health. Height and weight are noted and evaluated in comparison with the normal for age. The average 22-year-old American woman is 64 inches tall and weighs 138 pounds. In women, the trunk is proportionately longer and the legs shorter than in men. This results in a lower center of gravity; thus, women tend to be more agile and to more easily maintain their balance, but they have less speed and power than men.

Fatty deposits give women their characteristic contour. Locations of fatty deposits are hormonally and genetically determined. In women fat is most pronounced in the hips, thighs, buttocks, arms, waist, and breasts. The amount of body fat in a woman should not exceed 28 per cent of her total weight. There does not appear to be a desirable lower limit. Some women can be healthy while quite lean, whereas in others, if percentage of body fat becomes too low, steroid production decreases so much that ovulation ceases. Body fat above 28 per cent appears to interfere with the ability of the body to absorb nutrients and nourish itself. A common indicator of amount of body fat is skinfold thickness; this can be measured with the dominant arm flexed 90 degrees. The assessor pulls out the skin on the upper arm midway between the achromion and olecranon processes and measures its thickness with calipers. Average skinfold thickness is 14 to 22 mm for women. Without fat, skinfold thickness is 2 to 3 mm. In the female, over 30 mm skinfold thickness is considered obese.

As women age, subcutaneous fat is lost from the hands, arms, calves, thighs, and buttocks, and is increased on the abdomen. Also associated with aging is loss of muscle tone and bulk, resulting in a higher fat-to-lean ratio. There is loss of stature, narrowing of the shoulders, increased flexion of the hips, increased curvature of the thoracic spine, and backward tilting of the head.

Skin

The condition of the integument, including the hair, skin, and nails, is a particularly good indicator of overall health status. The skin is the largest body organ. It serves five purposes: it protects the body tissues from injury, drying, and invasion of foreign materials; it regulates body temperature; it provides a means for the excretion of sodium, chloride, potassium, lactate, glucose, and urea; it plays a role in the production of vitamin D; and it houses the receptors for sensation. Almost every generalized disturbance in body function is mirrored by changes observable in the skin, including disturbances affecting the collagen, capillaries, sebaceous and sweat glands, fatty metabolism, and neuroendocrine regulation.

In the assessment process, the interview should be designed to elicit systemic signs and symptoms associated with any abnormalities of skin's condition, patterns of occurrence and progression of abnormalities; and aggravating factors such as pressures at work, home, and exposure to foreign objects, heat, cold, sun, and epidemic diseases. On observation, abnormalities in skin color should be noted; in particular, cyanosis, erythema, jaundice, pallor, carotinemia, or areas of increased or decreased pigmentation. Skin turgor can be determined by picking up a fold of skin: sodium loss and consequent dehydration is manifested by a skin fold remaining more than thirty seconds. In determining skin texture, it should be noted whether the skin is dry, rough, or scaly, or shows deposits of salt or urate crystals. Temperature and smell of the skin should also be noted.

In women with poor nutritional status, regardless of whether there is wasting or obesity, there are accompanying signs in the skin. Skin color is usually pale, and in more extreme cases becomes thin and translucent. As the skin thins, it becomes friable. The skin, lacking protective mechanisms, becomes subject to dermatitis, more commonly on the scalp, underarms, and upper center of the chest and back, beneath the breasts and in the pubic and coccygeal areas. The skin may develop a "goose-flesh" appearance. Occasionally, there is a loss of pigmentation in the skin, particularly over the cheeks and under the eyes. On the face, lesions often develop in the angles of the mouth and eyes; the nasolobial folds may develop a greasy, yellow appearance.

In women under stress, there are changes in the hormone secretions that are designed to maintain physiologic balance. Stimulation of the adrenals increases the secretion of androgens and sets off a reaction, even in the mature woman, resembling that of the acne of adolescence. The androgens stimulate the sebaceous glands in the skin, resulting in increased oiliness and the development of lesions on the face, scalp, shoulders, upper chest, or back.

Degenerative changes in the skin, including wrinkling, telangiectasia, and keratoses, are ultimately a function of aging. Skin aging is greatly accelerated by conditions under which the skin is repeatedly damaged: dry climates, areas with high levels of dust and wind, and areas where there is repeated sun damage. Suntanning and sunburning are particularly damaging to fair-skinned persons who have minimal melanin pigmentation. Tanning darkens the pigmentation already present, while burning results in melanogenesis. When those with poor tanning ability repeatedly expose themselves to the sun in an attempt to increase tanning, severe damage to the connective tissue, particularly elastin and collagen may result, which evokes degenerative changes, with the accompanying thinning and tightening of the epidermis that typically gives a leathery appearance. There is a concomitant loss of collagen, elastic tissue, and other changes.[13] A striking example of the difference between damaged skin and undamaged skin can be seen in the faces of older women in some religious orders who wore traditional habits that covered much of their faces. The skin that had been covered is typically unlined, well nourished, and healthy, whereas that which has been exposed looks wrinkled and old.

Hair

The hair is a part of the integumentary system. In women, the condition of the hair is a particularly useful indicator of general health status, except when it has been damaged by dyes and permanents. The hair root and shaft are embedded in the hair follicles and are nourished by the sebaceous glands. Hair growth is regulated in the woman by testosterone, which is secreted by the adrenal cortex and the ovary. Hair distribution is also regulated by the form and amount of this hormone.

Hair growth occurs in three stages: in the anagen stage the hair growth is at its average, that is, 0.3 to 0.4 mm a day; in the catagen stage growth vacillates from activity to nonactivity; the telogen stage is a resting stage that may occur every several months to every several years. Scalp hair grows an average of 2.5 mm a week. The length it can attain is determined by breakage and by the rate of hair loss for the individual, and this varies from loss of 20 to 100 hairs per day. Body hair achieves maximum growth in three to four months. Growth rate and rate of shedding can be determined by history.

Patterns of hair distribution vary by ethnic origin; hair is darker, coarser, and thicker in darker-skinned women. In the woman, pubic hair is distributed as an inverted triangle with the flat edge on top. The hair thins and loses its pattern, extending down the inner thighs with age. It is not unusual to have a few coarse hairs around the areola of the breasts and a sparse line of darker hair from the umbilicus to the pubis. Excess body hair accompanies hypothyroidism and Cushing's syndrome; hirsutism and virilization are associated with excess testosterone production, usually a consequence of ovarian and adrenal neoplasms. Diminished hair growth occurs with aging, trauma, nutritional deficiency, and many endocrine disorders.

In cases of poor nutrition and excess stress, hair becomes dull, wiry, and brittle, and often it loses pigmentation. In those having a temporary period of poor nutrition, such as that following an illness or surgery, the hair grows out with a band or stripe of less-pigmented hair visible. At this time, too, many hairs may break off at the hairline and one can almost date the period of stress or malnutrition by observing the length of the broken hairs.

Nails

Like the skin and hair, the nails are indicators of general health status. The fingernails achieve full growth in about five and one-half months, and the toenails in about one year. Their condition often gives evidence of general health. During a period of illness or trauma, nail growth may be disturbed, causing characteristic transverse depressions called Beau's lines. Common abnormalities observed are spooning associated with anemia, clubbing associated with insufficient circulatory oxygen, transverse white lines due to damage during manicuring or low zinc intake, distal separation of the nails from contact dermatitis, and yellow, excessively curved nails from bronchiectasis and pleural effusion.

Mucosa

The condition of the mucosa provides an indirect indication of the body's tolerance of stress. The oral mucosa, particularly, is constantly exposed to mechanical, thermal, chemical, and microbiologic stressors and, in addition, is easily subject to observation. The mucous membranes of the lips and cheeks are normally smooth, moist, and shiny. The color should be greyish red. The membranes covering the gums are normally pale and glistening and, in health, should be firm, stippled, and sharply pointed between the teeth. While inspecting the mucous membranes of the mouth, the nurse should note color, integrity, swelling, bleeding, gingival recession, and metal absorption lines (thin, usually silver or blue lines of color parallel to the gum line consequent to the absorption of foreign metals such as lead).

GYNECOLOGIC EXAMINATION

Any discussion of the assessment of women's health would appropriately include the gynecologic examination. One difficulty in approaching the subject from an absence-of-illness point of view is that the normal range on almost all indicators is so broad as to be almost useless in the elimination of illness. In addition, norms vary widely according to age and family history. Women seldom discuss symptoms associated with the function of the reproductive system except in the most general terms, so most women and most caregivers have little knowledge of what constitutes the norm. Symptoms of gynecologic illness are closely associated with normal functions, and history taking is designed to determine the extent to which these symptoms deviate from the individual's norm.

The assessor usually ascertains the menstrual history of the woman to furnish a basis for comparison. This history would include age at menarche, patterns associated with menstruation, including interval between periods; duration, amount, and pattern of flow; and presence of pain, tension, nausea, premenstrual symptoms, and intermenstrual bleeding. The assessor also determines the dates of the last menstrual period and of the last normal menstrual period. Irregularities of pattern of flow should be explored, and symptoms associated with abnormalities should be noted. The woman's interpretation of the meaning of these irregularities and her knowledge of what factors might determine such changes are important data for planning intervention.

Pain accompanies many gynecologic disorders, and the assessor should learn its location, character, and associated symptoms. Pain may be present in the back, abdomen, pelvis, or vaginal area and may either be easily localized or so generalized as to be impossible to localize. Pain may be of sudden or gradual onset; it may be precipitated by identifiable events or related to onset of menses or ovulation. It may be associated with other symptoms such as fever, nausea, discharge, or bleeding. Words used to describe the severity of pain should be noted. "Knifelike," "gnawing," "dull," "aching," and "fullness" are typical descriptions of pain for different disorders, from infections to space-occupying lesions.

Change in the character of vaginal discharge is a source of concern to most women. The bleeding patterns associated with menstruation change in character with most gynecologic disorders as well as with age. In cases of reportedly heavy flow, an estimate of amount of flow, usually in terms of numbers of tampons or pads saturated, is helpful. Any consistent or heavy loss of blood would be accompanied by signs of anemia, such as pallor of mucous membranes, a constant feeling of being cold, or excessive fatigue. Normally, as women age menstrual patterns change, with an increase in cramping, increase in initial flow and in irregularity, and shortening of flow duration.

Nonbloody discharge may or may not be problematic. When women first notice the pattern of nonmenstrual vaginal discharge associated with the ovulatory cycle, they often interpret it as abnormal and seek advice. Too much discharge is abnormal, however, so its character, color, odor, consistency, and factors surrounding its onset should be noted.

Abnormalities associated with urination and defecation should be noted in conjunction with the gynecologic exam. Infections, tumors, and pregnancy each result in an interaction of symptoms among these three systems.

As part of the interview, a complete obstetric history, history of illness and surgery, a family and marital history, and a fertility history should be gathered. Historic factors associated with a few of the more common gynecologic events are briefly considered here.

Premenstrual syndrome is a name given to any combination of experiences that surround the beginning of menstruation. Hypotheses concerning its cause are many. It usually refers to the negative experiences accompanying menstruation that begin when the woman is in her late 20s that usually worsen until the woman reaches menopause. The symptoms include breast tenderness, abdominal or pelvic fullness, obsessive eating or craving of sweets, bloating, headache, nausea, bowel function changes, depression, fatigue, and irritability. Some women report that positive experiences occur at this time, such as periods of creativity, increased productivity, and increased energy. Premenstrual syndrome appears to be alleviated by regular exercise, a diet high in calcium, and an increase in fluid intake. It is aggravated by a diet high in sodium and caffeine and by a sedentary lifestyle.

Endometriosis is most severe when the woman is between age 30 and the onset of menopause. Symptoms are usually menstrual abnormalities, including dysmenorrhea, with particularly increased abdominal or back pain; and what women describe as a "deep ache." Pain gradually increases over time. Infertility is frequently associated with endometriosis. There is often a family history of the disorder.

Fibroid tumors are accompanied by excessive menstrual flow, irregular bleeding, and aching or fullness in the abdomen.

Gynecologic cancers are frequently postmenopausal and accompanied by abdominal fullness and aching, and occasionally by abnormal bleeding.

The menopausal syndrome is accompanied by signs of decreasing estrogen, such as diminished muscular development, thinning of the epidermis, decrease in vaginal lubrication, increased vaginal alkalinity and infection, and flattening of the labia. Women will often report "hot flashes." The assessor should note factors that trigger the hot flashes and the pattern of spread, as well as a description of the degree of lifestyle disruption.

The physical examination consists of a breast examination, height, weight, blood pressure, urinalysis, and an abdominal and pelvic examination. The abdomen should be observed for abnormalities in contour. Auscultation for bruits and abnormalities in circulation and for bowel sounds should be done before palpating the abdomen. Finally, the abdomen is percussed and palpated for size of organs, presence of masses, and characteristics of sound transmission indicating fluid, solid masses, and gas formation. The pelvic exam includes observation of the external genitalia, palpation of abnormalities of the escutcheon, vulva, clitoris, Bartholin's glands, Skene's glands, and

the urethra. The speculum is used to assist in examination of the vaginal walls and to note color, size, consistency, lesions, discharge, and lacerations of the cervix, the shape of the cervical os, and the character of the squamocolumnar junction.

The bimanual examination permits exploration of the size, position, shape, mobility, and consistency of the corpus and palpation of the parametria. The rectovaginal examination permits examination of the posterior corpus and uterosacral ligaments and the rectum. The reader is referred to a textbook on physical examination for the details on how to carry out such an examination.

It should be noted that some women, particularly athletes, are beginning to carry out menstrual extraction as a means of eliminating the inconvenience of menstruation. These women typically insert a cannula and withdraw the products of menstruation with suction. It is unknown what the dangers of this procedure will be. It has been suggested there will be an increase in uterine perforation and infection, but little actual data are available.

ASSESSMENT OF SOCIAL ROLE AND TASK

Much is known about sex-role stereotypes and the values placed on male and female roles, role tasks, and society's definition of what these should be. Society's standards, both as indicated by tradition and as dictated by those seeking to liberate women from them, have an impact on the woman's view of her performance and on her concept of her real and ideal selves. Since the woman herself is often unconscious of what her real and ideal selves are and of what her roles, role tasks, and level of role performance are, assessment is made somewhat more difficult.

Roles are the expectations associated with one's social position. In identifying those persons and groups of persons who are important in the woman's life, one can attempt to determine the expectations encumbent on the woman as a result of these relationships. The traditional female roles are wife, mother, homemaker, and labor force participant.

There are, of course, many other roles for each woman: grandmother, daughter, student, employer. For each of a person's roles there are expected behaviors determined by the persons involved in the relationship and learned through their socialization process. These behavior expectations may be very rigid and tied to stereotypes or may be loose and situation dependent. If, in the performance of role tasks, there is a discrepancy between actual or perceived performance and actual or perceived expectations for performance on the part of either or both of the persons in a relationship, there is role strain. To relieve the tension associated with role strain, either performance or expectation must change. If it does not, conflict will develop.

The patterns developed to handle strain and conflict are determined by social norms, or rules for conduct. If one's performance deviates from the rules, it can be labeled "deviant." Certain forms of deviance are labeled "sick." For example, a woman experiences strain in her housewife role and views her performance as less than that expected by both herself and her family. She tries to improve her performance but can never reach what she views as adequate performance. If, no matter how hard she works, she can never perform well enough, she becomes helpless and passive, going into a downward spiral of loss of self-esteem, of anger, and of depression: all "sick" behaviors. When expectations for role performance are rigid, flexibility is lost, and there are few situations in which adequate performance is possible.

In the process of assessment, one attempts to determine what the woman's expectations for performance are, including both her own expectations and those expectations she thinks others assign to her. This can usually be determined by straightforward questioning or by a combination of direct and indirect methods. Most indirect assessment methods involve projective techniques; for example, asking how a "good" mother would respond to a child in a given situation, or role playing a situation and comparing the woman's ideal with her view of her own circumstances. The range of responses available to a woman in a given situation can be a determinant of her health. One can assess this by presenting a fictional role situation, such as "Your husband calls you at 5:00 to say he is going out after work and is not sure when he will be home. You are going to a PTA meeting at 7:30. Describe three different ways you could respond, and then describe which response you would choose and why."

Often a fictional situation is not required for assessment purposes, as the real situation the woman presents is more than adequate. The woman with low back pain cannot perform the tasks associated with any of her roles. Her description of the strain associated and the response to changed or unchanged expecta-

tions will determine whether she is sick, given the social definition of health.

The response to role strain is the major focus of the assessment process, because the response is a major determinant of future performance. When a woman defines role behavior according to rigid sex-linked criteria, she loses a great deal of flexibility and can perform well only in situations in which stereotyped behavior is the expectation.

In order to determine the norms operating in a woman's situation, the caregiver might explore behaviors that cause the woman guilt. The experience of guilt is closely associated with acting contrary to expected norms. If these norms can be identified, the woman can restructure her situation to change either the norms or her behavior, thus reducing strain.

Social expectations for behavior are often tied to expected age-related levels of development and to age-related tasks. The emphasis on stages of growth and development in the social definition of health is based on the assumption that in order to grow, one must solve the problems encountered at one's stage in life. The problems are created through interpersonal interaction and are solved by the development of effective patterns of behavior. If the patterns of behavior are successful at solving the problems, the individual can advance to a new set of problems. Ineffective response patterns lead to behavior labeled "sick." Different views of growth and development present different views of the problems to be solved, so judgment about someone's level of performance requires knowledge of some theoretical frame of reference.

Through interaction with others and the performance of socially expected tasks, persons develop a concept of self. William James (1910) defines self as all that a person calls his, from his body and mind to his possessions (including his wife, children, and home).[14] Persons acquire knowledge about themselves through interaction with others and through the recognition of certain of their features by other people. At certain times and under conditions fostering self-awareness, persons focus inward and become more aware of their good and bad features, and of discrepancies between their real and ideal selves.[15] In this way, particular features of one's identity become salient, and a person uses them in future situations to determine his or her behavior.

A woman's concept of herself can be assessed by what she says about herself verbally and nonverbally. Verbal self statements can be assessed by noting the ratio of positive to negative self-statements or by noting areas discussed in positive and in negative self statements. One can attempt to elicit self statements by asking "What did you think about in that situation?" or "What do the people in your group think you are like?"

A particularly good opportunity for evaluating self statements occurs in situations when the caregiver is attempting to teach a woman to perform a new task. This might be a psychomotor task (such as self-administration of insulin), or a cognitive task (such as role playing the solving of a complex problem using a systematic process). During the carrying out of the assigned task, the assessor might ask the woman to talk aloud to herself. In giving oneself directions while carrying out a task, one frequently uses evaluative self-referent speech.

Nonverbal behavior is also an indicator of self-concept. A woman who uses hair dye to disguise graying hair and obtains a face lift, speaks in this way about her response to her aging self. One who fully invades the space of others is evoking assertion and power. A woman who sits slumped with arms and legs folded is thereby showing who she is and how she wishes to present herself. Note the messages given by the woman who "dresses for success" and the woman who dresses like her adolescent daughter; one may be ready for responsibility, while the other is not.

By evaluating the woman's behavior in the face of her own and of society's expectations of this behavior, the assessor can determine her level of health from society's viewpoint.

ASSESSMENT FOR THE ABILITY TO ASSUME AN ECONOMIC ROLE

The third view of health, that it is a state consistent with the system of capital accumulation, would require that the woman have a tolerance for competition and be capable of high productivity and of withstanding the anxiety and stress associated with effecting high productivity. These conditions would require that the woman acquiesce to being treated as an object by the system, on the one hand, and be capable of initiating action leading to greater production, on the other hand. This clearly puts a woman in an impossible situation, an alienating condition in which she is forced to separate herself from her experience. Alienation is the state that is the consequence of objectification, and this state interferes with

health. Assessment of health, then, would require assessment of tolerance for competition, productive capability, control of anxiety and stress, and absence of alienation.

Tolerance of competition can be assessed by determining (1) the extent to which the woman views herself as the source of her own acts and not merely the recipient of the acts of others, and (2) the woman's skills in asserting her beliefs. The alienated woman would not be in touch with her own beliefs or feelings in response to others, and in not knowing herself or even recognizing her experience, would be incapable of initiating acts to control it.

Capability for high productivity can be assessed by evaluating tasks required to bring forth the "product" in question and by determining the extent of the woman's skills in relation to these tasks. This would range from the neuromuscular ability to pull the appropriate lever to the communication skills required of the manager. Absence of skills for task would be equated with absence of health. The alienated woman would be unaware of skills required to perform desired tasks, and she would be unaware of her own skills; consequently, she would be incapable of high productivity.

Control of anxiety and stress require that the woman have skills in monitoring her internal state, determining factors leading to arousal, identifying and gaining the necessary information to allow her to control those factors in her situation that are subject to her control, engaging in actions that will control these factors, and altering the internal state of arousal. The alienated woman would be unaware of the factors producing anxiety and stress and of the signs of such reactions within herself. She would lack personal control, would feel helpless, and would likely experience stress-related illnesses.

Alienation, the separation of the person from his or her experience, is the consequence of the person being defined as an object and accepting this definition. It is a consequence of viewing life as a problem to be solved, rather than as a mystery to be lived. Its absence is manifested by a sense of harmony or unity with one's self and with the universe and by an ability to live in the present. The absence of alienation is manifested by autonomy, openness, and spontaneity. Interestingly, if one were to ask a woman to describe how she felt the last time she felt healthy, she would be likely to respond by describing this experience with words such as "peaceful," "together," "balanced," "energetic enough to do what I want to do," and "capable." These kinds of responses would indicate that most women have been in touch with their experience and recognize this state. Most are also able to describe when they deviate from this state by using such words as "anxious," "uptight," "preoccupied," and "phrenetic."

One can evaluate some aspects of health by determining how women deal with situations in which they find they are estranged from self. Unhealthy ways of responding are by dealing with oneself as an object; by acting against one's own self interest by withdrawing into daydreams, alcohol, drugs—worlds where reality does not demand action. Healthy ways of responding are by dealing with oneself as the source of change, by risk taking, by encountering painful experiences,[16] and by acting to change unhealthy social systems and to achieve what one perceives as one's state of health.

In conclusion, health is viewed from three perspectives: as the absence of disease, as the ability to carry out socially defined roles, and as the capacity to work productively. These perspectives permit a consideration of diverse indicators of the overall health status of women. No single viewpoint at present encompasses all these views, but philosophic and scientific development of any one of them may permit a single perspective to be useful to the practitioner. Health can be viewed as either an objective state or as an experience of a certain quality, but an assessment of the health of an individual woman requires an assessment of both.

References

1. Nathanson, Constance A. Illness and the feminine role: A theoretical review. *Social Science and Medicine,* vol. 9, 1975, pp. 57–62.
2. Tillich, Paul. The meaning of health. *Perspectives in Biology and Medicine,* Autumn 1961, pp. 92–100.
3. Tillich, Paul, ibid.
4. Hoke, B. Promotive medicine and the phenomenon of health. *Archives of Environmental Health,* vol. 16, 1968, pp. 269–278.
5. Tillich, Paul, op cit. pp. 269–278.
6. Tillich, Paul, ibid.
7. Parsons, Talcott. Definitions of health and illness in the light of American values and social structure. *In* Jaco, E. (ed.) *Patients, Physicians and Illness.* 3rd ed. New York: Free Press, 1979, pp. 120–144.
8. Kelman, Sander, The social nature of the definition problem in health. *International Journal of Health Services,* vol. 5, 1975, pp. 625–642.
9. Kelman, Sander, ibid.
10. Lovell, Mariann C. Silent but perfect partners: Medicine's use and abuse of women. *ANS,* vol. 3:2, 1981, pp. 25–39.
11. Rogers, Carl R. *On Becoming a Person.* Boston: Houghton Mifflin, 1961.
12. Carkhuff, Robert R. and Pierce, Richard M. *The Art of Helping: Trainer's Guide.* Amherst, MA: Human Resources Development Press, 1977.
13. Wintrobe, Maxwell M. et al. *Harrison's Principles of Internal Medicine,* 7th ed. New York: McGraw-Hill Book Company, 1974, pp. 283–284.
14. James, William. *Psychology: The Briefer Course.* New York: Holt, 1910.
15. Wicklund, Robert A. Objective self-awareness. *In* Berkowitz, L. (ed.) *Advances in Experimental Social Psychology 8.* New York: Academic Press, 1975.
16. Sarosi, Grace. A critical theory: The nurse as a fully human person. *Nursing Forum,* Vol. 7, 1968, pp. 349–363.

3

WOMEN'S HEALTH PERCEPTIONS IN A MALE-DOMINATED MEDICAL WORLD

MARY WEISENSEE

In this chapter, Mary Weisensee deals with women's perceptions of women's health, and the actual health risks and health care needs of women. She provides a revealing background of the impetus toward health care for women.

The study of women's health is full of contradictions and nearly void of solid data and findings. Women actively seek health services, engage in preventive health behaviors, and consider the psychophysiologic implications of health to a greater extent than men do. Yet women are perceived to be, not wiser and more responsible than men, but sicker and more dependent. Apparently, perceptions held by women and men about women's health have a profound and somewhat perverse effect on the growing cultural necessity for self-care and healthy practices.

Interestingly, women perceive themselves to be more ill than others; they utilize medical services more than men; they report more days lost to physical and psychologic symptoms. At the same time, they live longer than men, and they experience fewer chronic diseases. On the one hand, the presenting complaints of women are taken less seriously by physicians than those of men; on the other, women are prescribed far greater quantities of medications, particularly psychotropic drugs. In addition to describing the perceptions of women's health by women and by predominantly male physicians, this discussion poses many of the hypotheses for the differing perceptions and raises a call for judicious research.

Clues are introduced to the actual health needs of women and the role of health promotion in meeting those needs. Based on my preliminary research, few people engage in a total program of health care. They perform a few maintenance behaviors, seek annual dental check-ups, or emphasize one aspect of self-care without balance among others. While physical fitness, nonsmoking, and weight control appear to be more actively pursued in this decade, lip-service remains the primary activity of most Americans toward nutrition, safety, control of alcohol and caffeine, reduction of salt and sugar intake, and the consistent integration of physical, emotional, and spiritual components of self-care. Reliance remains heavy on ill care, remedial cures, drug therapies, and technologic treatments for ailments of lifestyle and mind-set. Taken as a whole, these findings will urge women to heighten their knowledge, self-perception, and level of positive action toward health.

ROLES OF THE TRADITIONAL SYSTEM

What has traditionally been accepted in western culture as health care in reality is medical "ill care." As stated by Richmond,[1] the role of medical care in an individual's life may complicate or inhibit health, in that:

. . . health professions are not conceptually well equipped to study health, that they have virtually no vocabulary or classification of functional capacity in health, and, while they have concentrated appropriately on the study and control of disease, they now must attend to positive health maintenance.

Oelbaum[2] acknowledges that even ". . . nurses accept but do not strive for this positive goal. Instead they concern themselves with illness . . . paying more attention to maladjustment and physical ailments than other areas of deprivation which influence well-being."[2] The dilemma is that, even with a growing commitment to self-care and improved health, the available technology and financial prerogatives lie with a health care establishment that is prescriptive, pathologically oriented, and directed by research and practices that are male dominated.

In a work devoted to women, it is especially critical to determine the interaction of the traditional medical model and women's perceptions of their well-being. Perception and interpretation are as influential on health as the presence or absence of pathology. "The body cannot distinguish between a real event and a well-imagined one".[3] If women are perceived by themselves and others to be more susceptible to illness, they will in fact function below their actual capacity.

PERCEPTIONS OF WOMEN' HEALTH BY MEDICAL PROVIDERS AND RESEARCHERS

Three facts are repeated throughout the literature on women's health. The first is that women use existing medical services more than men do. In 1977, visits to a physician by American women totaled 594,465, compared with 425,932 by men. Under age 18, male and female visits to physicians were about equal. In all other age groups, women consulted physicians more often than men, with the highest comparison in the 25- to 44-year age range.[4]

Second, women report being sick more than men, and they report more days of limited activity owing to physical or psychologic distress. Third, far more pharmaceutical prescriptions are written for women than for men.

From these three axioms, the nearly global conclusion has been drawn that women experience greater morbidity than men do. Painfully little evidence exists to substantiate the leaps from more frequent "visits" to more frequent "illness," from illness "reported" to illness "experienced," and from medications "prescribed" to medications actually "needed." Although many investigators have probed sex differences in health, "discussions

and analyses of these differences are poorly conceptualized, polemic, and not particularly informative".[5]

Nursing researchers have paid little attention to the health care needs of women based on genetic differences. According to Stevenson,[6] the largest women's health profession conducts twice as much research on the woman as childbearer and caretaker as on the woman as subject or object of health care.

Research and literature, when they do consider differences in health related to gender, have focused on illness, "ill behavior," and the use of various "ill-care" services. The central finding is that women perceive themselves to be sick more frequently than men. Riley and Foner[6a] examine the variables of sex difference and older age in relation to needs for health services, finding that there are greater numbers of women in the population and that they consistently exhibit higher morbidity rates than men.

Nathanson, in *Illness and the Feminine Role*,[8] asserts that there are insufficient data to evaluate the various explanations of women's high morbidity rates. Historically, three models have been used to account for gender differences in illness. These are:

1. Women report more illness than men, because it is culturally more acceptable for them to be ill; "the ethic of health is masculine."[7]
2. The sick role is relatively compatible with women's other role responsibilities and incompatible with those of men
3. Women's assigned social roles are more stressful than those of men, consequently, they have more illness.[8]

Several equally plausible explanations for women's morbidity have not been posited or examined:

1. Mothers are exposed more frequently to the symptomatically acute illness of their children
2. Proxy effects in surveys may distort the reporting of illness
3. Bias on the part of medical practitioners may define women's complaints as hypochondriacal or inconsequential, resulting in palliative treatments or repeat visits for recurring symptoms or both
4. Normal but exclusively female functions may have been assigned definitions as illnesses requiring medical intervention
5. Ways women demonstrate distress may be considered "ill behavior," while ways men exhibit distress are defined as something else

6. Women misunderstand the nature of their ills and overuse doctors
7. Men are genetically or biologically superior to women and therefore, are less susceptible to illness

Perceptions and Hypotheses Examined

In the absence of reliable data from medical research, the reader must turn to other disciplines and studies in order to test, by extension, the previous hypotheses. Much of the following discussion will treat the hypotheses in general terms, seeking only to identify promising arenas for further study and to eliminate those that have been repudiated by judicious research in other fields.

Mechanic[5] emphasizes the need for study of sex differences in health and cautions the reader to consider other variables when interpreting statistics on rates of the use of illness care services, since many diagnoses, referrals, and interventions are carried out by male physicians. He points out that male physicians are more likely to regard women as hypochondriacs. He cites data from the National Ambulatory Medical Care Survey indicating that physicians are likely to regard the principal problem reported by women as serious in only 17 per cent of the cases presented, compared with 22 per cent of the problems presented by men. Armitage and Schneiderman found that "men received more extensive workups than women" for all common complaints (e.g., headache and lower back pain).[9] When asked to describe their typical "complaining" patient, 72 per cent of the physicians surveyed referred to a woman; only 4 per cent referred to a man.[10]

Why do doctors take women less seriously? Mechanic[5] asserts that the perception might be either a biased or accurate reflection of the presenting patterns of women, with the role played by male and female socialization not demonstrated satisfactorily. Broverman's[11] research provides evidence that clinicians accept and thereby perpetuate sex-role stereotypes. Maccoby and Jacklin[12] conclude that social shaping is the most important factor in determining sex-typical behavior.

Dowling[13] proposes a major difference in socialization:

Males are educated for independence from the day they are born. Just as systematically, females are taught that they have an out—that someday, in some way, they are going to be saved. That is the fairy tale, the life-message we have introjected as if with mother's milk. We may venture out on our own for a while, we may go away to school, work, travel; we may even make good money, but underneath it all there is a finite quality to our feelings about independence. Only hang on long enough, the childhood story goes, and someday someone will come along to rescue you from the anxiety of authentic living.

Independent people who are in positions of autonomy or power tend to be "stress carriers,"[14] while dependent people in controlled or reactive positions tend to absorb stress. This evidence, along with that of Tangri,[15] that the overwhelming proportion of women is still employed in traditionally female, unprestigious positions, contributes to the conclusion that women are exposed to more stress and are socialized to perceive themselves as less able to meet the demands of independent living. Dual careers of homemaker and employee, single parenting, and vulnerability to assault constitute other unique demands on women. Depressed earnings, perceptions of inferior importance, and reliance on prescribed psychotropic drugs may uniquely impair women's resources to cope. Since stress is "the perception that one's demands outweigh one's resources,"[3] the relationship of women's stress to their health and to special needs for health care will merit extensive research.

Whatever the causes of greater use of medical services by women, the effects are not satisfactory. If a woman is conscious of health and tells a male physician that she only wants a check-up, she may be labeled as an overly concerned, "emotional," "crock" female.[16] Male physicians are educated to focus on pathology, microbiology, diagnosis, and treatment resulting in "cure." The areas of health and illness that are perceived by women to be important do not lend themselves to precise diagnosis and prescription. Nor are these areas esoteric enough to arouse genuine interest and concern: colds, low back pain, digestive upsets, bowel and urinary problems, fatigue, aches and pains, premenstrual syndrome (PMS), hormonal shifts, and a vast array of emotional problems associated with women's roles, which are misapprehended and misunderstood by many male physicians. These conditions rarely are life threatening, but they have profound influence on the quality of women's lives, relationships with family and friends, and self-concept. Whether the difficulty in acquiring responsive health care lies only in different definitions of what constitutes care or whether male bias and female patterns of presenting behavior create self-fulfilling negative stereotypes can only be surmised.

Clearer, however, is the more fundamental bias concerning what constitutes illness. Pregnancy and routine gynecologic exams are considered pathologic conditions and counted in the utilization rates for women. So is medical treatment for physical abuse, while the aggression and violence of the abuser are not, even when identified and treated. In one study showing greater incidence of mental illness among women than among men, "mental illness" was limited to neuroses and psychoses, not considering alcoholism, personality disorders, and acting-out behaviors—patterns all occurring more frequently in men.[17]

The perception that women are sicker than men is itself arguable. While women do report more disability from acute illness, men report more chronic illness, and there is no marked difference in long-term mobility loss.

The more tangible and physiologic the symptoms, the less difference there is between men and women.[5] Given the longer life expectancy of women, these findings point toward changing the current presumptions about women's morbidity. Pending unbiased research and measurements, and awaiting a concerted effort to counter the views currently held by medical professionals, women will continue to be tolerated, labeled, sedated, operated on, and ushered out the door.

Consider the common practices cited by Schiefelbein.[9] The nausea of pregnancy still is classified as a neurosis; even colic is listed under "psychologic disorders." Although 84 per cent of drug-using women in one study reported that a particular drug had been recommended to them by a physician, physicians claim that the women themselves demanded the prescriptions. Eight years after the discovery of cancer in "DES daughters," 5000 DES prescriptions were written in 1978 for pregnancy tests. In resisting the efforts of the FDA to inform women of the side effects of the drugs related to the female reproductive system, physicians claim interference with the doctor-patient relationship (a relationship based on the assumption that a woman is too stupid or too fragile to judge side effects for herself). Prophylactic hysterectomies sometimes are justified to reduce risk of cancer. In other cases, surgeons recommend alleviating the "drudgery of the menses" or the inconvenience to physicians of performing "unpleasant pelvic exams." One gynecologic text even suggests that "if menstruation can be abolished

. . . it would be a blessing not only to the woman but to her husband."[9]

Physicians continue to be assaulted by advertisements from pharmaceutical companies that seem to carry the message "shoot her up and shut her up with our product," as in the announcement for trifluoperazine HCl:[18]

You've talked . . . you've listened . . . but there she is again. Looks like chronic anxiety. Looks like a case for the use of Stelazine.

WOMEN'S PERCEPTIONS OF WOMEN'S HEALTH

It may be tempting to portray the mismanagement of health care for women purely as the result of misguided or misogynistic research, physicians, and profiteers. The fact remains that women do report more "days of limited activity due to feeling unwell" than men do.[5] Women perceive themselves to be ill more often than men.

I am conducting research to determine current health perceptions and practices by middle class adults in the Midwest. In the past, study has been limited to Federal projects on behalf of underserved populations and investigations of the attitudes of people already receiving traditional medical care through clinics and hospitals.[19] A principal assumption of my research is that 'people seek care on the basis of self-assessed need for it."[20] The findings (from my research) that are most pertinent to this discussion are presented in this section. Comparative responses from men and women are shown when relevant.

On the Ware Health Perceptions Tool, only one item reveals statistical significance based on gender: "Most people get sick a little easier than I do" ($X = 6.11$, $df = 2$, $p = 0.05$). The majority of males (75 per cent) indicate "true," while 25 per cent indicate "don't know" and 0 per cent indicate that the statement is "false" for them. In comparison, only half (52.6 per cent) the females state the item is "true," while 15.8 per cent answer "don't know" and 31.6 per cent indicate the statement is "false."[21]

Some other comparisons are significant at $p = 0.10$, which indicates a tendency, particularly in so preliminary an analysis (Table 3–1).

In a related questionnaire on health practices and attitudes, four items reveal differences in lifestyle or approach to health care between men and women.[21] Only two of the items in Table 3–2 are statistically significant in chi-square analysis–those concerned with

Table 3–1. **Ware Health Perceptions by Sex (1982)**

Item	Females (N=19)			Males (N=16)			Total (N=35)			x^2	df	p
	MT*	DK	MF	MT	DK	MF	MT	DK	MF			
Most people get sick a little easier than I do	52.6	15.8	31.6	75.0	25.0	—	62.9	20.0	17.1	6.11	2	0.05*
According to the doctors I've seen, my health is now excellent	73.7	10.5	15.8	100.0	—	—	85.7	5.7	8.6	4.91	2	0.09
When I'm sick, I try to keep it to myself	63.2	—	36.8	37.5	18.8	43.8	51.4	8.6	40.0	4.87	2	0.09
My health is excellent	63.2	15.8	21.1	93.8	—	6.3	77.1	8.6	14.3	4.91	2	0.09
I never worry about my health	33.3	5.6	61.1	62.5	12.5	25.0	47.1	8.8	44.1	4.50	2	0.11

Response key: MT = Mostly true; DK = Don't know; MF = Mostly false.
*Significant at the 0.05 level.

health and dental check-ups. Over twice as many women (78.9 per cent) as men (37.5 per cent) state it is true that they have health check-ups every year. The difference for dental check-ups is not so large between women (94.7 per cent) and men (62.5 per cent), with both groups reporting a much higher response rate of "true." Ninety-four per cent of women, but only 68.8 per cent of men, state that health is their most important asset. Interestingly, though, many more women (52.6 per cent) than men (31.3 per cent) smoke cigarettes, which will be addressed later in a discussion of women's health risks.

Taken together, these findings suggest that women feel more susceptible to illness, are more concerned about maintaining their health, and act on their beliefs regularly by consulting medical professionals.

Related research, although not conclusive, tends to support my preliminary findings. Regarding women's objective health, there is agreement that women have a longer life expectancy than men, and also that they use health care facilities more. Although women obviously have greater need of health facilities for prenatal care and childbearing, when hospitalizations for deliveries are deleted, utilization rates for women of 166 per 1000 still compare with 141 per 1000 for men.[4] Marieskind also reports unpublished data from an Ezzati survey, showing the principal reason for physician visits by women aged 15 and over to be "general, special, and administrative examinations (e.g., annual physicals, psychologic testing, prenatal check-ups, breast and pelvic examinations, etc.), accounting for 16.7 per cent of the visits."[4]

Thus, women apparently pursue preventive and psychophysiologic care. Yet, their perceptions regarding their own health and rationale for seeking care reveal an estimation of lesser health than others around them. Perceptions held by women and by those providing the care are influenced extensively by societal expectations, economic conditions, and entrenched assumptions and stereotypes of women's personalities.

Whatever the cause of self-perceived susceptibility, the effect is powerful. The ability accurately to perceive one's own state of health is an important aspect of properly managing it. In Dolfman's[22] model of health, the individual must determine the meaning of adaptation and normal function. Pender[23] highlights the importance of perception:

In discussing the determinants of health behavior within a humanistic context, perception emerges as a key concept. It is not the external event that directly affects behavior but the meaning an individual gives to any object or event.

Table 3–2. **Lifestyle Practices Comparing Males and Females**

Practice	Female (N=19)			Male (N=16)			Total			x^2	df	p
	True	DK	False	True	DK	False	True	DK	False			
I smoke cigarettes	52.6	—	47.4	31.3	—	68.8	42.9	—	57.1	.87	1	0.35
I have a health check-up once a year	78.9	—	21.1	37.5	—	62.5	60.0	—	40.0	4.61	1	0.03*
I have a dental check-up once a year	94.7	—	5.3	62.5	—	37.5	80.0	—	20.0	3.81	1	0.05*
Health is my most important asset	94.7	—	5.3	68.8	18.8	12.5	82.9	8.6	8.6	4.80	2	0.09

*Significant at the 0.05 level.

The concept is not new. Shakespeare said, "There is nothing either good or bad, but thinking makes it so." The prevailing medical model of trying to get health by searching for illness seems to parallel the assumption, "to get peace, prepare for war." For women's outward confidence and health to more closely approximate the apparent truth of their equal resilience and greater longevity, they first must relearn fundamental assumptions about their own state of well-being, comparative strength, and astuteness concerning their needs.

If perception dictates ill behavior and the search for remedies, perception equally can lead to healthy behavior and the quest for self-health care. Or, citing Oelbaum's assumptions, "Apathy toward the work of wellness is a precursor to disease."[2] Conversely, a perception of self as becoming healthier, more self-caring, and more wise in regard to one's well-being ought to be a precursor to behaviors that lead, in fact, to high-level wellness.[2]

Women's perceptions do appear to be changing. Those who disagree with the perceptions and values of traditional practitioners now are expressing dissatisfaction with the "ill care" system and are seeking alternative health care providers and settings. Women have been especially vocal in obtaining more humane and pleasant surroundings for the delivery and care of their babies. They find greater satisfaction with the care received from midwives and female nurse practitioners than from male obstetricians and pediatricians. Ten years ago, a British study showed that 90 per cent of nonprofessional care and advice came from women.[24] The current trend seems to be a formalizing of health care by and for women, based on these assumptions (and differing from those of the medical professions):

1. That women are healthy and functional
2. That their perceptions of health and need are valid and important
3. That their risks and health care needs are different from those of men
4. That one does not have to be ill to improve one's degree of health and capacity to function in the daily responsibilities of life
5. That women as consumers will decide which alternatives are appropriate, expensive, unpleasant, or upsetting, and will act accordingly
6. That women require greater access to the knowledge, decisions, and services that transform self-perception into self-care, and self-care into positive health

The response of the health care system, properly arrayed, will be to meet women on their own terms. "Program planners must research, acknowledge, and build upon the types of concerns expressed by the (clients) and not impose what expert opinion deems necessary."[25]

WOMEN'S HEALTH RISKS AND HEALTH CARE NEEDS

Part of the needed research involves disproving the mythology of women's physical and emotional inferiority, followed by a concerted effort to remove false assumptions from medical texts and advertising. Equally important is to identify and organize objective information about the risks and needs that actually do impact women's health. To start, "women's" research must supplant studies of "rats and men."[26]

Preliminary and inferred findings point toward the special concerns that women have (or need to develop) for their own health. This section will attempt to highlight what is known to date, as a means to impel the reader toward action.

First, women live longer than men. Conditions of aging related to lifestyle and long-term habits are more likely to cross the threshold of visible symptoms or limitations in women. Owing to longevity and lower remarriage rates after divorce or widowing, women are more likely to live alone in later life, demanding greater ability to care for themselves (or risk enforced surrender of self-determination to long-term care or confinement).

Second, women appear to be at greater risk of developing cancers. The American Cancer Society, in its protocol for early detection, recommends that women take part in all preventive screening, while mentioning men in only three. For example, "a cancer-related health check-up" is recommended for all women over 20 years of age every three years, and for all persons over 40 years of age every year.[27] These include pap test, pelvic examination, mammogram, breast physical examination, stool guaic slide test, sigmoidoscopic examination, and digital rectal exam, depending on age and personal history.

Preventive measures also include self-examination, based on accurate knowledge and skill, for breast cancer, sexually transmitted diseases, and conditions indicated by family history.

Third, smoking is of particular concern in

the prevention of lung cancer, which is approaching breast cancer as the most frequent cancer in women. It is also the carcinogen most under the direct control of each person who risks exposure. Yet, women are smoking in ever greater numbers. Recalling my preliminary comparison of 52.6 per cent women smokers and 31.3 per cent men smokers, substantiating evidence began to appear as early as the 1977 Health Interview Survey.[28] The percentage of men who smoke has decreased from 53 per cent in 1964 to 38 per cent in 1978, while the percentage of women has hovered around 30 per cent during the period. In absolute terms, the number of men who smoke has declined, while the number of women smokers has remained steady or increased, with some variation among studies. More important is the tendency of people to start smoking, since those who never smoked enjoy considerably less risk. Among teenagers in 1981, 10.7 per cent of males smoked (approximately the same as in 1978). However, 12.7 per cent of females report smoking (a significant increase from 1978).[29] In one statewide study, smoking by women aged 20 to 29 (37 per cent) also has surpassed the rate for men the same age (29.1 per cent). The report's authors conclude, "The large number of women in this age group who continue to smoke should be the focus of our public health energies."[30] At the current rate, smoking by women overall will exceed that by men within a few years.

Women also have more difficulty giving up smoking, for reasons that are unclear. This is the conclusion of a study by West to follow up on a population of smokers leaving a withdrawal clinic. Pechacek believes, "There's clearly a sex difference . . ." possibly rooted in the radically different social climate of females.[31]

Smoking is a serious health risk for women. Besides the risk of lung cancer, which is notoriously resistant to treatment, smoking during pregnancy is associated with retarded fetal growth, birth defects, and increased risk of spontaneous abortion, and prenatal death, as well as mild impairment and poor development during childhood.

Fourth, stress—or the biochemical, physiologic, and psychologic drain of stress—is linked to heart attack, hypertension, arthritis, allergies, accidents, and depression as a natural by-product of adapting to change. Some research is beginning to indicate that women do experience more stress than men. Cleary and Mechanic[32] find that men report fewer demands than working women or housewives. Women find the dual role of parent–wage earner to be more stressful than men do, since in even the most egalitarian of households, parenting of young children still reverts primarily to the female. More women than men are single parents with primary responsibility for children; they experience isolation, followed by anger, then guilt. Even when they are the sole support of the family, women earn 60 per cent of male salaries for comparable work. Decades of research have shown that isolation and deprivation can be sufficient in themselves to lead to physical and psychologic deterioration, even death.

Whether women actually are exposed to more stressors or whether they respond relatively more negatively to stress, has not been demonstrated adequately. Nor does the distinction matter, since stress stems from the perception that one's demands exceed one's resources to cope. To the extent that stress contributes to illness and accidents, women are at great and increasing risk as they take on multiple roles in a confusing and often biased environment.

Finally, the very history of greater reliance on the "ill care" system has resulted in greater exposure to radiation, psychotropic and addictive drugs, unnecessary surgical procedures (often with intrinsic side effects and risks), lingering conditions that do not receive serious consideration, and the psychologic burden of presumed morbidity.

This last "risk" is not a condemnation of technologic or technical advancements in acute care medicine. When required, there is no substitute. But it is a tool of only limited application on which women have relied too heavily for risks and needs that can be met better through preventive care, self-care, and personalized, positive health care. These are not luxuries for women. They are fundamental prerequisites for survival in modern life.

THE IMPETUS TOWARD HEALTH CARE FOR WOMEN

If the previous discussion lacked the motivational force to move the reader from awareness into action, the financial and personal advantages of positive health care might suffice. Prevention, self-care, and alternative ("high-touch") health services are more economical, more humane, and more effective than treatment, dependency on experts, and "high-tech" services.

As a basis for women's health care, the

health and self-care movement offers all these benefits. First is its focus on prevention, rather than on treatment, of disease. Second is the advocacy of lifestyle and habits that promote and prolong physical, spiritual, and emotional well-being. Third is its foundation in the dignity of each person and the parity of relationship between health advisor and client. This section outlines the assumptions and approaches that, once actively adopted, lead to ever-increasing functional capacity for virtually anyone. (Readers unfamiliar with the trends and concepts of self-care and wellness are referred to the appendix to this chapter for a glossary and preliminary readings.)

Prevention is a most congenial interface between medicine and health care, drawing on both. Immunizations have been developed for many acute diseases. Even so, people concerned with progressive health do complain of the complacency (or lack of information) on the part of physicians who do not discuss side effects, heed contraindications, or defer to the wishes of families when doubt exists. In Great Britain and other countries, immunization is recommended but not always advisable. Education, containment, and treatment are substituted to balance the risk of chronic side effects with the prevention of disease. An informed and active constituency, particularly parents, is required to help render the approach effective.

Early detection is now possible for many hidden diseases or systemic deficiencies, increasing survival rates dramatically. Paralleling the conquest of epidemics at the beginning of this century, the correction of organic defects has been the mid-century challenge. Cancer and heart disease are particularly good examples of longevity and freedom from illness resulting from detection. Tests such as the pap smear, proctoscopy, mammogram, and electrocardiogram, are conducted by skilled health care providers. Other procedures are so simple that anyone can learn to monitor his or her own vital characteristics: blood pressure, pulse, breathing, height, and weight. Other procedures previously too technical for self-testing (e.g., pregnancy, glucose levels, hemoblobin, pacemakers with wrist-watch monitors) are also now in general use. Again, the benefit requires more than available technology. Information about the woman's normal body functions, accurate information about significant variations, attention to the signs and signals from her physical and emotional monitors, and a heightened sense of responsibility to and for herself all make the difference between early and late detection of conditions. In addition, knowledge of the effects on her system of medications, nutrients, environmental hazards, and habits will determine the extent to which a woman can detect abnormal or unwarranted states of being.

Finally, informed confidence to deal with medical and health services in one's own best interest is essential to prevention and early detection. Physical examinations, check-ups, and consultations with health professionals are important. In the positive health model, however, these are conducted not primarily to diagnose illness but to reveal the dynamic pattern of ever-changing physical states. Discussion, self-awareness, teaching, and mutual assessment of the meaning of results by practitioner and client all weigh as heavily as laboratory tests and physical diagnosis.

Indeed, there is some confirmation that women do translate their perceptions of health and health care needs into behavior. Langlie[16] is one of few who have researched the area of prevention, following the prevention health behavior (PHB) model of Rosenstock.[33] Female gender is one of the variables having an effect on PHB:

Demographic characteristics may also influence PHB: younger adults, whites, and women appear to have higher utilization rates for preventive health service.

Langlie[16] found that Direct Risk PHB (related to tangible danger of illness or disease) is primarily associated with older age and female gender. Indirect Risk PHB (related to choice of actions with vague or long-term danger) is related to perceptions of control and being a member of a high socioeconomic status group.[16] There is insufficient evidence to conclude that women overall seek and engage in health and self-care to any greater extent then men do for indirect risks.

Evidence is mounting that choice of lifestyle, habits, and personal practices have a major impact on the quality and duration of health.[34–36] For women to improve the self-perceptions and overcome imposed perceptions of their health, it is essential that they cultivate both the "behaviors" and the "perceptions of control" that Langlie identifies.[16] A fundamental axiom of learning is that successfully engaging in activities can change underlying attitudes, as surely as attitudes influence behavior. In the case of fully developed personal health care, the starting point (perception or practice) matters not nearly as much as the actual doing.

The monumental task appears to be that of causing the choices and actions that lead to improved well-being. Kemper[37] acknowledges that, although many educational and persuasive tactics have been employed, "the state of the art is still relatively undeveloped. Little research has gone into determining the best approaches for promoting self-care." In contrast to illness, there is no concrete laboratory test that will result in a "diagnosis" of health for body, mind, or spirit (let alone a balance among them). The dilemma is that normal functioning in one arena does not always promote health in other aspects of functioning. Critical evaluation of untraditional approaches is difficult, as the body of knowledge on self-care is housed indiscriminately in those who are credentialed and those who are unqualified, in those who are ethical and those who exploit individuals who are vulnerable. Gaps in research and knowledge warrant caution in heeding the unqualified claims of research and testing for products or procedures that may have only short-term or cosmetic effect. Naive acceptance of promises for successful self-care or "do-it-yourself miracles" is a critical danger of which providers and consumers must be mindful.

Caution notwithstanding, certain assertions can be made about approaches to enhance health. First, self-care starts with self-awareness and knowledge of healthy functioning (Fig. 3.1). Several authors now publish tools to assist in the assessment of personal health and lifestyle. Ardell,[35] Travis,[36] and Hettler[38] have been mentioned as reliable sources given the current best knowledge about factors contributing to health. Others are Clark,[39] Pender,[23] and several others discussed in Doerr and Hutchins.[40]

Knowledge of health stems from independent investigation through literature, workshops, even public media. A rule of thumb for selecting resources is to choose approaches that are multidimensional and that are backed up by research or recommendation by health advisors of holistic philosophy, or both.[41]

Following awareness is the matter of choice—choice to change one's setting onself or choice not to change. Choosing is essential in self-care, not only initially but hourly and daily, as health is a process and not a static state. Everyone is a runner, a nonsmoker, or a concerned eater, only from urge to urge. Positive practices and lifestyles become habitual gradually, as they replace dependence and illness behavior.

Bridging the gap from awareness and choice to action depends on many factors both internal and external to the individual. Pender[23] states:

> Good health demands individual knowledge, motivation, responsibility, and participation in making choices related to health. Personal health behavior *can* be changed, but frequently this change must be made in the face of counterforces, advertising, peer groups, etc.

For many in our society, habits and short-term problems block the vision of long-term planning (Gresham's Law). Setting priorities is complicated for an individual who may have many conflicting goals, demands, health needs, desires, and acquired or genetic risks. Some may attempt to accomplish an unrealistic number of changes at one time or have inadequate motivation and support to follow through consistently on an attempted change. Hubbard[42] cautions:

> The real dilemma is the contest between the value assigned to health and the value assigned to competing activities which may be antagonistic to health.

According to Northcutt,[43] less than half the adults in the United States are functional, or competent, with regard to their own health.

The study conducted by Yankelovich and co-workers[44] for General Mills found that 60 per cent of the respondents were "concerned" (very health conscious), while 40 per cent were

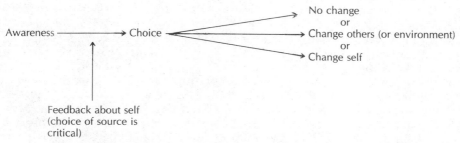

Figure 3.1. Awareness model of change. (Adapted from Hall, J. by Ward.[55a])

"complacent" (not health conscious), based on two criteria:

1. Taking good health for granted versus not taking health for granted and really working at it
2. Dealing with health problems on a crisis basis versus taking a preventive approach to health care

Yankelovich and co-workers conclude that the majority of Americans accept in principle, although they may not practice, the concept of prevention. There is agreement that health check-ups are a good thing in concept, but a majority question whether they are necessary when one is feeling well. The three major factors that prevent these families from seeking regular health check-ups are denial, fear, and money.[49] In the data collected by Drury in 1974,[4, 45] the primary reason for women of all ages not to seek health care is excessive cost (49.5 per cent).

According to Yankelovich and associates,[44] there is conflict between the old and new family health perceptions. In most families, the wife still is the family health officer, and "parents appear to be neglecting their own health in the interest of their children's."[44] One obviously implied problem is a misapprehension by parents of desirable role modeling for children. Far more appropriate than the sacrifice of health is the enhancement of it by parents as a positive model for later life. The reader is referred to the original study for a more in-depth analysis.

Self-care means action, but it does not mean self-denial or belittling. Just as the habits of illness are cumulative and the rewards of the sick role reinforcing, so are the habits of positive health. Acquiring a healthy holistic lifestyle is a building process, not a destructive one, a positive effort to replace some or all negative habits. There are no absolutes; everything one does can help or hinder. Just as crash dieting does not make one nutritionally healthy, so an occasional drift into cookies or coffee does not make one a nutritional failure. Every cigarette not smoked is a success, regardless of the choice one makes about the next one. Counting successful or positive actions and forgetting about one's imperfections are parts of perceiving oneself as healthy. The impact of perceptions on health already has been discussed.

In general, a plan for health would include some of the following elements and actions:

1. Seeking a balance among physical, emotional, and spiritual health. One cannot participate in one area at the expense of the others (running instead of socialization). Balance is multidimensional, complex, and unachievable with a unidimensional approach.
2. Seeking to reduce exposure to risk from stress, environment, and internal messages of low self-esteem or illnesses image.
3. Seeking personal and professional support systems for choice and change, recognizing that people become healthier in sharing with others than in isolation.
4. Establishing a means of rewarding self and others for healthy practices and self expression.
5. Seeking a balance among privacy and togetherness, work and play, thinking and feeling, selecting and letting go, and so on.
6. Recognizing barriers and systematically planning goals that will overcome them.

On the positive side is the fact that most people are "in real life abundantly healthy."[46] People have a miraculous capacity to absorb minor collisions with daily life and to rebound fully. Changes toward greater self-care need to be only minor in many cases. Further, the practices that have been cited in this discussion are inexpensive and self-perpetuating once adopted. Also, women in particular appear ready and able to exercise self-care and responsibility, once freed of misperceptions and stereotypes regarding their own health and wisdom.

IMPLICATIONS FOR FURTHER WORK

Clearly, there is a need for additional research in the areas of health and preventive care, beginning with the most basic:

Many of the factors, conditions, and circumstances leading to disease are known, but there has been little research conducted with well people to discover what makes them healthy.[47]

The first challenge is to search for the factors enhancing or blocking the causes of positive health, self-care, and preventive health care, in order to present the health seeker and health care provider with reliable information on which to base choice and change.

Second, much work is needed to resolve the dilemma facing most health practitioners: the discrepancy between what people understand and what they are willing to pursue in terms of learning, choice, and action. A major problem with health prevention programs is that providers often perceive needed changes in lifestyle that are not recognized as priorities by clients. On the other hand, even when cognitively and verbally in accord, people often are neither ready nor motivated to activate the change in their lives. Researching the factors that cause people to move from awareness through choice to action is called for by Sehnert:[48]

   . . . points of reference such as confidence, anxiety, loneliness, apathy, high or low energy level, time, the process of decision making, human contact, location of activity, quality of life, money, and so on, are as yet, not well researched.

Rosenstock proposes that "emotions may have greater value in accounting for behavior than cognition."[28] These factors likely have great implication for interventions with clients. Persons professing to believe in health promotion will contribute to the research and assist in the matter of closing the gap between intention and action. In the meantime, health promotion may continue to appear faddish, spasmodic, and disjointed, as agencies offer primarily those resources which consumers are ready to use.

Third, although this discussion has focused on the variable of sex, it may be equally crucial to study the variable of age when investigating women's health. Women carry their cumulative state of health through approximately seven more years of life than do men. Half are widowed by age 56, and thereafter are alone to face the effects on health following some of life's major changes and losses (widowhood or divorce, menopause, retirement, economic deprivation, and loss of purpose). Finances, living arrangements, companionship, transportation, social activities, family, the will to live, and many other factors have implications for women's health and health care in later life.

Fourth, the whole arena of women's health, perceptions, practices, and health services merits intense study. Since most research focuses on illness and disease, rather than on health and prevention, and since most pathologic diagnoses are made by male physicians, further longitudinal research must be conducted on issues such as these: What do individuals do to remain healthy; what risk factors are most consequential for women and which are most directly related to self-care or preventive practices; what differences emerge from a premise of positive health rather than that of illness; what different conclusions result from a premise of psychophysiospiritual sources of health and illness than from that of pathologic microbiologic causes? Certainly, massive research is needed concerning the

stressfulness of women's roles: are they more stressful, and if so, why? Extensive work is needed to identify the necessary and sufficient conditions for maintaining and improving the health of women.

Fifth, the most urgent, concrete findings and proactive advocacy are required to validate the perceptions and practices of women relative to their own health and to engender more realistic notions about women's health and health care among providers of that care. Decisive steps are needed to counteract the messages entrenched in and marketed to physicians concerning women.

Drawing once again from the full-color advertisements showing furrowed brows and wringing hands, this time the concerned physician affirms:

Many times it is not relevant for the primary physician to get at the underlying cause. So I am confident that antianxiety agents are the treatment of choice in most cases. Even if you can't get to the cause, you can control the symptom.[48a]

Finally, it is left to women—the most powerful consumers of health and medical care—to change, find, or develop the approaches and services of health care, such that the evolving needs of this decade are met. As stated in the *New England Journal of Medicine*:

A new era is beginning wherein neither the prevention of death from epidemics nor the correction of physiologically measurable abnormalities will be the principal medical challenge. The central objective of the coming era will be the maintenance or improvement of individual patient functioning while he or she performs usual activities.[49]

The important question is, who will decide what constitutes healthy "functioning" and the appropriate means to achieving it? A perception by and of women as healthy, competent, informed, and equally responsible will be an essential cornerstone.

What Is Health?

There are many conflicting, misunderstood, and misinterpreted definitions of health, and as many conceptions and perceptions as there are writers. Each has a personal theory of what health is and how to improve it. Many approaches are unidimensional rather than holistic, in that they advocate the elimination of or addition to one's lifestyle of a single practice: running, megavitamins, a specific nutritional change. This confusing advice tends to leave the consumer bewildered and without direction, seemingly faced with a choice among competing alternatives. Should I run, meditate, take vitamins, avoid physicians or traditional or even nontraditional health care providers? The reader can be made to feel responsible for personal health or guilty about its lack without knowing what to do. In his book, *Take Care of Yourself*, Vickery and Fries[50] state,

You (the patient) can do more than any physician to maintain your own good health and well-being. With the exception of those diseases which are prevented by immunization, surprisingly few diseases can be prevented by the physician.

Health is not a simple term to define, let alone an easy state to achieve. It is more than a concern with physiologic functioning or absence of disease. Complexly interwoven with the individual's life and owing to genetic makeup, health is not distributed equally among all individuals. Even one's perception of health is influenced by economics, politics, fashion trends, environment, cultural roles and expectations, psychologic norms, the art or science of standard health care, and available technology during a particular time and place of existence.

Traditionally, health has been defined as the absence of disease. More recently, attempts have been made to describe health as a positive state in its own right. The starting point for most authors, whether accepting or critical of it, is the World Health Organization's definitions stated in its preamble: "Health is a state of complete physical, mental, and social well-being and not merely the absence of disease or infirmity." Antonovsky[51] evaluates the latter as "impossibly abstract, philosophically utopian and misleading, and static." Callahan[52] states:

It is a dangerous definition and it desperately needs replacement by something more modest. Its emphasis on "complete physical, mental, and social well-being" puts both medicine and society in the untenable position of being required to attain unattainable goals . . . Health may be, most of the time, a necessary condition for well-being, but it is not a sufficient condition. By even suggesting that medicine can succeed in such a goal—which is tantamount to making medicine the keystone in the search for human happiness—there is posited for it an impossible and illusory task.

McGrory[53] asserts:

As an absolute, health does not exist. Since any definition is limited by the criteria used to measure

the concept and since the criteria for measuring health are vague, the definition of health will remain vague until more precise measurements are established.

Several authors have begun to publish measurable criteria for lifestyle assessment in the attempt to name the processes and choices by which a person moves toward integration and balance of physical, emotional, and spiritual well-being. As early as 1972, Belloc and Breslow[34] demonstrated that better health is related to seven basic practices:

1. Three meals a day rather than snacking
2. Eating breakfast regularly
3. Moderate exercise, two or three times a week
4. Seven or eight hours of sleep per night
5. No smoking
6. Moderate weight
7. No alcohol or used in moderation

Ardell,[35] in *High Level Wellness*, proposes five dimensions as a framework for assessing one's lifestyle: self-responsibility, nutritional awareness, stress management, physical fitness, and environmental sensitivity.

The Wellness Inventory, developed by Travis,[36] contains 12 areas for individual assessment, including:

1. Self-responsibility and love
2. Breathing
3. Sensing
4. Eating
5. Moving
6. Feeling
7. Thinking
8. Playing and working
9. Communicating
10. Sex
11. Finding meaning
12. Transcending

This assessment tool provides the individual with a scoring wheel that can be compared with the other scores to determine balance for the individual. Although descriptions of a healthy lifestyle rather than definitions, these measurements reveal two essential elements. First, health is multidimensional and dynamic—a process rather than a state. Second, the personal practices that increase one's health all are within the possibility of self-care by an individual, family, or peer group, given adequate commitment and resources.

In fact, a study from the University of Wisconsin[38] reveals that 53 per cent of a person's health depends on lifestyle and 21 per cent on environment, support, and other factors within the control of lay people collectively. Only genetic factors (16 per cent) and existing medical protocol (10 per cent) are outside the daily influence of most people.

The theme is emphasized by Blockstein:[54]

> . . . the greatest untapped manpower resource in this country is the individual consumer. Needed is an informed and "activated" citizen who can take his [sic] own initiative in personal health approaching and utilizing the health care system properly for all services required in his [sic] personal health management program.

Norris[55] adds:

> The person on the street today knows more about health, disease and health care than the average physician did at the turn of the century.

Self-responsibility, knowledge, choice, commitment to self-care, and mutual support are the milestones of health. The beginning of a conscious pursuit of well-being lies in becoming fluent and comfortable with the traditional and emerging vocabulary of health care.

The following glossary has been adapted and developed, serving as a guide for my research at this point. It must, however, be recognized that working definitions will be expected to change as more is learned about the health promotion and self-care areas.

GLOSSARY

Health: A wide range of states, ranging from "a relatively passive state of freedom from illness in which the individual is at peace with his environment, a condition of homeostasis" to "a dynamic condition of change in which the individual moves forward, climbing toward a higher potential of functioning, a condition of wellness."[56]

Direct risk: Activities involving putting oneself in "direct potential for producing injury or disease."[16]

Indirect risk: Behavior not generally believed to be hazardous in and of itself. The perception that one has some control over one's health status and that benefits of preventive action are high and costs are low.

Health: A multidimensional complex process including all that an individual is, desires, and comes in contact with.

High-level wellness: "An integrated method of functioning which is oriented toward maximizing the potential of which the individual is capable, within the environment where he is functioning."[56]

Healthy individual: "Central to the concept of health is the idea that a healthy individual is one who is able to function in his role in society."[57]

Self-care: "Those processes that permit people and families to take initiative to take responsibilities and to function effectively in developing their own potential for health."[55]

Patient education: "Has an illness orientation, focuses on coping with the immediate situation and suggests that someone—not the consumer—is going to control the process."[58, 58a]

Self-care education: "In contrast, does not assume sickness, thereby assigning a generic meaning to care—that is to look after."[58, 58a]

Health education: "Stimulating or providing experiences at times, in ways and through situations leading to the development of the health, knowledge, attitudes and behavior that are most conducive to the attainment of individual, group or community health."[59]

Health maintenance: "Any behavior or activity which results either in the prolongation of life expectancy or in an increase in the quality of life, whether or not this was originally intended as a main objective."[60]

Disease prevention: "Specific behaviors or activities which are intended to prevent either the experience or the spread of specific disease."[60]

Self-help groups: "The essential point of self help groups—in health or in any other field—is that members feel themselves united by a common bond of disadvantage. The type of disadvantage may vary widely but each is characterized by a need for help and support which is not available in any existing service, professional or otherwise."[60]

Health care: A broad term including medical care and nursing care, as well as the interventions of other members of the interdisciplinary team, social workers, pharmacists, psychologists, and other traditional and nontraditional practitioners of the healing arts.

Medical care: Pathology (disease)–oriented care with the diagnosis and treatment of the pathologic complaint and alleviation of the symptom as the goal.

Nursing care: Focus on assisting the individual to attain his or her optimum level of physical, social, and spiritual state of health in any situation.

Preventive care: Measures taken by an individual to attain or maintain his or her optimal health.

Curative care: Measures taken to alleviate some symptoms that are interfering with the optimal state of health.

Lifestyle: All of one's behaviors, collectively.[38]

Health perception: The meaning that an individual gives to health.

Lifestyle practice: Engagement in an activity that enhances positive health avoidance of an activity that is detrimental to health (e.g., "I do not smoke").

I wish to acknowledge the assistance of Bob Ward in revision of this chapter.

References

1. Richmond, J. Human development. In Jones, B. (ed.) *The Health of Americans* Englewood Cliffs, NJ: Prentice-Hall, 1970, p. 7.

2. Oelbaum, C.H. Hallmarks of adult wellness. *American Journal of Nursing,* Vol. 74, 1974, pp. 1623–1625.

3. Molberg, A. Address to American Society for Health Care Education and Training of the American Hospital Association. Duluth, MN, July 1983.

4. U.S. National Center for Health Statistics. *Physician Visits, Volume and Interval Since Last Visit*: U.S., 1975. D.H.E.W. Public Health Service, Office of Health Research, Statistics and Technology, Hyattsville, Md, Series 10, NO1128, April 1979, Table II, p. 25.

5. Mechanic, D. Sex, illness, illness behavior, and the use of health services. *Journal of Human Stress,* Vol. 2, Dec. 1976, pp. 29–40.

6. Stevenson, J.S. Women health research: Why, what, and so what? *CNR Voice,* Ohio State University School of Nursing, Fall 1979, pp. 2–3.

6a. Riley, M.W., and Foner, A. *Aging and Society,* Vol. 1. New York: Russell Sage Foundation, 1968, p. 211.

7. Philips, D.L., and Segal, B.E. Sexual status and psychiatric symptoms. *American Sociological Review,* Vol. 34, 1969.

8. Nathanson, C. Illness and the feminine role: A theoretical review. *Social Science and Medicine,* Vol. 9, February 1975, pp. 57–62.

9. Schiefelbein, S. The female patient, heeded? Hustled? Healed? *Saturday Review,* March 1980, pp. 12–16.

10. Corea, G. *The Hidden Malpractice: How American Medicine Treats Women as Patients and Professionals.* New York: Morrow, 1977.

11. Broverman, I.K., Broverman, D.M., and Clarkson, F.E. Sex-role stereotypes and clinical judgments of mental health. *Journal of Counseling and Clinical Psychology,* Vol. 34(1), 1970, pp. 1–7.

12. Maccoby, E., and Jacklin, C. *The Psychology of Sex Differences.* Stanford, CA: Stanford University Press, 1974.

13. Dowling, C. *The Cinderella Complex.* N.Y.: Pocketbook, 1981.

14. Ford, D.L., and Bagot, D.S. Correlates of job stress and job satisfaction. In Adams, D. (ed.) *Understanding and Managing Stress.* San Diego: University Associates, 1980.

15. Tangri, S. Determinants of occupational role innovation among college women. *In* Mednick, M., Tangri, S., and Hoffman, L. (eds.). *Women and Achievement.* New York: John Wiley and Sons, 1975.

16. Langlie, J.K. Social networks, health beliefs, and preventive health behavior. *Journal of Health and Social Behavior,* Vol. 18, Sept. 1977, pp. 8, 244–260.

17. Grove, W.R., and Tudor, J.F. Adult sex roles and mental illness. *American Journal of Sociology,* Vol. 78, January 1973, pp. 812–835.

18. Kiefer, T. The 'neurotic woman' syndrome. *The Progressive.* Madison, Wisconsin: The Progressive Inc., Dec. 1980, p. 28.

19. DeRoos, E.K., and Coder, R. Assessing low income health concerns. *Health Education,* Vol. 36, 1977, pp. 29–31.

20. Ware, J.E., Davies-Avery, A., and Donald, C.A. *Conceptualization and Measurement of Health for Adults in the Health Insurance Study,* Vol. V. General Health Perceptions, Santa Monica: Rand Corporation on HEW Grant, 1978.

21. Weisensee, M.G. *Health Perceptions and Wellness Practices.* Unpublished report, University of Minnesota School of Nursing, Minneapolis, MN, 1982.

22. Dolfman, M. Toward operational definitions of health. *School Health,* Vol. 44(4), 1974, pp. 206–209.

23. Pender, N. *Health Promotion in Nursing Practice.* Norwalk, CT: Appleton-Century-Crofts, 1982.

24. Elliot-Binns, C.P. An analysis of lay medicine. *Journal of the Royal College of General Practitioners* Vol. 23, 1973, pp. 255–264.

25. Barry, P.A., Pezzullo, S., Berry, W.L., DeFriese, G.H., and Allen, J. *Self-Care Program: Their Role and Potential.* Chapel Hill, NC: Health Services Research Center, University of North Carolina, 1979.

26. Lutter, J. Body image, body fat. Lecture by President, Melpomene Institute, at Coffman Union, University of Minnesota, Minneapolis, April 11, 1983.

27. American Cancer Society. *Guidelines for the Cancer-Related Check-ups: Recommendations and Rationale.* July-August 1980, pp. 195–196.

28. Moore, E.C. Woman and health. *Public Health Reports,* Suppl., Sept.-Oct. 1980, p. 11.

29. Richmond, J.B. *Smoking and Health.* A report of the Surgeon General. Washington, DC, DHEW 79-50066, Jan. 1979.

30. Minnesota Department of Health. Smoking: Health Risks. Minneapolis, MN, February 1983.

31. Murray, L. Medical advances (Smoking: Why it's harder for women to quit.) *American Health,* Vol. 1, Sept.-Oct. 1982, p. 60.

32. Cleary, P., and Mechanic, D. Sex differences in psychological distress among married people. *Journal of Health and Social Behavior,* Vol. 24, 1983, pp. 111–121.

33. Rosenstock, I.M. Why people use health services. *The Milbank Memorial Fund Quarterly,* Vol. 44, 1966, pp. 94–124.

34. Belloc, N.D., and Breslow, L. Relationship of physical health status and health practices. *Preventive Medicine,* Vol. 3, 1972, pp. 409–421.

35. Ardell, D.B. *High Level Wellness.* Emmaus, PA: Rodale Press, 1977.

36. Travis, J.W. *Wellness Inventory,* 2nd ed. Mill Valley, CA, Wellness Resource Center, 1981.

37. Kemper, D.W. Medical self care: A stop on the road to high level wellness. *Health Values,* Vol. 4, 1980, pp. 63–68.

38. Hettler, B. *Life Style Assessment Questionnaire* (2nd ed.). Stevens Point: University of Wisconsin, 1980.

39. Clark, C.C.: *Enhancing Wellness.* New York: Springer Publishing Co., 1981.

40. Doerr, B.T., and Hutchins, E.B. Health risk appraisal: Process, problems, and prospects for nursing practice and research. *Nursing Research* Vol. 30, Sept./Oct. 1981, pp. 299–306.

41. Tubesing, D.A. *Wholistic Health*. New York: Human Sciences Press, 1979.

42. Hubbard, W.N. Health knowledge. *In* Jones, B. (ed.) *The Health of Americans*. Englewood Cliffs: Prentice-Hall, 1970.

43. Northcutt, N., et al. *Adult Functional Competency, A Summary*. Adult Performance Level Project, Extension Division, University of Texas, Austin, March 1975.

44. Yankelovich, Skelly, and White, Inc. *Family Health in an Era of Stress*. Minneapolis, MN: General Mills American Family Report, 1978–1979.

45. Drury, T.F. Unpublished data from the 1974 Health Interview Survey, Division of Health Interview Statistics, Washington, DC, 1979. (Quoted in Marieskind, H.I., op. cit.)

46. Thomas, L. On the science and technology of medicine. *In* Knowles, M. (ed.) *Doing Better and Feeling Worse*. New York: W.W. Norton and Company, Inc., 1977.

47. Warr, W. Toward a higher level of wellness: Prevention of Chronic Disease. *In* Anderson, S., and Bauwens, E. (eds.). *Dynamics of Chronic Health Problems*. St. Louis: C.V. Mosby, 1981.

48. Sehnert, K. *How to Be Your Own Doctor, Sometimes*. New York: Grosset and Dunlap, 1975.

48a. Werkman, S. Avoiding problems in short-term management of anxiety. (An interview conducted by Borland, Coogan Associates). Chicago: Abbott Laboratories, 1980.

49. Tarlov, A.F. The increasing supply of physicians, the changing structure of the health-services system, and the future practice of medicine. *New England Journal of Medicine,* Vol. 308, May 19, 1983, pp. 1235–1244.

50. Vickery, D.M., and Fries, J.F. *Take Care of Yourself.* Philippines: Addison-Wesley Publishing Company, Inc., 1976.

51. Antonovsky, A. *Health, Stress and Coping*. San Francisco: Jossey Bass Inc., 1979.

52. Callahan, D. Health and society: Some ethical imperatives. *In* Knowles, J.H. (ed.). *Doing Better and Feeling Worse*. New York: W.W. Norton and Co., 1977, pp. 23–34.

53. McGrory, A. *A Well Model Approach to Care of the Dying Client*. New York: McGraw Hill, 1978.

54. Blockstein, W.L. Developing a model for consumer health education. *Critical Issues in Continuing Education in Nursing,* Madison, Wis. October 1971, pp. 43–57.

55. Norris, C. Self care. *American Journal of Nursing,* Vol. 79, 1979, pp. 486–489.

55a. Ward, B. *Change Model*. (Adapted from Hall, J.) National Training Laboratory, 1974.

56. Dunn, H. What high level wellness means. *Canadian Journal of Public Health,* Vol. 11, 1959, pp. 447–457.

57. Belloc, N.D.: Relationship of health practices and mortality. *Preventive Medicine,* Vol. 2, 1973, pp. 67–81.

58. Levin, L., Lowell, S., Katz, A.H., and Holst, E. *Self-Care*. London: Croom Helm Ltd., 1978.

58a. Levin, L. Patient education and self-care: How do they differ? *Nursing Outlook,* Vol. 25, 1978, pp. 170–175.

59. Dalzell-Ward, A.J. *A Textbook of Health Education*. London: Tavistock Press, 1974.

60. Williamson, J., and Danaher, K. *Self Care in Health*. London: Croom Helm Ltd., 1978, p. 109.

4

OLDER WOMEN'S HEALTH CARE

LINDA McKEEVER
IDA MARTINSON

Linda McKeever and Ida Martinson give an in-depth look at the older woman. The chapter begins with the factors that influence the health care of older women, and six commonly held myths are identified. The chapter concludes with an examination of the four major health conditions that affect older women—osteoporosis, coronary heart disease, breast cancer, and gynecologic problems.

The fastest growing population segment of the United States is the woman age 65 and over. In 1981, 15.8 million older Americans were women. This statistic accounts for 60 per cent of the 26.3 million persons age 65 and over.[1, 2] In 1978, 112 million people, or 51 per cent of the population in the United States, were women; and of these, 13.5 million were women age 65 years or older (58 per cent of the over age 65 population).[3] It is projected that by the year 2035, 33.4 million people will be older women and 22.4 million will be older men.[3] These powerful statistics are influencing this nation to look at the implications an older population will have on institutions and society in general. Nurses are in an advantageous position to influence the health care of older women by identifying the specific health needs of this population, by identifying actual and potential stressors that influence health status, by enhancing programs for prevention and self-care, by constructing improved programs for the chronically ill and those needing long-term care, by dispelling myths that add to the stress older women face, by advocating the health needs of older women, and by interpreting these health care needs to legislatures and social institutions. As a profession dominated largely by women, it is most appropriate that nurses attend to the needs of women. By

improving health care for women, we improve health care for humankind; and by not forgetting the older woman, we ensure our own future.

It is useful to view older women within a framework of stress and coping. So many psychosocial factors contribute to compound the stress these women face. The prejudices of ageism and sexism serve to increase the vulnerability to stress and to make management of stress more difficult. Widowhood, financial status, socialization of women, chronic illness, and the aging process itself become more difficult to deal with in a society that devalues one who is old and female. Nurses can intervene in these processes by reducing stressors that might lead to future problems; also they can reduce stress itself by working with patients and strengthening their coping processes. It is with this framework in mind that factors influencing the health care of older women will be presented.

FACTORS THAT INFLUENCE THE HEALTH CARE OF OLDER WOMEN

Age-related categories that define who is old vary according to eligibility categories and according to who collects and who describes research data. Many sources speak of the older woman as age 65 and over, whereas others designate "older" as age 50, 55, or 62, and over. It is common for many to associate the onset of old age with menopause, at or around age 50; and it is not uncommon to hear college professors speak of the older woman as the 35-year-old student returning to school, or gynecologists referring to the elderly primipara who is in fact 30 years old. Many persons speaking or writing about older women include mid- and late life, because these women often share many of the same characteristics that make them vulnerable to stress. Matthews[4] challenges the notion of old age being defined by biology, but rather advocates its definition as a social category molded by social and historical forces. For example, being old could be associated with health and physical ability rather than with age. Goffman[5] says that old-ness is a stigma, a discrediting attribute. Matthews[4] discusses the relationship of uncertainty to being old. "The overriding source of uncertainty, however, is related to self-identity. The lack of a rite of passage that places people in the age category 'old' and the lack of norms and expectations that prescribe 'old' behavior in American society combine to place old persons in ambiguous social positions: how are they to view themselves in relation to their age?"[4] How do we know when we get old? There are no rites of passage and depending on the meaning for individual women, old may begin at menopause or at retirement, but what is clear is the element of uncertainty. In this discussion, older women will be defined statistically as those 65 and over, but health concerns and psychosocial problems know no age boundaries and may include women in midlife. Age is only relative. Also, an attempt will be made to address stressors that are specific to older women and not the problems common to older men and women that can be found in books on aging or gerontology.

Profile of the Older Woman: At Risk for Stress

Who is the older woman? We know she is growing in numbers, but what about her health and socioeconomic status? What stressors influence her life, and how does she cope with the situation in which she finds herself?

Mortality rates among females remain substantially lower than among males, resulting in women continuing to outlive men. Women born in 1981 can expect to live 77.9 years, 7.6 years longer than males born the same year.[1] It has been speculated that differences in life style between men and women account for men's higher death rate. As women's roles and lifestyles change and become more comparable to that of men, it has been expected that mortality rates would be more equal. Research has documented an increase in lung-cancer deaths in women but has not clearly demonstrated an increase in cardiovascular or suicide rates.[7] Evidence is not yet available to accurately predict whether women's lifestyle and role changes will alter their mortality rates.

In 1981, marital status statistics for women age 65 and older revealed 5.7 per cent were single, 38.6 per cent married, 51.3 per cent widowed, and 4.4 per cent separated or divorced. Older women are four times as likely to be widowed than are older men owing to their increased life expectancy over men and to the cultural tendency to marry men older than themselves. Research on widowhood has identified psychosocial cultural factors that influence the experience as well as the process of grief and grieving and coping with the loss.

Widowhood is one factor that influences the living arrangements prevalent among older women. In 1981, 42.4 per cent of older women lived alone, compared with 15 per cent of older men living alone.[1] Social isolation and loneliness are possible risks for older women who live alone. Of the 5 per cent of the elderly population living in institutions, 74 per cent are women.[3] This is a powerful statistic and has great implications for nursing in long-term care facilities. Many elderly live in substandard housing in urban neighborhoods that may put their safety at risk. The geographic distribution of older women has implications for the social institutions in the areas where these women live. More than half the population of older women live in New York, California, Florida, Illinois, Ohio, Pennsylvania, and Texas, with New York and California accounting for the greatest proportion.[6]

Generally, at present, most older women are not employed and if they were employed during their lifetime, their earnings were less than their male counterparts and their retirement benefits are only 76 per cent of that which men receive. Most older women are poor, and their poverty is more profound than that of men. Older women have fewer employment opportunities compared with men, owing to the stigma of old age assigned to women, little educational training, and poor self-concept. Economically, many older women of today have been dependent on their husbands, and many have not learned to handle finances. This fact makes it difficult for all older women lacking financial experience. Those women who were widowed and left with adequate resources may lack the knowledge to manage their resources successfully.[8] Another employment issue is the fact that many of today's older women were unpaid workers in their own home and are not entitled to social security or retirement benefits.

In summary, Butler and Lewis[8] characterize the older woman as widowed, poor, living alone in substandard housing, receiving little medical care, and enjoying few employment opportunities. Vulnerability to stress is increased, and coping alternatives are reduced by virtue of age and sex. Although this picture of older women may be true for most, it is also untrue for many. The ease of stereotyping older women must be guarded against. Besides, the older woman of tomorrow may exhibit much more diversity as she reflects the changing status of women today.

Older Women Neglected

Older women have been neglected by society in general and have remained relatively invisible, adding again to their vulnerability to stress and lack of confidence. Fuller and Martin[9] have identified several reasons why older women have been neglected by researchers and writers in the past. Researchers, in their search for universals and similarities in research findings, have frequently avoided differentiating their findings in terms of sexual differences. Findings are therefore reported as generalizable to the whole older population. This has created great difficulty in understanding the specific differences between older men and women in our population. Also, scientific theories that have been proposed to explain development have often not accounted for age and sex differences. Most developmental theories have emphasized child growth and development, with little or no mention of adult growth and development. An exception to this is Erikson's developmental theory, which does account for adult developmental stages but does not account for sex differences.[9a] There is a need for current lifespan theories to account for sex differences in development.[10, 10a] The normative-crisis model of lifespan theories of development, of which Erikson's is an example, presumes that men and women develop on the same time schedule. There is no research to substantiate that this is true, and Rossi[10] cites examples to refute this idea. Neugarten[11] is a proponent of the timing of events model of development, which assumes that there is no overarching plan to adult development. Rossi says that "the phasing and the shifts in self-definition are structured largely by age norms rooted in culture and society, not in biology."[10] Attention needs to be paid to the differences in development between men and women to better understand their idiosyncrasies. Caution needs to be paid to developing lifespan theories that do not reflect and incorporate the current change in women's status and roles.

Other reasons that older women have not been studied include the relative invisibility of the older woman in society, the fact that large numbers of older women did not exist until recently, the male-normal method of statistical analysis, and the fact that researchers and funders of research rarely are older females.[9] As the population has become older and the older population has become larger, more emphasis has been placed on the study of aging. Older women, as the majority subgroup in gerontology, must receive their proper amount of attention.

The older woman has been neglected not only by researchers and writers, as well as the society in general, but also by the early women's liberation movement. Lewis and Butler[12] attributes this neglect to the prejudice of ageism. "Ageism can be described as a process of systematic stereotyping of and discrimination against people because they are old, just as racism and sexism accomplish this with skin color and gender."[12] The stereotype of ageism allows us to categorize older people as different from others. Older people are victims of this prejudice as well as believers in it, thus defining themselves like the stereotype or spending energy to convince themselves they are not a part of it.[4] Older women deal with the prejudices of ageism as well as the prejudices of sexism, making them particularly vulnerable to stress and coping with it.

Prevailing Myths Contribute to Stress

Myths abound around the aging population in general, creating a climate of discomfort and stress. Myths also prevail about and have contributed to society's negative image of the older woman. A myth is not a representation of objective reality. Myths are products of the bourgeoisie and are always a distortion but are hailed as universal truths, according to Barthes[12a]

Payne and Whittington[13] describe six myths that pertain to older women:

Myth Number 1. Older women have more health problems than older men. Statistics have shown that women in general tend to report more illness than men and have more days of restricted activity and disability owing to illness than men.[14] These statistics are obtained by self-report and are not corroborated by medical exams, prompting the question of whether women actually have more illnesses than men or just report more illnesses. When the rates of heart disease and hypertension were determined by evaluation of medical history alone, the women were diagnosed with higher rates of both diseases than were the men. Evaluation by medical exam alone revealed equal rates of heart disease and hypertension among the men and the women. This result makes this myth as well as the validity of self-report suspect. It has been stated that women are more likely than men to report symptoms, to be sensitive to symptoms, and to believe they are more susceptible to disease.[14] Women have higher rates of chronic diseases, while men have higher rates of fatal diseases. Women over 65 had 6.8 physician visits per year in 1980, compared with 5.9 visits for men. More men are hospitalized than women in the over 65 age group.[1] The myth that states older women have more health problems than men needs to be questioned in light of the fact that women do live longer and are apt to report illness more frequently than men.

Myth Number 2. Older women are usually widowed or never married. Statistics in 1981 revealed 5.7 per cent of older women were single and 51.3 per cent were widowed. The combined total of never married or widowed is 57 per cent, which accounts for a significant proportion of women 65 and over. However, this does not account for 43 per cent of the population who are married or are separated or divorced, and it subtly ignores the fact that all those widowed were formerly married.[1]

Myth Number 3. The older woman is both sexually inactive and sexually uninterested. Masters and Johnson[15] have reported that older women may achieve orgasm and can have a positive sex life. The regularity of intercourse and availability of a socially sanctioned sex partner are variables that influence the ability to engage in sexual intercourse.

Myth Number 4. The older woman is a happily married "wife for life," who, even in widowhood, retains a sense of personal identity based on that of her sainted husband. This myth is evidence of the double standard that still persists even among those in the older population. Men are expected to remarry and most frequently do. They do not remain "husband for life." Older women have identities of their own and many individual accomplishments. As women's roles change, this myth will dissolve.

Myth Number 5. The older woman often resembles a pleasantly plump "granny," who spends her time in a rocking chair knitting or sewing. It seems that older women are getting younger, especially as we ourselves are getting older. Older women are often employed, involved in a variety of activities and organizations, and have little free time. Visualize some older women you know, and this myth dissolves.

Myth Number 6. Older women participate in few voluntary associations other than the church. Older women can be found in a multitude of nonpaying and paying jobs. In fact, many women have been volunteers for much of their life, and consequently they receive no retirement benefits or social security. In 1982, 22 per cent of women over 65 were volunteers, compared with 2 to 4 per cent of older men.[1]

Health Needs of Older Women

White[3] and Moore[2] state that stroke, visual impairment, asthma, and mental and nervous conditions are more common among older women than among older men. Logically, these conditions are likely to be more common in the population that lives longer. Diabetes may also be more common in older women, because diabetes often accompanies obesity, a problem more common to women than men throughout the life-cycle. Mental and nervous disorders may be more common in elderly women who are widowed and isolated. However, in reviewing the literature, little is said as to why these conditions are common to older women, and most sources do not make any distinctions between the sexes in regard to incidence or specificity. Four major health conditions will be discussed here that affect or have implications for the health of older women: osteoporosis, coronary heart disease, breast cancer, and gynecologic problems. Nursing implications for older women exhibiting these health needs will be made.

Osteoporosis

Osteoporosis is defined as a loss of bone mass and occurs in both sexes as part of the normal aging process. There is no chemical change in the bone, and calcium and protein ratios are not altered, but the rate of bone absorption is greater than that of new bone deposition.[16] Older women have three to five times the incidence of osteoporosis that men have until age 80, when the incidence becomes equal between the sexes.[3, 17] Men and women reach their peak bone mass at about age 35 and either remain at a plateau or begin a decline at that time. Menopause has been statistically linked to the time that bone mass loss accelerates among women, and osteoporosis has been thought to be influenced by declining estrogen.[18] Osteoporosis results in thin, brittle bones that are three times as likely to fracture in women than in men.[3, 19] Bones most vulnerable to fracture in this population include the proximal femur and wrist. Lower thoracic and first lumbar vertebrae are susceptible to compression fractures and often result in kyphosis and back pain.[17] Osteoporosis is usually painless but may be accompanied by osteomalacia, which may cause pain. Fractures frequently occur with a minimum of stress to the bone and not infrequently in the course of normal activity. Gorrie[16] cites studies that show that one in four women over age 60 will suffer spinal compression fractures due to osteoporosis, with an increase to one in two women by the age of 75. Hip fractures are common in women, doubling in incidence every five years after age 60 and resulting in death 3 months following injury for 16 per cent of these women.[20] Diagnosis of osteoporosis is based on roentgenologic evidence.

Successful treatment and methods to prevent osteoporosis have remained elusive. Controversial theories about the course and treatment of osteoporosis abound. Nurses need to be aware of these controversies and to keep in touch with the growing body of research that will substantiate or refute current theories of cause and treatment.

Heaney[21] documented that bone loss occurs earlier in women who have had oophorectomies, giving support to the fact that it is the time since menopause rather than biologic age that is more strongly related to bone loss. Fractures due to osteoporosis usually occur about a decade after menopause in 25 per cent of women.[22] This link with menopause has focused much research on the effects estrogen deficiency has on bone mass.

Estrogen deficiency has been documented as increasing bone resorption sites, decreasing calcium and mineral content of bone, and decreasing osteoblasts needed for formation, resulting in loss of bone mass.[16, 23] Estrogen has been prescribed in the past as an antidote to slow aging, to control or limit menopausal symptoms, and to prevent or treat osteoporosis. However, a link between estrogen and endometrial carcinoma has been made, and the risk of endometrial cancer is four to eight times greater for estrogen users than for non-users.[24, 25] Estrogen replacement therapy (ERT) for osteoporosis is not contraindicated as a treatment modality but must be evaluated in terms of risk to the patient compared with possible benefits. There is greater possibility for postmenopausal women to suffer from osteoporosis than from endometrial cancer, but those women who are at increased risk for uterine cancer must be identified. Mass treatment of women with ERT is contraindicated because of this new research and because 20 per cent of postmenopausal women produce enough estrogen from their adrenal glands to warrant no effects from estrogen deficiency.

Complex processes involving vitamin D, parathyroid hormone, kidneys, and intestinal absorption act to balance the 1:1 ratio between calcium and phosphorus in adults. There is indication that the calcium:phosphorus ratio may be the most significant causative factor in osteoporosis.[26] As adults age, the intestines have a reduced ability to absorb calcium, and the dietary tendency is to ingest foods high in phosphorus, which include breads, cereals, soft drinks, meat, and potatoes. This tends to shift the calcium:phosphorus ratio toward higher levels of phosphorus and lower levels of serum calcium stimulating the parathyroid hormone to be released, which in turn stimulates bone to release calcium to restore the calcium levels in the blood. Foods that are typically thought to contain high amounts of calcium (e.g., cheese, milk, green vegetables) are also high in phosphorus and may not restore a negative calcium balance easily. There is also a need for vitamin D to facilitate the body's use of calcium, and deficiency of this vitamin may also lead to bone loss. The older woman who has decreased intestinal absorption of calcium coupled with vitamin D deficiency may be at increased risk for osteoporosis. Vitamin D supplements may be indicated in this population. Sunlight, a source of vitamin D, should be included as well. Calcium supplements are indicated for many patients and are recommended by many authorities for women beginning at age 25. The postmenopausal woman requires 1.4 gram per day of calcium, which is higher than the minimum daily requirement and which may be very difficult to maintain through dietary intake alone.[26]

High-protein diets, which may be ordered for patients to maintain to reach desired weights or for wound healing, have been found to stimulate bone loss.[27] Acid is a breakdown product of nitrogen and is buffered by calcium and excreted by the kidney, contributing to calcium loss and potential bone loss.

Lack of exercise is also considered a contributing factor in the development of osteoporosis. Fogel and Woods say that "the amount of calcium deposited in the bone is determined by the load the bone must carry; therefore, the more the bone is used, the denser it becomes."[18]

Nursing Implications. Nurses are in a unique position to influence women concerning their health. Health practices that include diet and exercise need to begin in early life and be reinforced as women continue to develop. Nutritional advice early in life is essential to establishing adequate intake of calcium. Women in their middle years frequently decrease their intake of milk and cheese to control weight and cholesterol levels. A switch to nonfat dairy products may be more appropriate to maintain calcium levels and still prevent weight gain and added cholesterol. Calcium supplements, as well as vitamin D supplements for facilitation of calcium use, are commonly being recommended to women in the middle years. Exercise needs to be included to promote the health of women at an early age. Exercise can help in weight control, provide a feeling of well-being, reduce stress, and establish a critical bone mass that can be preserved by maintaining an exercise program throughout life.

An example of nursing's effectiveness can be seen in a situation that occurred recently. A 47-year-old female nursing faculty member recently identified herself as being potentially at high risk for osteoporosis, owing to approaching menopause and a family history of osteoporosis (in her mother, two aunts, and one sister). She has now begun to take calcium daily, exercise more than before, and drink lowfat milk at all beverage opportunities, especially while traveling. During her frequent cross-country flying, a quart of lowfat milk is consumed instead of coffee. Her change in habits began by frequent discussions with a nursing school colleague who had a clinical and research interest in osteoporosis.

Nurses also are in a position to educate the woman being treated with estrogen. The nurse must know the risk of estrogen to her patient and must interpret this risk as well as understanding the proper method of taking estrogen. What to do if side effects of estrogen therapy occur must be discussed with the patient.

Nurses must keep current on research that refutes or supports the current controversies as to treatment and cause of osteoporosis. Women of all ages need information to help keep their bodies healthy, and nurses can facilitate the delivery of information, strengthen or influence coping strategies, and work with patients toward reduction of stress and risk.

Coronary Heart Disease

Most studies concerning coronary heart disease (CHD) have focused largely on men. Gillum[28] states that most of these studies have used all-male samples and a few have used male/female samples to compare differences between the sexes, but none have used all-female samples for their study. Studies that make comparisons between men and women emphasize the male findings. Heart disease has been characterized as a male disease and, because of its high mortality rate among men, it has received little attention within the female population. Although at younger ages men have a higher incidence of CHD than women, these differences disappear as both men and women age.[29] For men, heart disease typically occurs during middle- to old age. Women have a lower mortality rate than men from heart disease, but when the

female rates are considered separately, and are compared to the rates of other diseases that are usually associated with female mortality at young ages, the importance of heart disease mortality for women becomes much more striking. For example, the coronary disease mortality rate for white women at 45-54 years is 58.5/100,000 and in the 55-64 age category it is 226.7. Among non-white women at these ages the rates are even higher, 148.2 and 421.8 respectively. The incidence of breast cancer by comparison is 73/100,000 and the breast cancer mortality rate is 25 per 100,000. It is clear that coronary heart disease is a serious threat to black women after age 45 and to white women after 55 years old.[29]

There has been recent concern that as women's roles change, as traditional male occupations open up for women, as women change their lifestyles to patterns more similar to those of men, diseases associated with the stress of the male lifestyle will become more of a threat to women's lives.[30, 31] Studies have not shown clear evidence that coronary heart disease is on the rise among women nor will such changes, if they exist, likely become evident until some time in the future.[7] Data reported by Haynes and Feinleib[30] from the Framingham Heart Study[6] revealed that working women had the same rates of coronary heart disease as housewives. However, when work was broken down as to type, it was found that women in clerical positions had twice the rate of heart disease as did housewives. "The most significant predictors of CHD among clerical workers were suppressed hostility, having a nonsupportive boss, and decreased job mobility."[30] These findings may give clues that the type of occupation may be a risk factor for the development of heart disease in women and that these high-risk occupations may not be the same for men.

Although heart disease has been culturally constructed to be a male's disease and although women as part of this culture do not identify heart disease as being equally distributed between the sexes, it is interesting to note that prevalence data indicate that rates of heart disease are nearly equal for men and women. The National Center for Health Statistics[32] reported that women surveyed reported nearly the same number of heart conditions as men did in 1972.

The rise in incidence of cardiovascular disease among women coincides with the time of menopause. It has been postulated that estrogen decline is therefore related to cardiovascular disease increases. This link has not been clearly substantiated by research. Gordon and colleagues[33] suggest that estrogen may provide protection against coronary heart disease, but how this is done is not known. Shoemaker and associates[34] report that menopause is not related to coronary heart disease and that estrogen treatment does not provide protection from cardiovascular disease. Further evidence reveals that this increase in incidence of heart disease that coincides with menopause does not exist in other countries.[34]

Despite these statistics that document heart disease as being prevalent in the population of women, and especially in older women, the popular stereotype of the disease victim is male, hard-driving, type A personality, middle-aged, and upwardly mobile. This stereotype has obscured the observance of heart disease in women. Monteiro[29] suggests that this view of heart disease has affected women's assessment of their own symptoms of heart disease, the treatment instituted for heart disease in women, and the characteristics of cardiac rehabilitation programs that have been developed.

Monteiro[29] summarizes research indicating that women take longer to decide on what action to take when experiencing heart symptoms than men do, thereby jeopardizing their survival. Women tend to discount heart symptoms possibly because they believe that heart disease is a man's disease, thus delaying the decision to seek emergency care. Monteiro also suggests that treatment differences occur between men and women with heart disease, basically because health care providers also see heart disease as male and may treat women less aggressively or take longer to initiate treatment. A 65-year-old housewife reported to the Emergency Room screening nurse that she had been having chest pain for the past eight hours. She had treated herself for indigestion with baking soda, but the pain persisted. She stated she now thinks the pain is more than indigestion because she is sweaty and much more short of breath. This patient was diagnosed with an myocardial infarction (MI) and admitted to the coronary care unit (CCU). Her delay in seeking treatment might have cost her her life, and if the emergency room personnel had compounded this delay by a slow diagnosing process or nonaggressive treatment plan, the outcome might have been tragic.

"Although there are relatively few studies that provide separate analysis for male and female cardiacs, evidence from studies of other aspects of myocardial infarction recovery lends further support to the hypothesis that women are treated differently in such programs."[29] Rehabilitation programs for persons with coronary heart disease have been typically designed for men, with the intent to return the man to work and an active life. These programs may not be appropriate for older women who likewise need rehabilitation.

Nursing Implications. Nurses are in a position to recognize that heart disease exists as a major disease among older women, despite the male stereotype perpetuated in the American culture. By recognizing the prevalence and incidence of heart disease among women, nurses can be advocates for those women who come to medical attention with the risk for heart disease or with symptoms of the disease itself.

By working with women, nurses can help modify or reduce existing risk factors for heart disease. Hypertension detection and control, weight reduction, low-cholesterol diets, exercise, and stress reduction programs are important strategies to lower CHD risk. Exercise and nutritional programs for weight control and optimal cardiovascular performance started early in a woman's life may reduce risk during the older ages. Smoking cessation programs are also important. Many of these strategies are characteristics of a lifestyle that should be started early in a women's life.

Nurses must teach women the signs and symptoms of heart disease, when and where to seek treatment, and to be aware that CHD is a major illness for women as well as men. Nurses must be willing to be advocates for older women who present themselves to health care facilities with signs and symptoms of heart disease. Nurses and physicians belong to the same culture that perpetuates the "maleness" of heart disease that may obscure a quick and clear diagnosis. Alert and knowledgeable nurses may be able to intervene in this process and facilitate appropriate and aggressive treatment when needed.

Nursing can also institute rehabilitation programs designed for older women or modify existing male cardiac rehabilitation programs for older women's use. The institution of specific exercise plans that are more conducive to older women's participation is one example of this modification, as most programs are oriented to traditional middle-aged, male exercises such as jogging. Traditional cardiac rehabilitation programs have been designed to return men to work. This male emphasis may not be conductive to the participation of older women. Coeducational groups may not be appropriate when dealing with exercise programs for middle-aged men and older women, or when dealing in areas concerning psychosociosexual problems following an MI.

Breast Cancer

Breast cancer is the leading cause of cancer incidence and death for females in the United States today. One of every 12 women by age 75 years will develop breast cancer within her lifetime. Breast cancers occur in women most frequently between the ages of 30 and 80. Since breast cancer incidence increases with age, especially at or near menopause, it is interesting to note that this incidence increase has not been directly linked to menopause, although it has been postulated, and that estrogen is contraindicated for women with known or suspected breast cancer or estrogen-dependent tumors.[14]

Annual death rates from breast cancer also increase with age. For example, in 1981 it was reported that death rates for white women from breast cancer were 41 per 100,00; nonwhite women's rates were 43.5 in the 45 to 49 year age group, increasing respectively to 92.3 and 82.4 per 100,000 in the 60 to 64 year age group.[22a] The five-year survival rate for stage I breast cancer (early detection) is 87 per cent and drops to 45 per cent for women with stage II cancer.[35] Because of better survival rates in stage I breast cancer, early detection programs have been instituted that advocate breast self-examination on a monthly basis and mammography for high-risk patients. I suspect that many of our older women have not been taught breast self-examination and are seldom examined by the medical establishment for breast cancer. An example of this occurred recently during geriatric teaching rounds at a large, metropolitan teaching hospital. An 84-year-old woman was admitted with a pulse of 40 and the need for a pacemaker. Her history included a right mastectomy six years earlier owing to cancer. She had been followed monthly for years as an outpatient for congestive heart failure. Her present admission physical revealed left nipple discharge, nipple inversion, and dimpling. Early detection of breast cancer was not made in this woman's case, even though she was seen frequently by the health care establishment. In our striving for specialization, it is easy to become blind to other risks of health problems that may occur in our patients but that are not in our area of specialization. This is easy to do with the population of older women, who are stigmatized because they are old as well as because they are women. Furthermore, the organs of reproduction and sexuality have lost their youth and reproductive function and are, therefore, not examined as frequently by the health care establishment. Since 75 per cent of all breast cancers are discovered after the age of 40, the older woman should be targeted for education and risk assessment.

Women at high risk for breast cancer are usually age 40 to 70 and have a family history of breast cancer. However, Kelly[36] makes the point that family history of breast cancer does not necessarily indicate high risk. It is the type of family history that influences the risk for breast cancer. "Risks to first-degree relatives (mothers, sisters, or daughters) of patients with breast cancer can vary widely depending on the age at diagnosis (pre-menopausal or post-menopausal) and laterality (unilateral or bilateral) of affected women and the pattern of breast cancer in the family (occurrence in one generation or two)."[36] Kelly uses the example of first-degree relatives of women with bilateral breast cancer who were diagnosed premenopause and had a risk 8.8 times that of women with no family history of the disease. Relatives of women with bilateral disease diagnosed postmenopause had a risk of 1.2 times that of women with no family history of breast cancer. Kelly[36] also states that the risk for breast cancer is increased for the woman whose family has other types of cancer.

Other risk factors besides family history for women in the high-risk group include (1) prior history of benign breast disease; (2) a reproductive history that may include early menarche, late menopause, never pregnant or first child born after age 35, and sexual activity initiated late or never; (3) race and ethnicity predominantly northern European, Jews of European descent, or affluent blacks; (4) obesity due to diets high in animal fats and protein; and (5) living in large metropolitan cities, especially in the Northeast United States. All women should be screened for breast cancer risk, and older women should not be a neglected part of this group.

Treatment modalities for breast cancer have changed most recently from the overwhelming use of the radical mastectomy to simple, less debilitating surgery often followed by chemotherapy. Fogel and Woods[18] give a good description of the current detection and treatment modalities, as well as preoperative and postoperative needs of these women.

Nursing Implications. Nurses can alert older women to the increased risk for breast cancer and the need for monthly breast self-examination and yearly medical follow-up. About 90 to 95 per cent of all breast cancers are discovered by women themselves. Older women's breasts are easier to examine than younger women because the glandular tissue is replaced by fat.[22] This should encourage women whose breasts were cystic in earlier years to feel more confident in their ability to detect unusual lumps. Breast examinations should become a part of the plan of care for all women in long-term care facilities, home health agencies, senior citizen and day care centers, and acute care facilities. Nurses should never assume that the breasts of older women were examined routinely on hospital admission or even at their last physical examination.

Screening women for risk factors also helps identify those at increased risk and who need-

mammography or more frequent follow-up examinations. Nurses can be aggressive and screen older women wherever they find them, rather than wait for them to present for a "proper" appointment or, worse yet, after having detected a lump that may have progressed beyond stage I.

Nurses can influence the attitudes of other health care providers by being up-to-date with facts and current research and by insisting that older women's basic health care is not neglected.

Gynecologic Problems

Cancer is often considered a disease of aging and its diagnosis creates additional stress for its victims. Cancer of the genital tract is not uncommon among postmenopausal women. Adequate screening, prevention, and treatment of the older woman is an expectation. According to Fogel and Woods,[18] cancer of the cervix is ranked third in incidence after breast, colon, and rectal cancers in women. Two per cent of women by the time they are 80 will develop cervical cancer, although the peak incidence of cervical cancer occurs most frequently between ages 40 and 49. The incidence of cervical cancer levels off at menopause, when the incidence of endometrial cancer rises.[22] Notelovitz[37] states that the incidence of cervical cancer peaks at age 60. Because the rise in incidence of endometrial cancer is common among women between the ages of 50 and 70, Pap smear specimens from this group should include endocervical, cervical, and vaginal pool samples.[22] However, the American Cancer Society[38] reports that pap smears are not effective in detecting endometrial cancer and may have below 40 per cent reliability in actual detection. Glowacki[39] reports that approximately 10 per cent of those women who bleed vaginally after menopause do so because of endometrial cancer. Therefore, all vaginal bleeding from postmenopausal women needs follow-up to determine its source and cause.

Cancer of the ovary is not common, but the mortality rate from the disease is extremely high.[39] Incidence is most frequent in women aged 40 to 65, and the risk is about 1 per cent for a woman developing this type of cancer in her lifetime. Cancer of the vulva occurs as a disease of older women, usually between the ages of 50 and 70.[18] These cancers of the genital tract point out the need for periodic inspection of the vulva and cervix, pap smear of the cervix and vaginal vault, and bimanual examination of the ovaries and uterus of the older woman to detect abnormal changes as early as possible. Nurses can teach the older female population the need for preventive and health maintenance examinations, as well as advocate that these examinations not be neglected by the health professionals that come into contact with older women.

Atrophic vaginitis is a common condition experienced by many postmenopausal women as the result of naturally declining levels of estrogen. As estrogen declines, the epithelium of the vagina decreases in glycogen content, causing an alkaline environment that is favorable to the growth of bacteria and subsequent infection. The decline in estrogen is responsible for the atrophy of the vagina and vulva, resulting in the narrowing and shortening of the vaginal structure and pelvic relaxation that predisposes the patient to uterine prolapse, cystocele, rectocele, or enterocele.[40] Estrogen is also responsible for the maturation of vaginal epithelium, and as the hormone declines in production the vaginal walls become thin, easily traumatized, and less expansible with decreasing lubrication during sexual excitement.[22]

Symptoms common to the older woman with atrophic vaginitis include vaginal dryness, dyspareunia, pruritis, vaginal discharge, tenderness, and burning. Vaginal spotting following douching or sexual intercourse is not uncommon.[41]

Estrogen replacement therapy can reverse these atrophic changes. With estrogen treatment, the vaginal epithelium matures and thickens, and glycogen returns to the cells causing the vagina to return to a normal acid pH, thereby encouraging normal vaginal flora. Vaginal dryness, itching, burning, and the associated dyspareunia disappear. The vagina regains some of its elasticity, making sexual intercourse less difficult.[22]

Systemic (oral) estrogen or topical estrogen cream is frequently prescribed. Topical estrogen creams must be prescribed with care, because the precise dosage is difficult to monitor and the medication is absorbed systemically at a rapid rate. Martin and associates[42] found that absorption after 12 hours was at the level of the follicular phase in ovulating women. ERT is therefore prescribed cyclically, with drug-free intervals every two to three months.

Oral estrogen has the same effects on the vaginal mucosa as does topical estrogen cream. Oral estrogen is usually prescribed when vasomotor symptoms of menopause are severe. Oral estrogen is administered cyclically (21 days out of 28) and is often supplemented with the addition of progestogens that decrease or prevent endometrial hyperplasia.[43] The use of progestogens is thought to decrease the risk of developing endometrial carcinoma, which is directly linked to ERT. The smallest dose of estrogen for the shortest period of time is a common rule of thumb in ERT, applying to topical estrogen preparations as well.

An active sex life seems to contribute to less vaginal atrophy and to fewer atrophic symptoms. It is also true that abstinence is associated with vaginal shrinkage. The symptoms of vaginal atrophy with decreased lubrication can lead to dyspareunia and less sexual activity. This actually compounds the problem, for less sexual activity contributes to shrinkage and dryness of the vaginal tissue. Those who maintain regular sexual activity will maintain vaginal tone and lubrication into old age.[15]

Nursing can take an active role in educating older women about ERT. Frequent follow-up is necessary for women receiving estrogen. Nurses can advise older women regarding the advantages of remaining sexually active into the older years, while balancing the risks that may be associated with that sexual activity.

Estrogen decline in the postmenopausal woman also influences the tissues of the urethra, often resulting in dysuria and urinary frequency. Urinalysis is usually normal, and symptoms decrease and disappear with estrogen replacement therapy.[22] Leakage of urine is common, especially when coughing and sneezing. It is important to rule out other causes of dysuria or incontinence. A urinalysis can rule out cystitis, and cystometric studies may be necessary to rule out incontinence due to anatomic changes that can occur in aging pelvic tissues and organs. Sometimes a urethral stricture can occur, facilitating residual urine and subsequent urinary tract infection. Treatment with antibiotics for infection, antispasmodics for relief of urinary incontinence, and estrogen either orally or vaginally may be indicated for estrogen-depletion urethritis.[44]

Gynecologic health and care should not be disregarded because a woman has successfully passed the menopause. Nursing may be the most appropriate discipline in facilitating the gynecologic health of older women through education, through clinics specifically designed for older women and their health, through programs offered at long-term care facilities, and through senior centers and home health agencies. A West Coast long-term care facility is reaching out to the elderly women in the community by providing a pap smear and breast examination clinic monthly at various senior citizen centers. Many of the elderly women have never been taught breast self-examination or have thought it was unimportant to continue at their age.

CONCLUSION

As the population of older women increases, more importance will be placed on the health needs of this unique and vulnerable group. The stress of stereotyping, prejudice, and myths surrounding older women needs to be reduced, so that society and health providers can identify the health risks and needs of this population as well as institute equality of treatment. Nursing is in an excellent position to take the forefront in constructing systems of care that would provide much of the necessary health care needed by this group. Of prime importance is adequate research on this population to define health risks, validate interventions, and ultimately raise the level of health enjoyed by older women.

References

1. Factsheet on Women. *Women and Aging.* Community Services, American Council of Life Insurance, Fall 1982.
2. Moore, E. D. Woman and health. *Public Health Reports Supplement,* Sept.-Oct. 1980.
3. White, R. (ed.) The surviving majority: Older women and their health. *Mendocino Medicine and Gazetteer,* vol. 6, December 1981.
4. Matthews, S. H. *The Social World of Old Women: Management of Self-Identity,* vol. 78. Beverly Hills: Sage Publications, 1979.
5. Goffman, E. *Stigma.* Englewood Cliffs, NJ: Prentice-Hall, 1963.
6. Dawber, T. R. *The Framingham Study.* Cambridge: Harvard University Press, 1980.
7. Johnson, A. Recent trends in sex mortality differentials in the United States. *Journal of Human Stress,* vol. 3, 1977, pp. 22–32.
8. Butler, R. N., and Lewis, M. I. *Aging and Mental Health: Positive Psychosocial Approaches.* St. Louis: C.V. Mosby Co., 1977.
9. Fuller, M. M., and Martin, C. A. (eds.) *The Older Woman: Lavender Rose or Gray Panther.* Springfield, IL: Charles C Thomas, 1980.
9a. Erikson, E. H. *Childhood and Society.* New York: W. W. Norton, 1950.
10. Rossi, A. S. Life-span theories and women's lives. *Journal of Women in Culture and Society,* vol. 6, 1980, pp. 4–32.
10a. Datan, N., and Ginsberg, L. H. (eds.). Life-Span Developmental Psychology: Normative Life Crisis. New York: Academic Press, 1975.
11. Neugarten, B. L. Time, age, and the life-cycle. *The American Journal of Psychiatry,* vol. 136, 1979, pp. 887–894.
12. Lewis, M. I., and Butler, R. N. Why is women's lib ignoring old women? *International Journal of Aging and Human Development,* vol. 3, 1972, pp. 223–231.
12a. Barthes, R. *Mythologies.* New York: Hill and Wang, 1972.
13. Payne, B., and Whittington, F. Older women: An examination of popular stereotypes and research evidence. *Social Problems,* vol. 23, 1976, pp. 488–504.
14. Giele, J. Z. (ed.) *Women in the Middle Years: Current Knowledge and Directions for Research and Policy.* New York: John Wiley and Sons, 1982.
15. Masters, W. H., and Johnson, V. E. *Human Sexual Response.* Boston: Little, Brown, 1966, pp. 223–247.
16. Gorrie, T. Postmenopausal osteoporosis. *Journal of Obstetrics and Gynecological Nursing,* vol. 11, 1982, pp. 214–219.
17. Harvey, A. M., Johns, R. J., McKusick, V. A., Owens, A. H., and Ross, R. S. (eds.) *The Principles and Practice of Medicine,* 20th ed. New York: Appleton-Century-Crofts, 1980.
18. Fogel, C. I., and Woods, N. F. *Health Care of Women: A nursing perspective.* St. Louis: C.V. Mosby Co., 1981.
19. Johnson, R. E., and Specht, E. E. The risk of hip fracture in postmenopausal females with and without estrogen drug exposure. *American Journal of Public Health,* vol. 71, 1981, pp. 138–144.
20. Sandler, R. B. Etiology of primary osteoporosis: An hypothesis. *Journal of the American Geriatric Society,* vol. 26, 1978, pp. 208–213.
21. Heaney, R. P. Estrogens and postmenopausal osteoporosis. *Clinical Obstetrics and Gynecology,* vol. 19, 1976, pp. 791–804.
22. Martin, L. *Health Care of Women.* Philadelphia: J.B. Lippincott Co., 1978.
22a. DeLorey, C. Health care and midlife women. *In* Baruch, G., and Brooks-Gunn, J. (eds.). *Women in Midlife.* New York: Plenum Press, 1984, pp. 277–302.
23. Lindsay, R., Hart, D. M., Aitken, J. M., et al. Long-term prevention of postmenopausal osteoporosis by estrogen: Evidence for an increased bone mass after delayed onset of estrogen treatment. *Lancet,* vol. 1, 1976, pp. 1038–1041.
24. Antunes, C. M., Stolley, P. D., Rosenshein, N. B., Davies, J. L., Rutledge, A., Pokempner, M., and Garcia, R. Endometrial cancer and estrogen use: Report of a large case-control study. *New England Journal of Medicine,* vol. 300, Jan. 1979, pp. 9–13.
25. Ziel, H. K., Finkle, W. D. Increased risk of endometrial carcinoma among users of conjugated estrogens. *New England Journal of Medicine,* vol. 293, 1975, pp. 1167–1170.
26. Jowsey, J. Why is mineral nutrition important in osteoporosis? *Geriatrics,* vol. 33, 1978, pp. 39–52.
27. Albanese, A. A., Lorenze, E. J., and Wein, E. H. Osteoporosis: Effects of calcium. *American Family Physician,* vol. 18, 1978, pp. 160–167.
28. Gillum, R. F. Ischemic heart disease mortality declining since 1940. *American Journal of Public Health,* vol. 72, 1982, p. 213.
29. Monteiro, L. A. Who has heart attacks? Gender related perceptions of myocardial infarction. Paper presented at the Medical Sociology section session, American Sociological Association Meetings, San Francisco, September 1982.
30. Haynes, S. G., and Feinleib, M. Women, work and coronary heart disease: Prospective findings from the Framingham Heart Study. *American Journal of Public Health,* vol. 70, 1980, pp. 133–141.
31. Nathanson, C. A. Sex roles as variables in preventive

health behavior. *Journal of Community Health,* vol. 3, Winter 1977, pp. 142–155.

32. National Center for Health Statistics: Division of Health Interview Statistics. Reprinted in Breslow (ed.). *Annual Review of Public Health,* vol. 1, 1980, p. 18.

33. Gordon, T., Kannel, W. B., Hjortland, M. C., et al. Menopause and coronary heart disease—The Framingham Study. *Annals of Internal Medicine,* vol. 89, August 1978, pp. 157–161.

34. Shoemaker, E. S., Forney, J. P., and MacDonald, P. C. Estrogen treatment of postmenopausal women: Benefits and risks. *Journal of the American Medical Association,* vol. 238, Oct. 1977, pp. 1524–1530.

35. Napoli, M. Breast cancer: A critical look at early detection. *National Women's Health Network Newsletter,* vol. 3, May-June 1982, p. 4.

36. Kelly, P. T. Refinements in breast cancer risk analysis. *Archives of Surgery,* vol. 116, March 1981, pp. 364–365.

37. Notelovitz, M. Gynecologic problems of menopausal women: Part 1. Changes in genital tissue. *Geriatrics,* August 1978, pp. 24–30.

38. American Cancer Society. 1980 Cancer Facts and Figures. New York, 1979.

39. Glowacki, G. Postmenopausal gyn problems. *Hospital Practice,* vol. 6, May 1977, pp. 107–113.

40. Ryan, M. (ed.) *Ambulatory Care in Obstetrics and Gynecology.* New York: Grune and Stratton, 1980, pp. 317–426.

41. Gardner, H. L., and Kaufman, R. H. *Benign Diseases of the Vulva and Vagina.* St. Louis: C.V. Mosby Co., 1969, pp. 1–223.

42. Martin, P., Yen, S., Burmier, A., et al. Systemic absorption and sustained effects of vaginal estrogen creams. *Journal of the American Medical Association,* vol. 242, 1979, p. 2699.

43. Notelovitz, M. When and how to use estrogen therapy in women over 60. *Geriatrics,* vol. 35, 1980, p. 113.

44. Smith, P. Postmenopausal urinary symptoms and hormonal replacement therapy. *British Medical Journal,* October 1976, p. 941.

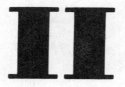

II

BIOPSYCHOSOCIAL FACTORS IN HEALTH AND ILLNESS

The second section covers those factors that contribute to women's stress and health, beginning with female sexuality, continuing with special areas of interest such as the lesbian woman, childbearing dilemmas, communication patterns, the problems of dependency and alcohol abuse, and how sexism can affect women's mental health, ending with the chapter on health of low income women.

5

FEMALE SEXUALITY
ROSEMARY HUERTER

Rosemary Huerter provides an overview of female sexuality in this chapter. She identifies and discusses the major factors in determining a person's sexuality—gender identity, gender role, and biologic sex. The physiology of sexual stimulation is described for both women and men. Case studies illustrate both the problems and their resolutions.

Few areas in women's lives have been left unstressed. In few areas have women been under more severe or sustained stress than the area of sexuality. Historically, a woman's sexuality was bound up with her economic worth. A virgin was more desirable for marriage, not because of moral or religious scruples so much as the notion of the virgin as "undamaged goods."

These stresses may be related in part to the menstrual and childbearing functions of women. They may also be related to the supposed weakness of the female. Whatever the reasons, societies have maintained four characteristics related to sexual behavior control.

The first characteristic is some form of marriage. Marriage ensures several things. One is the continuation of the race. Although different cultures have held differing views of children being born to unmarried mothers, and sometimes this has been encouraged, the usual view is of some kind of family bond for the upbringing of the child. In addition to this there is the assurance of access to sexual partners; marriage takes certain people out of the arena of sexual competition and establishes kinship and the obligation of kinship.

A second characteristic of societies is the agreement that forced sex is prohibited in one's own group. It was permissible for conquering armies to rape the conquered, for masters to rape slaves, or simply for members of one tribe to rape women of another tribe. In some of the biblical stories that tell of revenge for rape,

the rapist was of the same tribe as the woman. This characteristic has become less important in our present society. Statistics reveal increasingly that women are being raped by people they know, including husbands in marital rape.

A third characteristic of sexual behavior control is the existence of taboos related to the eligibility of sexual partners. The incest taboo has been fairly universal throughout history. Some primitive tribes allowed marriage only within the group; others allowed marriage only outside the group. Today some religious groups still look with disfavor on any exogamous relationship, particularly in marriage. Only recently has the idea of interracial marriage been tenable in most parts of the United States.

A final characteristic of control in the area of sexual behavior is the existence of some form of exception to most rules. Because it was recognized that inflexibility breeds trouble, there were always methods of circumventing the rules. Exceptions to the incest taboo in ancient Egypt are well known. This may have been for the sake of keeping wealth in the family, but it still represents an exception. In our society, divorce is one method of breaking the ties of kinship and its obligations. The time-honored custom of kissing under the mistletoe is another exception that allows more intimacy between men and women than they might otherwise enjoy.

Although all four characteristics supposedly apply to both men and women, there has been more pressure on women than on men to conform. The famous "double standard," which still regulates much of our sexual thought and ideals, is a perfect example of this. Men were encouraged to become sexually experienced, whereas women were expected to wait for marriage. A man who had many sexual partners was thought to be a great guy and was looked up to by his peers. A woman who had many sexual partners was considered "fast," "loose," or a whore. Although the women's movement has been instrumental in breaking down some of these barriers and prejudices, the conditioning that most women have received from parents and society will remain with them for a long time. The final equalizing of the sexes with regard to sexual expectations will come only through a concerted effort made by both men and women.

In the past women were generally told about their sexuality by men. They were taught to distrust their own feelings and ideas and to look to men for answers to their sexual problems. Even when women began to enter the professions that related to women's sexuality, e.g., medicine, anthropology, and sociology, women were trained by men and often repeated what they were taught by these male teachers. Fortunately, this is changing. Women are beginning to say, "I know something too; in fact, when it comes to my body and my sexuality, I know more than any man could possibly know."

It is hoped that this chapter is an affirmation of this budding attitude and a reinforcement for women that they do indeed "know something too"!

WHAT DETERMINES A PERSON'S SEXUALITY?

How do women get to be women? Gender identity, gender role, and biologic sex are the main factors. Some parts of the answer to this are obvious; others are a little more subtle. Six factors determine whether we are female or male: (1) the chromosomes we get from our parents, specifically the X or Y we get from our fathers; (2) the gonadal structure we develop while in utero; (3) the hormonal activity and output of our bodies; (4) hormonal spurts at puberty; (5) sex assignment and rearing; and (6) how we feel about being female or male.

At the time of conception we receive the chromosomes from our parents. The mother contributes an X chromosome, whereas the father contributes either an X or a Y chromosome. If the father gives an X chromosome, the child will be a girl; if he gives a Y chromosome, the child will be a boy. For the first 6 weeks there is no further sexual differentiation. About 6 weeks after conception, if the chromosomal structure is XY, the conceptus will begin to develop testosterone, and the sexual differentiation of a male will occur. If the chromosomal structure is XX, no testosterone will be produced, and the gonadal structure of a female will develop. If the chromosomal structure is that of a male, but for some reason testosterone is not produced, the differentiation will not occur and gonadal female structures will continue to develop.

After the initial development of gonadal structures between the sixth and twelfth weeks, there appears to be little or no additional sexual differentiation. This is regarded as one critical period in the development of the sexuality of a person.

The interrelationship of the six factors that make us either male or female is understood relatively well. Whether one is more causally dominant is not as well understood. A considerable body of evidence suggests that the lack of testosterone in a conceptus that is genetically male will result in the lack of gonadal development appropriate to a male. The tissue masses that eventually differentiate into clitoris/penis, ovaries/testes, and labia/scrotum are present in both the female and the male conceptus. Whether estrogen is necessary for female differentiation is not clear, but if there is no testosterone present the fetus will develop as a female, regardless of the chromosomal structure.[1]

At some point in early childhood, probably before the age of 2 years, further differentiation of female and male occurs. By the age of 2 years, children know whether they are "boy" or "girl." Their understanding of what this means is still undeveloped, and their sexual identity will continually be modified and added to. The first 2 years of extrauterine life are crucial in the development of a sexual identity. Thus, the sex assignment, and rearing of the child in accordance with the sex assigned, are of prime importance during these early years. When the genitalia are not clearly differentiated and the sex of the child is unclear, researchers who deal with gender-identity disorders estimate that if a sex reassignment is to be made it should be done before the age of 18 months.[2] A child reared for 2 years as a boy and then declared a girl (or vice versa) will have not only his or her confusion to deal with, but also that of parents and other family members. The earlier a sex reassignment is completed, the better the chance that the child will adapt satisfactorily. However, I know of a case in which a girl decided much later that she had always felt like a boy and underwent a successful sex change in late childhood. This is not to be confused with the changes undergone by a transsexual person.

A final factor that determines whether we are female or male is how we ourselves feel about being the sex we are. Children who are loved and wanted as either the girl or boy that they are will probably grow up feeling comfortable with their sex. The parent who wants a girl and gets a boy, or vice versa, may be instrumental in making the child feel that there would be something inherently better in being the other sex. Something so fundamental and basic as our sexual selves, if not accepted by persons significant to us in our early childhood, will likely have serious repercussions in our adult life and practices.

PHYSIOLOGY OF SEXUAL STIMULATION

Basic to an understanding of sexuality and sexual functioning is an understanding of the sexual response cycle. Masters and Johnson in their research on the physiology of sexual stimulation identified four phases: excitement, plateau, orgasm, and resolution. Both women and men experience all four phases, but the patterns differ. Masters and Johnson also identified three patterns of orgasm for women and one pattern for men.[3] The four phases will be discussed briefly.

Excitement develops from any source of physical or psychic stimuli. If stimulation is adequate, the intensity increases rapidly.

Plateau is a consolidation period that follows the excitement phase if stimulation is continued. Sexual tension becomes intensified and reaches a level at which orgasm is experienced. Both the excitement and the plateau phases can be interrupted or terminated altogether by distracting stimuli.

Orgasm is the involuntary climax of sexual tension. It involves only a short period of time in the cycle, usually not more than a few seconds. It usually cannot be prolonged, although some women have a pattern of peaking and declining, with multiple orgasms occurring from one cycle of excitement and plateau. Once orgasm has begun there is no way to

stop it. As mentioned previously, Masters and Johnson identified three patterns of orgasm for women. In the "minimal" type, the feelings are not very intense, the peak of the orgasm is low, and resolution requires a moderate amount of time, about 20 minutes. The second is a multiple type, in which the peak of feelings is higher than in the minimal type, and the peak repeats itself. Resolution is more prolonged than in the minimal type. The third type of orgasm is one in which there is a high intensity of feeling and a rapid resolution of these feelings.[4]

Resolution is the phase during which changes occur that restore the pre-excitement status. Some women may be restimulated and again begin the excitement phase immediately. Men have a refractory period, however, and cannot be restimulated until the resolution phase has been completed. In general the resolution phase lasts as long as the excitement phase. Sexual tension dissipates slowly.

Sexual response is a total-body response and not just a reaction of the genitals. In fact, as the saying goes, "The brain is the primary sex organ." Research has revealed electroencephalographic changes at orgasm. Much research has been carried out on the effects of sexual stimulation on the rest of the body. Table 5–1 reviews the physiologic changes that occur during each phase.

FEMALE SEXUALITY AND MYTH

Some time ago I presented a female sexuality workshop to a group of nurses at work in the profession. One concern was to discover their knowledge level. As a preparation for this workshop, a list of myths about sexuality was developed. To my surprise (and horror) it was relatively easy to gather a large number. The result was a document entitled "The Ninety-Nine Most-Cherished Myths in Sexuality." Although many researchers have made inroads in clarifying the area of myth, there are still many misconceptions. Sometimes it seems that we dispel one myth only to have it replaced by another. An example is the outmoded Victorian idea that women do not enjoy sex and submit to it only for the sake of having children. We replace that idea with the notion that all women must enjoy sex, have sex all the time, and furthermore have multiple orgasms, and we are no farther ahead than we were 50 years ago.

Some of the more prevalent myths attached to female sexuality follow.

Table 5–1. **Physiologic Changes of Sexual Response**

Female	Male
EXCITEMENT	**EXCITEMENT**
Genital	*Genital*
swelling of clitoral glans	rapid erection of penis (may come and go)
elongation of the clitoral shaft	tensing and thickening of scrotal skin
enlargement of the clitoral shaft	elevation of scrotal sac; testes elevated toward perineum
vaginal lubrication	shortening of spermatic cords
vaginal expansion, both length and width	
vaginal vasocongestion	
possibly uterine elevation	
changes in labia in effort to open vaginal introitus	
Extragenital	*Extragenital*
nipple erection	nipple erection
increase in breast size	tensing of abdominal and intercostal muscles
engorgement of areola	
"sex flush"—redness and rash over breast and epigastrium	
increase in heart rate and blood pressure	
PLATEAU	**PLATEAU**
Genital	*Genital*
retraction of clitoris against symphysis, under clitoral hood	increase in penile circumference at coronal ridge
vasocongestion of outer third of vagina and labia minora	deepening of color at corona
further increase in depth and width of vagina	increase in testicular size, sometimes as much as 50%
full elevation of uterus	testes elevated closer to perineum (indicative of impending ejaculation)
vaginal tenting due to cervical rise	secretion from Cowper's gland; contains active spermatozoa
engorgement of labia majora	
color change in labia minora, from red to wine-colored	
some secretion from Bartholin's gland	
Extragenital	*Extragenital*
continued nipple erection and turgidity	sometimes nipple erection and turgidity
sex flush possibly over whole body	sex flush, late in phase, occasionally
muscle contraction—facial, abdominal, intercostal (both voluntary and involuntary)	further voluntary and involuntary contractions
occasionally, voluntary rectal contractions to increase stimulation	hyperventilation late in phase; pulse rate increased to 100–175; blood pressure elevated, usually higher than in female
hyperventilation; pulse rate increased to 100–175; increased blood pressure	
ORGASM	**ORGASM**
Genital	*Genital*
contractions of uterus, starting at fundus and spreading downward	expulsive contractions of entire length of penile urethra
	contractions of secondary organs such as the vas deferens, epididymis, seminal vesicles, and prostate
	closure of internal bladder sphincter
Extragenital	*Extragenital*
sex flush intensified	sex flush in some men
involuntary spasms and contractions of muscle groups	occasionally "goose bumps"; spasms of various muscle groups, especially rectal sphincter
increase in respiratory rate	increase in respiratory and heart rate similar to woman's
rapid heart beat, possibly an increase	blood pressure elevation more pronounced
high blood pressure, possibly an increase	
RESOLUTION	**RESOLUTION**
Genital	*Genital*
return of clitoris to normal position, 5–10 seconds after cervical contractions cease	superimposition of refractory period (unable to restimulate to excitement) on resolution phase; may be as short as 10 minutes, but appears to definitely exist
return of other genital structures to normal in 10–30 minutes	rapid loss of vasocongestion of penis; detumescence to 1.5 times normal size
Extragenital	*Extragenital*
rapid loss of sex flush	return of vital signs to normal
slower return to normal of vital signs	occasionally sweating of palms of hands and soles of feet
some persistence of myotonia	
widespread film of perspiration	

☐ *Myth 1.* Women should satisfy men in sexual encounters, since women's needs are secondary to those of men. A slightly more up-to-date version of this is that each partner should be concerned with the sexual satisfaction of the other and that sexual pleasure is the responsibility of the partner.

Somehow this myth has survived a great deal of exploration. The original version implies that a woman's sexuality is just a cut below a man's. His feelings must be tended to; his needs must be met. If a woman's needs happen to be met and her feelings tended to, that is fine. But the man is the more important partner.

Sometimes the consequences of a woman violating the norm presented by this myth are serious. She may be accused of being unfeminine, selfish, and even castrating.

Lucy, married at the age of 20 years, believed the mores of her generation as taught by her mother. Her husband, Bob, was a professional man, educated and socially aware. For nearly 15 years, both of them subscribed to the idea that sexual pleasure was primarily for the man and that Lucy's part in the marriage was to please Bob. When he had repeated extramarital affairs, Lucy blamed herself, saying, "I am not concerned enough about him. I do not satisfy him adequately." She never considered her own satisfaction, or the lack of it, nor did Bob ever give it any thought. In her quest to find an answer Lucy attended one of my seminars. During this seminar it was suggested that each partner in a relationship was entitled to some pleasure and consideration and that each was responsible for her or his own pleasure. A consequence of this was that each partner had a right to ask for certain things, and each had the right to refuse certain things that were not pleasurable for her or him. Most important, it was stressed that women were not responsible for their partner's pleasure or lack of it.

Lucy had never heard such ideas proposed before, but the more she thought about them, the more they seemed to apply to her. She readily acknowledged that living by the ideals she had been taught had not resulted in happiness for herself. Nor had this lifestyle resulted in happiness for her husband. She had always blamed herself for everything that was wrong in the marriage, particularly in the sexual area. Also, Bob had obliged her by blaming her. She decided to make some changes in her life. If Bob could be part of this change, she would be happy; if not, she would have to find some other way to work the situation out.

She began by telling Bob about the seminar and what it had meant to her. He agreed intellectually that it would be acceptable to make some changes. She initiated this by telling him during lovemaking the things he did that she liked. He responded with astonishment at first, then with anger. "After 15 years are you telling me how to do it?" he demanded.

"No," she told him, "after 15 years I'm telling you what things you do that I like."

Her next step was to ask him to continue a particular activity that she found pleasurable. He had frequently asked the same from her and had never thought that it was anything but the way it should be. Her change in this regard left him unsettled and wondering if he had been inadequate during the previous years of the marriage. He was unable to ask her directly about his adequacy, and her sensing of his need for verbal reassurance on this point did little to allay his worry. Finally, one night Lucy initiated sexual activity. Bob failed to achieve an erection, blamed Lucy for this, and then proceeded to tell her how wonderful she had always been and how she had changed. It took them many months to work this out, and there are still parts that are unresolved. Lucy has made it clear to Bob that she will no longer settle for his half-hearted attempts to satisfy her or for his assumption that their sexual activity is primarily for his pleasure. He is trying to change, but there are still times when both think they would do better to separate and start over with someone else.

Possibly the most positive outcome has been that, when Bob had another extramarital affair, Lucy was able to say that he was responsible for his own behavior, that if he was unhappy about something in their relationship she would be willing to work with him on it, but that she would not be blamed for his unfaithfulness.

The current version of the myth—that each partner should be concerned with the other and is responsible for the other—is more subtle and on the surface looks good. Yet in such a situation someone nearly always comes out second. Lovemaking is such an intensely personal experience that concentration on self is inevitable. If the partners adhere to the credo that each should concentrate on the other, the person with the better skills will be more successful. In general women have been taught to be more concerned about others, and men are socialized to be more self-concerned. It's not difficult to imagine who concentrates harder on the other person.

☐ *Myth 2.* Women are slower to arouse sexually than men.

This is a very old myth. Books are still available telling adolescent girls that boys will become sexually aroused when girls in the same situation will remain calm and cool. In fact, it will take a great deal of stimulation for girls to become aroused sexually. The same books indicate directly or imply that "holding the line" or "giving in" is the responsibility of the girl.

There are two things wrong with this myth. One is that the girl who is easily aroused is led to feel that she is unusual, perhaps abnormal. The second is that there are enormous variations in both men and women, and within the same person over a period of time. Some women, because of adverse experiences that they may have had, need hours to be aroused. Some men may have had experiences that led to impotence and cannot be aroused at all. Variation in the individual may be such that what is arousing one day may make little or no difference the next. Very few people, female or male, go through life with only one pattern of arousal.

Ellen and Fred had been married 6 months when they came to see me about a "problem." According to both of them in separate assessment sessions, Ellen was swift to arouse, often climaxed before Fred did, and seemed to be aroused sexually more frequently than Fred. When questioned, both said that Ellen never discontinued intercourse after orgasm but was happy to continue until Fred had climaxed. She enjoyed intercourse even after her climax and was never in any hurry for Fred to finish. When asked what they thought the real problem was, neither could identify it. Nonetheless, they had been having intercourse less and less frequently, and they were not as satisfied as they had been at the beginning of the marriage.

Further discussion sessions finally revealed that Fred believed a "real woman" should not be so easily aroused, that if she was easily aroused she should wait for the man to become aroused, and in fact hold back until he was ready. His reading, his locker-room buddies, and hints from his father had led him to believe that women could be satisfied sexually only if the man worked hard at it. There was something unusual, if not pathologic, about a woman who was so easily aroused as Ellen. When it became apparent to Fred that this was his expectation and when he was able to understand that there are wide variations in both sexes, he and Ellen were able to work out the problem.

☐ *Myth 3.* Women who are raped ask for it, and secretly every woman wants to be raped.

Probably no one knows how such a myth came to be. The linking of sex and violence is not new to our generation or culture. Susan Brownmiller, in her book *Against Our Will: Men, Women, and Rape,* has explored the history of rape thoroughly. She concludes that wars, pogroms, riots, and revolutions have always been an excuse for men to rape women. Although she further explores many cases of rape, there seems to be little evidence that women actually want to be raped.[5]

During a class I taught on sex and the law, one student devised and carried out a project on rape. His major emphasis was on the treatment of the victim by the police and the experience from a legal point of view. He interviewed several rape victims and asked a variety of questions designed to assess the victim's perception of the experience.

The structure of the interviews was not geared to this myth, but two of the victims alluded to it. "No one asks to be raped," one woman stated. "I was minding my own business, coming home from work. It wasn't even dark, and the clothes I was wearing weren't seductive. I was just there. If I had been old, or ugly, or even crippled, he would still have raped me."

Another victim stated: "The sexual act itself was no big thing. It was nothing unusual. People always think it is something special and that all girls fantasize about being raped. It wasn't like that at all. The actual intercourse just made the whole thing more humiliating."[6]

This myth is all the more incredible since no one who is robbed or mugged is ever asked if they want to be robbed or mugged. Rape is the only crime in which the victim rather than the offender is under fire. Rape is basically not a sexual act but an act of violence. Most women do not want acts of violence committed against them.

☐ *Myth 4.* When people engage in lovemaking, men automatically know what to do and do not need directions from the partner.

This myth makes about as much sense as saying that people are born knowing how to walk. It can be easily observed that children learn how to walk only through trial and error, and usually with the help of some person or object.

There is no validity to the assertion that one person can know "instinctively" what another person likes or dislikes, still less that anyone can know what feels good to another. Living with this myth is often damaging and ends with one of the partners feeling put upon. If the man thinks he knows what the woman likes and acts accordingly, she may feel strange if she doesn't like it. After all, he is supposed to know these things. On the other hand, if the woman tells the man that he is doing something she doesn't like, he may feel that he has failed, since he is supposed to know. Some things feel good to one person and not to another. Some things feel good to a person at one point in life but not so good later. People are not known for their ability to read each other's minds with any degree of accuracy. Clear communication between partners about sexuality, sexual performance, and sexual likes is essential to a happy relationship.

Marian complained that Chad had no sensitivity to her sexual needs. He wanted to use "funny" positions and liked to manipulate her breasts during lovemaking, especially in the early stages of excitement. She found the positions tolerable but got almost no stimulation from breast manipulation and in fact usually found it distracting. I asked her if she had ever mentioned this fact to Chad. "Of course not," was her reply. "He ought to be able to figure that out. I squirm enough. Besides, men ought to know."

Chad and Marian had been sexually active with each other for 6 months of their 8-month relationship. They discussed other aspects of their relationship: where they went together, what kind of books each read, what kind of gifts were exchanged, if any, and what kind of food they ate. Marian liked Chinese food; Chad preferred Italian. The ensuing conversation went something like this:

Marian: In fact, I fixed him a big meal of spaghetti and clam sauce just last night.

Interviewer: And did he like that?

M: He loved it. It's his favorite meal.

I: How do you know it's his favorite meal?

M: He told me so.

I: You mean you didn't just know that?

M: Of course not. How would I know such a thing?

Marian seemed to hear her own words. Finally, a look of wonder and amusement crossed her face. "Is that what you were trying to tell me?" she asked. "We don't know what other people like unless they tell us?"

She started telling Chad what she liked and what was not pleasant to her. She also stopped trying to convey her message nonverbally through squirming. Their relationship and sexual experience have improved immensely.

☐ *Myth 5.* Children, especially little girls, should not be told about sex. It just puts ideas into their heads.

Of all the myths pertaining to human and female sexuality, I believe that this one is the most dangerous and damaging. In classes and seminars women repeatedly tell of the pain and anguish they experienced as a result of not being prepared for menstrual periods and not knowing about male sexual development, penile erections, the sexual feelings that girls experience, or having babies. Children are constantly exposed to books, magazines, newspapers, and television. The amount of material in these media that is directly connected with sexuality is staggering. Children probably do not even need these stimuli to be curious about sex and interested in the subject.

At the age of 5, Mona crawled out on the roof and looked in the window at her mother taking a bath. She asked, "Is that where I sucked as a baby?" Her mother was angry and told her to get down from the roof immediately. In relating this story some 40 years later, Mona was convinced that concern for her safety was less important to her mother than the question she had asked. The fact that her mother had never answered the question, had never discussed any aspect of sexuality with her, and still acts as though sex and sexuality do not exist has reinforced Mona's original feeling: Sex is bad; don't talk about it.

If children do not learn about sexuality from the media, they are likely to hear about it from their peers, and such information is not always accurate.

When Sharon was 10 years old, she had a friend who was 12. The friend, Wilma, showed Sharon a sanitary napkin one day and tried to explain how it was used. "But why do they bother?" Sharon asked.

"Because they bleed," Wilma told her.

Sharon tried to think where the blood came from. She was aware that there were two openings but did not know about the vagina. Finally she asked, "Why do they bleed? Where does the blood come from?"

"Oh, they scratch themselves with their fingernails somehow. And then they bleed," was Wilma's knowing response.

Children are full of curiosity about all their worlds, and the world of sexuality is no exception. Wynne still laughs when she remembers her young niece asking if Wynne could have a uterine transplant to enable her to have babies after a hysterectomy. If you can get a new heart, why not a new uterus?

Many parents believe that the sexual education of children is the prerogative of the schools, whereas the schools say that it is the responsibility of the parents. The ideal situation is neither but rather a cooperative plan whereby both parents and schools take the responsibility of educating the child for this important aspect of life.

Even when there are attempts at education on the part of the schools, there may be serious gaps in the curriculum. A very small survey of sex education in junior and senior high schools was conducted by one of the students in my class. Obviously the sample was restricted and may not be representative of all schools in the area or country. Nonetheless, the student's findings may be significant, even with the restrictions in sample. The basic questions she wanted to research were: What are students taught in schools about sexuality and when are they taught it? What do students like about the suitability of the topic for their age? If a particular topic pertaining to sexuality is not included in the curriculum, do students think it should be?

The questionnaire was answered by 25 juniors and seniors in one high school. The topics included were menstruation, intercourse, conception, contraception, abortion, and masturbation.

All students in this sample thought that all the topics should be covered somewhere in the school sex education curriculum. However, less than 20 percent had received any information about abortion, and less than 10 percent had learned about masturbation from the school curriculum. All students in the sample had been given some explanation about the menstrual cycle and the resultant ability to conceive, but only about 50 percent had received any information about intercourse from the school curriculum. About 30 percent had been given information about contraceptives.

When information had been given on any topic, the age varied from seventh grade (ages 12 to 13 years) for menstruation to twelfth grade (ages 17 to 18 years) for information about contraception. Considering that many girls begin their periods earlier than the age of 12 years and that by the junior year in high school (eleventh grade) a considerable number of young adults of both sexes are sexually active, this would appear to be inadequate. Students need information about menses before the period starts, not a year later. By the time most students in this sample had received information from school programs, the need for the information as a preparation for an event was long past. The students recognized this and pointed it out to the investigator.[7]

The age of menarche has dropped in the past generation. Ages 12 or 13 years might have been early enough for parents or schools to begin discussion of menses 20 years ago. Today there is a likelihood that at least one girl in the 11 year age group will have started her periods. Once she has, there is little basis for the expectation that the other girls in her circle of friends will remain ignorant of the fact. Even if they did, what purpose would be served? If menstruation is a normal function, as people like to say it is, there are more reasonable ways to educate little girls about it. An ideal setting would be a household in which having menstrual periods is such a part of the routine that girls (and boys) would always know about them. Girls would then be prepared, and the onset of menses would not be a worry nor a shock to them.

☐   *Myth 6.* Women are not interested in sex following a hysterectomy or menopause.

For many women the opposite is true. Once the possibility of pregnancy is eliminated a woman can often be more relaxed and interested in sexual intercourse than she was previously. Part of the unspoken basis for this myth comes from the idea that women are sexual primarily in order to bear children, and, when they are no longer able to bear children, they are not interested (should not be interested) in sex.

Also, women have been led to believe that having a hysterectomy will automatically lead to a decreased hormonal output, and this in turn will cause a lessened sex drive. Although a total hysterectomy involving removal of ovaries, fallopian tubes, and uterus will result in loss of hormones, in many instances an estrogen replacement therapy can be used. Many hysterectomies are not total, and the presurgical hormonal level is maintained.

Menopause is the gradually decreasing functioning of the ovarian hormone and occurs simultaneously with other changes that are apt to begin at about the late forties and early fifties. The danger of this myth is that rather than each person being considered individually, an artificial norm is created and everyone is expected to conform to it. Such expectations create pressures on women to be something other than what they are and end by stifling women's self-expression and spontaneity.

When Polly first became aware that her

periods were changing, she expected that her interest in sex would diminish. Her mother had never discussed the menopause with her, and she had no idea what to expect. The accompanying physical phenomena of menopause bothered her a great deal. She found that many nights she was unable to sleep. She was often irritable, and she found herself identifying with victims of tragedy, even though she did not know the people involved. Once, for example, she read a short news item about a Kansas family who had been left homeless by a tornado. Polly cried nearly half an hour over this newspaper article, although she did not know the Kansas family. Such behavior was completely foreign to her usual cheerfulness.

However, her interest in sex continued and, as she became aware that she had been released from the concerns about pregnancy that she had experienced earlier in her marriage, sexual activity and enjoyment increased. Her relationship with her husband was strengthened by this, and she was given support from him during those periods when she was unable to sleep or felt depressed over other people's troubles.

STRESSES PLACED ON FEMALE SEXUALITY

As mentioned earlier in this chapter, all societies have had ways of regulating sexual behavior. These regulations pertained to both men and women, but emphasis often has been on conformity by women, whereas men have had more freedom to violate these restrictions.

Many would argue that the double standard is dead, but it is alive and well in America. One has only to read "Dear Abby" and many other newspaper articles to see evidences of it. Not long ago on the radio a news item began, "Today a 55 year old grandmother was arrested for. . . ." No one ever states that a man who has been arrested is a grandfather. Infrequently a man's marital status is mentioned or possibly the number of his children.

We are becoming more aware that female sexuality involves a great deal more than mere childbearing functions. Obviously we haven't discovered sex in our generation, but we may be in the process of rediscovering it. A study initiated in 1890 was recently published in *Psychology Today*.[8] This study indicated that not all Victorian women were repressed and hated sex. Nor did all of them have unwanted and unlimited hordes of children. Many women cited in the study used some form of birth control and apparently found it effective,

since many of them had fewer children than women in similar circumstances in the early 1970s.

In this section, some of the specific problems women face in their sexual lives will be discussed.

One of the major stresses placed on a woman's sexuality is the attitude that sex is mostly for men. Women are still socialized to believe that men are "out for just one thing," and that, of course, is sex. Sex will not do a woman any good except to give her a reputation (usually bad) or a bunch of children. Neither of these things is very desirable.

Vicki's mother made frequent reference to the "bestiality" of men. Vicki determined never to have to submit to such demands, decided she would never marry, and further cut herself off from the necessity of relating to men sexually by entering a religious group. When she discovered that this way of life did not completely protect her either from her own feelings or from the advances of men, she became profoundly depressed. She left the religious group and then a year later rejoined it. She repeated this pattern of behavior once more and was finally advised that her destiny lay elsewhere. The last time I saw her she was still fighting the attitudes her mother had instilled in her.

A second problem women encounter is that they are raised to be sexually dependent on men. They must learn all the "womanly skills" and then await the time when the prince will come and arouse the sleeping beauty within them. If he never comes, a woman often believes it was because she was not good enough. If he comes and she does not like something he does, she dare not rebel. After all, he might go elsewhere, to another woman, to divorce, or, worse yet, to playing poker with his buddies. Thus, women believe that they must endure much for the sake of having a man to satisfy their sexual needs. If the man does go somewhere else, whatever will a woman do?

One of women's needs is to become sexually autonomous. This may include developing the freedom to say no when they do not want sex; it may mean initiating specific sexual acts and relationships; or it may mean finding ways of satisfying their sexual needs through masturbation or other means. It certainly means getting to know themselves and their sexual needs and being able to say what these needs are.

In one of my classes a series of films on some means of sexual satisfaction other than intercourse was shown. After the film on masturbation, most of the women said that they did not engage in this activity. Some of them had at one time but had discontinued the practice when they had developed a sexual relationship with a man. One of them said, "Why should I bother to do that when I have a man to take care of me? I resent having to take care of myself." Yet when questioned whether they thought their partners masturbated, and if so what they thought about it, all of them said they assumed their partners masturbated at least occasionally, and it seemed acceptable to them.

Still another problem that faces women is that of guilt. Women more than men are still socialized to believe that sex is wrong. Lois, a woman now in her mid-forties, relates that in her childhood, she had such a strong feeling that sex was wrong, she believed it was sinful even in marriage. "I was raised a Catholic, and I really thought that after having sex my mother confessed before going to communion." Neither parent ever said this directly; it was simply an impression Lois had. She never thought her father confessed his.

Rarely do parents say directly that sex is wrong or bad. The nonverbal message gets through, however, and children are often confused by it. This is particularly true if there is a double message involved. If sex is beautiful, why don't parents want their children to know about it? On the other hand, if sex is dirty, why the constant admonition to save it for someone you love? These attitudes cannot fail to have effects on people for many years. Old conditioning comes back to haunt even those who consider themselves enlightened or liberated. Some of the best literature on the market about sexuality still refers to sexual jokes as "dirty jokes."

Another problem is the attitude toward intercourse during the menstrual period. In the past many religions and cultures prohibited intercourse during menses. But why does the proscription remain? Men who do not have intercourse during their partner's period state that it is because menses is messy. This is a strange and interesting response; the implication seems to be that semen is not messy or—what is worse—if semen is messy that it is just too bad.

When a woman is having a period she is often experiencing physiologic changes that are not particularly pleasant or reassuring. She may feel sluggish or bloated due to hormonal changes or concerned about odors that might be generated due to menses. If during these times a woman's outside resources fail her or reinforce her feeling of undesirability and questionable cleanliness (messiness), no wonder she becomes hard to live with.

Another problem women encounter is lack of information. In teaching classes in human sexuality, I have observed that many women are still not adequately prepared for their first period, either by their mothers or through the schools. If there is no open communication between mother and daughter about menstruation, one can be sure that it is all downhill from there on. A mother who does not discuss menstruation with her daughter will not discuss male sexual development, wet dreams, necking, petting, intercourse, orgasm, conception, delivery, birth control, or masturbation. Daughters are forced to seek other avenues of information.

These other avenues may be satisfactory, but often they are not. Peer groups are usually the first source, and they are usually notoriously inadequate as far as facts are concerned.

Adulthood may not remedy this problem. In the book *Our Bodies, Ourselves,* many women tell of their experiences with doctors.[9] Presumably obstetricians and gynecologists are highly knowledgeable about female sexuality and female sexual functioning. After all, they deal with this every day of their professional lives. Yet this has not been the experience of many women. They have found that these doctors are cold, impersonal, sometimes ignorant of all but the most basic anatomic and physiologic facts, and often unsympathetic with the problems of their clients. My experience in counseling echoes this. Only in recent years has material on human and female sexuality been incorporated into medical school curricula.

Other sources of information include school programs; reading and experience. In recent years lectures, seminars, and workshops about sexuality have become widespread for professional groups and often for other groups as well. These can be a tremendous help to people but cannot meet everyone's needs.

At one workshop where I conducted a small group discussion, during an opening exercise each participant told a little about herself or himself and what each hoped to get from the experience. One man stated that he came mostly out of curiosity. He was a Canadian, and nothing of this sort was available in Canada. He wanted to know what went on at such a workshop. Whether he learned anything and whether he was disappointed we never learned. At the first break he disappeared and never returned.

Books can be of real benefit, but there are two problems in their use. One is accuracy of content. For a person well versed in the field of sexuality inaccuracies may be easy to spot. For the majority of people, however, glaring falsehoods may not be noticed. A second problem with books is the interpretation. For example, think of the many interpretations given to that very sexual book, the Bible. Few ancient books discuss sex as freely as this one does, but centuries of interpretation and reinterpretation have now given it the reputation of being repressive of sex. One of the favorite passages of the antihomosexuals is from the Book of Genesis. Lot, visited by two angels, is beseiged by male inhabitants of Sodom. The implication seems clear that the natives of Sodom want the visitors in order to "abuse " them. Lot refuses and gives them instead his daughter (a virgin of course). No thought of pity ever seems to be given to the poor girl who could be subjected to gang rape at her father's whim. People use the story to "prove" that homosexuality is sinful. It might be just as easy to use the story as an example of hospitality. It seems probable that some 40 centuries later there is no complete certainty about what the story was initially intended to convey.

Women have another problem with their sexuality. They are often raised to believe some funny things about themselves. Two important examples of this are the attitudes they learn about erotic literature and about masturbation. These attitudes may be a result of the idea discussed earlier that sex is mostly for men. Pornography is supposedly a male preserve, for only men are sexually aroused by pictures of nude women. Nude men would be offensive to women, so the theory goes. Reading a book with erotic content would be of no use to a woman; such matters are only for men. Yet erotic literature can be helpful to both men and women, as far as arousal is concerned. Apart from the exploitative nature of pornography as in movies or "girlie" magazines (would magazines featuring pictures of nude males be called "boyie" magazines?)—if it is arousing, it can be helpful. Erotic literature is sometimes a help in achieving orgasm also, by helping people concentrate on sexual matters and reducing distractions.

Masturbation is another area that remains a seemingly male prerogative. At puberty, if women are told about periods and conception, they are rarely ever told about the clitoris and its function in sexual pleasure. Since the penis is visible and boys learn early how good it feels to stroke and handle the penis, most males discover masturbation on their own, early in life. Most women, on the other hand, do not discover masturbation until much later, some not until they are well into adulthood. Unless they read about it, their discovery, too, is accidental. While most parents try to discourage both sexes from masturbating, the usual attitude is that "boys will be boys, but girls should not."

Karen told about an experience that occurred at 4 years of age. Her mother was horrified to find her fingering her genitals in the bath tub. "I don't ever want you to do that again," she said. "Promise me you won't." Karen promised, not knowing for sure what she had been doing that was so terrible and not knowing what she was really promising. Twenty years later she was still confused.

All too often parents refer to masturbation as "that," as though the activity is so terrible that it cannot even be named. Many women are confused by the proscription, not knowing just what is so terrible about their genitals.

Adela was raised by strict parents and had little information about her sexuality. Although she had no remembrance of any prohibition against masturbation, she assumed it was placed on her at an early age. She never remembered masturbating as a child. She grew to adulthood repressed and unsure of herself and remained sexually inactive until well into her thirties. When she was 36 years old she had the opportunity to do some nude solitary swimming. After several weeks of this she discovered that whenever she swam by the inlet stream of the pool the quick rush of water was especially pleasant. She experimented with the water on various parts of her body, including her genitals, and had her first orgasm this way. She described the experience as overwhelming, and she began to cry. She had read enough to know intellectually what was happening to her, but nothing had prepared her for the emotional response she felt. Later when she was no longer able to use the pool she experimented with other forms of water, such as the hose, the shower, and the bathtub. She finds this to be her most intense orgasmic response.

Still another problem women have is to see their concerns as unique, as never having been experienced by another person. This comes in part from a mistrust of other women and a consequent inability for women to open up to each other. When Corrine was first asked to do a self sexual history in one of my classes, she went about it in a half-hearted way. After several days of fighting with herself she finally wrote as much as she dared. The idea of writing about her sexual self was very threatening. Even verbally sharing her sexual past or present feelings with others seemed incomprehensible to her. When she ventured to say this timidly in the group, she found her feelings echoed by most women there. Most of them had complied with the assignment because they were accustomed to having someone tell them to do an assignement.

When women start to discuss their sexual past with other women, they frequently find a commonality not previously suspected. In one group, Denise said that there were a couple of things she was unable to talk about; in fact, she was unable to write them down. No one pressed her for any details or even hints about what these experiences were. Instead, those who felt comfortable started to talk about their experiences, and soon the rest joined in with, "Oh yes, that happened to me too." About halfway through the group session Denise interrupted another woman to say, "I can't believe this. Why did I ever think it was such a big deal? At least four of you have had the same experience I did." And she proceeded to tell the entire story to the group. For the first time in her life Denise was able to put her past sexual life and experience into the perspective of a common bond with other women.

A further difficulty with women's sexual experience is the tendency to see the problems as unique to women. Women do not see them in the context of human problems. Many times women are embarrassed about their bodies; they think that they have too much of one thing and not enough of another. But they seldom connect these feelings with the anxiety of the man who measures his penis every day or flexes his muscles before a mirror. Nor do they often see their concern about being preorgasmic or turned off by certain acts as being related to a man's frustration if he is too tired to have an erection or is not interested in cunnilingus. Nearly all sexual problems are human problems and are not specific to either sex.

What, then, can women do to alleviate some of these stressors on their sexuality? Women need to become comfortable with their sexuality. They need to know themselves as sexual

persons and to value the sexual part of themselves as much as they would the ability to fly an airplane, dance gracefully, bake a lemon meringue pie, or sculpt a statue. Most of the foregoing discussion has pointed to the fact that women's socialization is not aimed at these goals. It is, in fact, aimed at preventing them from finding any large measure of comfort or value in their sexuality. However, there are some things that women can do.

The first step is to write your sexual history. Begin with childhood: What thoughts and ideas did you have about sex then, what attitudes and ideas did your parents convey to you, what kind of childhood sexual play did you engage in, who were your friends and what did they contribute to your concepts of sexuality? Try to remember what your mother told you in preparation for your menstrual periods and dating or any other talks you might have had with her. Move from there to your first experiences with dating, kissing, necking, petting, intercourse, and masturbation. Recall any same-sex experiences as well as opposite-sex encounters. Try to remember not only the experience but your feelings at the time. Bring yourself up to date with your sexual experiences: going steady, engagement, marriage, honeymoon, divorce, widowhood, remarriage—whatever is appropriate to your life circumstances. This exercise helps you see where you are now and gives you some insight into why you are at this particular place.

In writing her self sexual history, Donna realized that her unwillingness to become close to any woman was connected with her attendance at a slumber party some years before. Many of the girls were just entering adolescence and were aware that they would soon be dating and kissing boys. During the slumber party most of the girls practiced hugging and kissing each other in an attempt to see what it felt like to kiss another person romantically. Donna participated in this activity but felt so guilty about it that she soon withdrew from this group of friends and never developed any other friends among the girls at school. In exploring this experience she was able to acknowledge that her greatest fear was that she was a lesbian. She married when she was very young in an attempt to prove to herself that she was heterosexual. Once she learned how common the experience was she was able to relax and become friends with other women.

It is important to write the history rather than to just think about it. There is something salutary about seeing your own history written by your own hand. And once the basic history is complete additions can be made as recollections occur.

Remnants of the past shape the present attitudes and behavior of many of us. Many of the half-remembered bits of information, parental prohibitions, and repressions from other authority figures still affect us. We often do not take the time to look at these attitudes from the vantage point of childhood. Consequently, we go through life with ideas and attitudes that are left over from our childhood. Only by examining these ideas are we able to determine which ones are appropriate in adult life and which need to be replaced by more mature concepts. Carrying this load of childhood ideas is a great waste of energy.

The second step is taking time to know yourself sexually. This may mean locking everybody out of your room for an hour a day while you get in touch with your body. It may mean experimenting with new positions or behaviors in lovemaking. It may mean masturbating with a new object or motion. It may mean just starting to masturbate. It may mean abstaining from intercourse for a time. We need to overcome the early conditioning to let everybody else come first and, if there's any time left over, then do something nice for ourselves. When we take care of ourselves, when we tell the world by our behavior that we are valuable and worth taking care of, others will respect this and take care of us too.

Jill's mother, Bette, made herself a slave to everyone else. If Bette needed something and one of the children wanted something, Bette would always go without. The result was an unhappy woman with selfish children and a pushy husband. "She was always giving up something for someone," Jill recalls. "As a result she never had any of the things she wanted. And she continually told us how much she had sacrificed for us. Now that we are all grown wouldn't you think we would repay her for all those 'sacrifices'?" None of the children ever visited her or took her a gift. Jill often forgot her mother's birthday and had not sent her a Mother's Day card for 3 years. The children never expected Bette to want anything and took her at her own evaluation, which was

"I am not worth anything; I am not worthy of any consideration."

In the area of sexuality specifically, women need to learn to say no when they don't want sex and to initiate it when they do. It is all part of the pattern of taking care of themselves.

The third step is to actively work toward incorporating a degree of positive regard for your sexuality. If your past has been mainly negative toward your sexual self (and that is true of most women), the time to start changing this is yesterday. Read about the experiences of others, talk to other women, and, more than that, trust your own experience. If you feel unhappy or put off by a given situation or behavior, do not try to pretend that those feelings do not exist or that these feelings are wrong. They are your feelings, and you have a right to them. If you want to do something about the situation or feeling, do it—not because your next-door neighbor tells you that you must or because you read a book that said you should, but because you want to, and for no other reason. Every person has a right to a fulfilling, happy sexual life. But you will not have such a life by doing what comes naturally, in most cases. It has to be worked for, and the achievement is up to you.

References

1. Woods, Nancy Fugate. *Human Sexuality in Health and Illness.* St. Louis: C. V. Mosby Company, 1975, chap. 2.
2. Money, John, and Arhardt, Anke. *Man and Woman, Boy and Girl.* Baltimore: Johns Hopkins Press, 1972, p. 13.
3. Masters, William, and Johnson, Virginia. *Human Sexual Response.* Boston: Little, Brown & Company, 1966, chap. 1.
4. Masters, William, and Johnson, Virginia, ibid.
5. Brownmiller, Susan. *Against Our Will: Men, Women, and Rape.* New York: Simon and Schuster, 1975, chaps. 4, 5.
6. Johnson, Scott. *Three Perspectives on Rape.* Unpublished manuscript, 1976.
7. Horner, Gail. *Sex Education in the School System.* Unpublished clinical study, 1976.
8. Gaylin, Jody. "Those Sexy Victorians." *Psychology Today,* December 1976, pp. 137–141.
9. Boston's Women's Health Book Collective. *Our Bodies, Ourselves.* New York: Simon and Schuster, 1975, p. 15.

6

LESBIANS
ELIZABETH MORRISON

Elizabeth Morrison writes of the lesbian in relationship to the health care system and includes basic information on the life styles of lesbians and their relationships. The chapter concludes with the process of acknowledging one's sexual/affectional preference as a lesbian.

Lesbians are women who prefer women as affectional/sexual partners. As women, they face all the pleasures, joys, problems, and pressures that every woman faces, with a few important exceptions. Elsewhere in this volume, stressors and stress-related issues for women are explored. This chapter focuses on stressors specific to lesbians. For purposes of this discussion, stress is the result of an external factor or stressor that leads to perceived anxiety, tension, or pressure. Stress is a fact of life for every individual in our society and a certain level or amount of stress can provide motivation and add a charge of excitement to daily routines. However, accumulated stress can lead to physical, emotional, or social dysfunction, or a combination thereof. The importance of understanding stress lies in being able to manage it effectively, not in eradicating it; eradication is impossible, but reduction may be a reasonable goal.

Many stressors affecting the lives of lesbians are related to the concept of homophobia, the irrational fear that heterosexuals have of homosexuality and homosexuals. The origins of homophobia are unclear, but it exists in religious doctrine, in the legal system, and in cultural myths. The discriminatory effects of homophobia evoke a certain level of fear in lesbians, which results in a degree of guardedness in their relationships with friends, family, and systems with which they interact. The guardedness is problematic in that hiding or passing as heterosexual protects the lesbian, but it also helps perpetuate myths and stereotypes. Lesbians who hesitate to comment on or to contradict negative images of lesbians for fear of being caught tacitly reinforce the misconceptions of others. Lesbians' fear of the consequences of homophobia persists even in light of changing images of gay people in the media and the efforts of gay rights activists. Attitudes change slowly, and research evidence indicates that attitudes of heterosexuals toward homosexuality are negative.[1, 2] It is interesting to note that while both heterosexual men and heterosexual women have negative attitudes, women are less homophobic than are men.[1, 2] Given that the overwhelming majority of nurses are women, nurses are in a position to meet the health care needs of the gay clients whom they encounter.

This chapter presents an overview of what is known about lesbian experience with the health care system, an overview of research related to lesbian life styles, and examples of some of the decisions lesbians must make in the coming out process. Each section illustrates some of the stressors with which lesbians cope.

LESBIANS AND THE HEALTH CARE SYSTEM

Stressors affecting lesbians in the health care system are related to attitudes of health care professionals and to how lesbians perceive they are treated if they acknowledge themselves as lesbians. Dulaney and Kelly maintained that physicians, psychologists, and social workers were all homophobic, that is, had negative attitudes toward homosexuality and homosexuals.[3] White found that although psychiatric nurses viewed homosexuality as pathologic, increased education led to increased tolerance of homosexual behavior.[4] Dritz acknowledged that many physicians are homophobic and may reject patients if patients do disclose their sexual preference.[5]

Dardick and Grady sampled homosexuals by means of a questionnaire to "explore the experiences of homosexual persons with their primary health providers."[6] Forty-nine percent of the female respondents and sixty-three percent of the male respondents reported they had disclosed their sexual preference to their primary health care provider and further reported that the disclosure had led to increased satisfaction with health care. Of those who had not disclosed their sexual preference to health care providers, fear of rejection was the major reason offered. McGhee and Owen also sampled homosexuals to determine satisfaction with health care.[7] Thirty-one percent of the women who had told physicians about their lesbianism perceived a negative reaction from the physician. Another survey to identify factors influencing gynecologic care of lesbians reported 18 percent of the respondents had told their physicians and 40 percent had not told because they thought they would receive a negative reaction.[8]

Two major issues which emerged from the above studies were confidentiality[8] and the assumption of heterosexuality.[6, 8] Lesbians were concerned that their sexuality would become a part of their medical records and could result in legal consequences. In many states homosexuality is illegal, and homosexual behavior may be used as grounds in child custody battles. If the nurse has the information that a client is a lesbian, it may be possible to negotiate the data that go into the medical record. The client's sexuality may or may not be relevant to patient care. If it is relevant, the nurse could inform the patient of the need for documentation; if not relevant, the nurse need not document the information.

The automatic assumption of heterosexuality is another stress-producing issue for lesbians. Some report that they have been harassed about contraception if they acknowledge they are not using any method of birth control.[8] Others object to assessment forms that list relationship options as single, married, divorced, or widowed as a form of discrimination against alternatives to heterosexual relationships.[6] Lawrence stated that homophobia and the assumption of heterosexuality may lead to ignoring or discounting the partner of the hospitalized homosexual.[9] The recommendation was made that nurses include homosexual partners in planning and implementing nursing care.

It is encouraging to note that many lesbians do disclose their sexual orientation to health care providers despite the risks involved, and that some report increased satisfaction with the care they receive as a result of such disclosure. Yet many lesbians still choose not to acknowledge their preference for women; these people may be receiving less than satisfactory care because nurses and other health care professionals are unaware of important information. Given that nurses are interested in providing holistic care and an atmosphere in which self-disclosure is safe for clients with alternative life styles, it is useful to explore our own assumptions and attitudes about lesbians. Many nurses with whom I have worked relate that their most satisfying emotional relationships are with other women, but they react negatively to the idea of sexuality between women. In the process of thinking through their reactions, they discover that the resultant negativity is based on stereotypes and misconceptions about lesbians and lesbian life styles. The section to follow presents current information from the theoretic and research literature.

LESBIAN LIFE STYLES

Lesbians Do Not Hate Men

The image of the lesbian as someone who dislikes or hates men persists in spite of the fact that many lesbians have been or are married, have children, and report close relationships with men.[10] As noted, lesbians prefer other women as affectional/sexual partners. The preference for one's own sex does not necessarily involve the rejection of the opposite sex. Perhaps the origin of this myth lies in the belief that homosexuality is an aberration. Lesbianism has not been considered a psychiatric diagnosis since 1973, but the stigma of lesbianism as a disease may still exist. Part of the concept of lesbians as ill involved either their rejection of men based on their alleged inability to relate to men or their adoption of masculine characteristics in an attempt to identify with men. However, research indicates that heterosexuals and homosexuals are indistinguishable with regard to psychologic and social functioning[11] and that there is no demonstrable connection between homosexuality and any mental disorder.[12]

The etiology of homosexuality is debated at length in the literature. Physiologic research suggests that homosexuality can be divided into primary and secondary types.[12] Primary homosexuals have no impulse to engage in sexual contact with the opposite sex, have had no sexual contact with the opposite sex, and are resistant to aversive conditioning to change their sexual orientation. Secondary homosexuals have experienced the impulse to engage in sexual contact with the opposite sex, have had heterosexual contacts, and are willing to undergo aversive conditioning to change their sexual orientation. MacCulloch and Waddington proposed a hormonal hypothesis that "leads to the prediction that primary homosexual females will show a male LH response and that the response will be normal in secondary female homosexuals."[12] The implication seems to be that some lesbians are born lesbian and others choose lesbianism as a life style. Concern about physiologic research has been expressed: "the motive and purpose of etiological research go hand in hand with the common discrimination against homosexuals in our society. It aims at preventing homosexual development by means of an endocrinological prophylaxis."[13]

Other researchers have focused on family dynamics as an explanation for homosexuality. A difficulty in assessing the implications of familial research for lesbians is that much of the research focuses on male homosexuals with results generalized to women. For example, Pillard and colleagues reviewed and synthesized all family studies relative to homosexuality.[14] They concluded that "there is substantial evidence from twin and family studies and from the pilot data we have gathered that male and probably female homosexuality is a disposition which runs in families." A cross-cultural study that compared the parental backgrounds of homosexual and heterosexual women concluded that family dynamics played a part in the lives of some but not all lesbians.[15] It seems that all lesbians are not alike. Genetic, familial, social, and political factors all may contribute to the development of a homosexual preference of life style.

Lesbians Are Not Sexually Promiscuous

Lesbians are no more sexually promiscuous than heterosexual women.[10] An associated stereotype is that lesbians are unable to form commitments. The fact is that most lesbians are involved in ongoing relationships and seldom engage in casual sex.[10] It is accurate that male homosexuals are more sexually active than any other group of people.[10] Perhaps the problem is that generalizations are made from male homosexual behavior to female homosexual behavior, thereby inaccurately equating lesbianism with promiscuity. Richardson proposed that one of the reasons homosexuality is equated with promiscuity is the relative importance placed on homosexual sexuality as compared with the relative unimportance placed on heterosexual sexuality.[16] People are curious about what lesbians do to each other sexually and not so curious about how they relate to each other. People are curious about how heterosexuals relate to each other and not so curious about what they do to each other sexually.

Lesbians engage in more relationships than heterosexual women,[10] perhaps because their relationships are not socially or familially sanctioned. The lack of positive sanctions results in a lack of support for lesbian relationships and a paucity of available resources when there are relationship difficulties. When lesbians experience problems there is little encouragement to work things out; the encouragement is in the direction of splitting up and moving on. When heterosexual partners experience problems, there is encouragement to work things out and to seek help when appropriate.

Lesbians Are Not Recognizable by the Way They Dress and Act

In general, lesbians are indistinguishable from other women. Lesbians are not confined to any one social group, race, or occupation. The ony way to know whether a woman is a lesbian is if she acknowledges herself as one.

Many women in our culture look "masculine." The cues that lead to the label of "masculine" are usually nonverbal—for example, body build, manner of dress, and gait. Cultural characteristics of femininity dictate that a woman should be petite, at least in relation to men; should be slender, if not thin; should dress seductively; should wear makeup; and should roll her legs from the hip while walking. Not many women conform to the feminine ideal, but most manage to conform in part to cultural expectation. The women's movement has assisted many women, both homosexual and heterosexual, to identify how stressful it is to live up to a youthful, beautiful image at the cost of one's individuality. Women who look masculine may be gay, may be straight, or may have decided not to continue to conform to an image they found personally discordant.

Some lesbians do look masculine. In a study of lesbians and body build, Perkins found that gay women who defined themselves as psychosexually dominant, that is, they had adopted a traditionally male role in their relationships, were "(1) significantly taller with broader shoulders and narrower hips, (2) significantly more muscular with greater arm and leg girth, (3) significantly fatter, and (4) significantly less linear than psychosexually intermediate and passive groups."[17] These data also support the idea that lesbians are as diverse and as individual in body build as heterosexual women.

Lesbian Relationships Are Not Dramatically Different from Heterosexual Relationships

Lesbians form relationships with women who have anxieties, doubts, fears, strengths, and assets instead of with men who have anxieties, doubts, fears, stengths, and assets. Relationships have their advantages and disadvantages regardless of the gender of the individuals involved. Satisfactions, issues, and problems are inherent in every relationship. When the satisfactions are greater than the dissatisfactions, the relationship is said to be a good one, and when the dissatisfactions are greater than the satisfactions, the relationship begins to erode.

However, differences in the kinds of issues faced by lesbian couples and by heterosexual couples can be found. There are no legal, social, or cultural sanctions for lesbian couples. The advantage of the lack of sanctions is relative ease of dissolution should the couple decide to end the relationship. There are no socially prescribed rules in lesbian relationships as there are in heterosexual ones. The advantage is a more flexible arena for division of household labor, economic input, and social interaction. The disadvantage is that when problems or conflicts arise, lesbians have more limited resources than do heterosexual couples.[18] One of the difficulties lesbians encounter is where to turn for help. A heterosexual couple in distress can call on family, friends, church, and the health care system. Lesbian couples may not have acknowledged the nature of their relationship to those people who might provide support, such as family and friends, or they may think that acknowledging their relationship to a pastor, a counselor, a nurse, or a physician will evoke condemnation and rejection rather than the support and assistance with the problem-solving they seek.

One obstacle to understanding lesbians and lesbian life styles is the lack of unbiased research available.[19] Only within the last 2 decades has research on women become an acceptable scholarly endeavor, and there is a growing body of knowledge about women, by women, and for women. Lesbians, by virtue of the way they structure their lives, are not inclined to volunteer for research, nor are they particularly amenable to research conducted by men who have a tendency to define women from a male perspective.[19] Therefore, much of what is known about lesbians and the lesbian community is based on findings from small, self-selected samples. The women who have chosen to participate in research may or may not be representative of the lesbian population. Owen cautioned that it is as inaccurate to assign similar life styles to homosexuals as it would be to assign similar life styles to heterosexuals.[20] When dealing with individuals it is important to assess them in the context of their life experiences. Part of the life experience of every lesbian are the decisions involved in coming out or passing as heterosexual. The section to follow illustrates some of the stressors evoked when dealing with those decisions.

COMING OUT

Coming out, that is, acknowledging one's sexual/affectional preference as a lesbian, has been sorted into four stages: "coming out to oneself (signification), identifying oneself to others who are gay, identifying oneself to someone nongay, and going public."[18] The latter two parts encompass the stages of coming out, preplanning, and dealing with the consequences. Although preplanning may ameliorate the consequences, reactions of others are often initially negative and it is useful to plan strategies for handling predicted responses.

The preplanning stage involves defining why the lesbian wants to come out, with whom she wants to come out, how she will go about disclosing, and the timing.[21] Preplanning also includes anticipating the reactions of others and defining behaviors to deal with their reactions. Examples of how the process of coming out was handled in a family context, both with and without preplanning, will be helpful.

Nancy is a 21 year old student who has lived

away from home since she began college at age 18. She states she has been a lesbian since age 16 and is currently living with another woman with whom she has a good relationship. Nancy is aware that there is increasing pressure from her family, particularly her father, to find a man and get married. She has three older sisters, all of whom were married by age 22, and she knows she is expected to do the same. She also knows she can withstand the pressure but believes she is being dishonest by not sharing her life style with her parents and siblings. She claims that over the past few years she has put too much distance between herself and her family because she has been afraid of telling them she is a lesbian. She misses the closeness with her family and decides she wants them to know about her. She thinks it would be most appropriate to begin with her next older sister. They have had a close relationship, and Nancy feels most comfortable talking with her. She plans to re-establish contact with her sister, to talk more about herself, and to find out more about her sister.

After 6 months of regular contact, Nancy says the time is right and plans some time alone by taking her sister to dinner. In terms of the actual statements she makes, Nancy wants to avoid a "demand bid" situation wherein her sister is forced to respond.[22] She handles the situation by telling her sister, over time, about her relationship with her "room-mate," finally stating that the two of them are lovers and that she is satisfied and happy in the relationship. Nancy's prediction was that her sister would be accepting of the information because Nancy was obviously content with where she was. Her prediction was accurate, and during the next year Nancy discussed her life style with all the other members of her immediate family. Her biggest surprise was that her mother said she had known for a long time but had not wanted to upset Nancy by bringing it up.

Sharon is a 28 year old secretary who lives at home with both parents and two younger brothers. She has been struggling financially for years and contributes to the support of her family. A new job with a raise in salary is finally enabling her to move out of the family home into her own apartment. She has been seeing the same woman for about 3 years, and both of them agree that Sharon needs time by herself, on her own, before they discuss living together. As the time for Sharon's move approaches, tension increases in the family sys-

tem, and family members become irritable with one another. One evening a heated argument develops between Sharon and her parents. During the course of the argument Sharon begins shouting she is a lesbian and they can like it or lump it. Sharon's father throws her against a wall, cracking three ribs, and beats her before telling her to get out of the house. Sharon leaves and has not seen or talked to her parents or brothers since the incident.

Although preplanning does not automatically produce acceptance, there is a much greater likelihood that acceptance will occur if the individual takes time to read her family system, to work on her own anxiety about coming out, and to formulate useful strategies based on her knowledge of how her family functions. The lesbian must then be prepared to deal with the emotional fallout in the family. One reaction is to appear to accept a lesbian relationship but to devalue it or to consider it a passing phase.[22] Many parents feel like failures and wonder aloud at length where they have gone wrong. Some consider lesbianism an illness and insist on treatment or hospitalization for a "cure." Others can accept the idea in the abstract but refuse contact with the partner in a relationship. Still others have violent negative reactions and disown the lesbian, while a certain percentage seem to accept the information, incorporate it into the ongoing family patterns, and have little difficulty adjusting.[18] All lesbians who have come out in their families report some period of adjustment for themselves and their family members.

It is useful to know that many communities have groups for parents of gays to assist them in dealing with the knowledge their child is gay. It should be recognized that coming out may be a difficult time for both families and lesbian.

Lesbians have friends who are gay and friends who are straight. Coming out to straight friends is more stressful than coming out to gay friends. The decision-making process previously noted is helpful in planning the disclosure process. The consequences of identifying as a lesbian with friends are both more and less risky than identifying as a lesbian with family members. Even though there is an emotional attachment to friends, usually the emotional intensity present in family systems is absent.[21] Therefore, the anxiety about disclosure is lower. Although friends are sometimes startled by the news and can be rejecting, more often they are supportive and accepting.

Resolution of sexuality between friends is predictably an issue, whether the friend is male or female, homosexual or heterosexual. The lesbian should be prepared for a sexually oriented response. Female friends may wonder if they are being asked for sex, may want to engage in a sexual encounter, may become hostile or seductive, or may be willing to discuss the implications of the information and the effects it will have on the friendship. Male friends exhibit similar reactions, with the unfortunate addition of attempted sexual assault in an effort to "prove" to the lesbian that all she really needs is a good experience with a man. The lesbian should also be prepared for the possible dissolution of the friendship and her grief at the loss if that does occur. Some lesbians report that as they become more comfortable with self-disclosure, they find it easier to tell others in a nonthreatening way and are available to assist other lesbians with the process. The lesbian can discuss with her gay friends her ideas about how to more effectively cope with the reactions of her straight friends. However, the final decision rests with the individual.

Deborah had been married for almost 3 years before divorcing her husband 5 years ago. She married her former boss after discovering she was pregnant; she subsequently miscarried and has no other children. Since her divorce she has been sexually involved with three men and two women. She has decided that her sexual/affectional preference is for women, but she is not currently engaged in any ongoing relationship. She has two friends, both women, whom she has known since high school, and the three of them spend a great deal of time together. Deborah has not informed them of her lesbian relationships but has told them about the men in her life. She is now seriously considering coming out to them since she believes she has made an important life decision. She seeks assistance in exploring ways to go about relating her decision to her friends. Deborah is guided through the preplanning phase of coming out and reviews the advantages and disadvantages of disclosure. Based on her assessment of her relationship with each of her friends, she chooses not to tell them she is adopting a lesbian life style. She discovers that the friendships have always revolved around the premise of heterosexual relationships and that her participation in those friendships is also based on the premise of heterosexuality. The probable disruption of the friendships, the risk, is greater than the benefit of disclosure, in her opinion.

This example illustrates the importance of assisting individuals to arrive at the best option for them at any given time, based on the information available. The coming out process is a continuous one, each relationship is different and each must be evaluated separately. Coming out does not happen all at once, if ever; it takes time and care. In the context of the nurse-patient relationship, nurses may become involved with helping lesbians to more comfortably disclose their identity and to predict the consequences of such disclosure. Nurses may find it useful to investigate community resources available to gay clients as referral or adjunctive services. The National Gay Health Education Foundation Inc., P.O. Box 834, Linden Hill, New York 11354, publishes the *National Gay Health Care Directory* which lists facilities that serve the gay community.

References

1. Price, J. H. High school students' attitudes toward homosexuality. *The Journal of School Health,* 1982, vol. 52, pp. 469–474.
2. Young, M., and Whertvine, J. Attitudes of heterosexual students toward homosexual behavior. *Psychological Reports,* 1982, vol. 51, pp. 673–674.
3. Dulaney, D. D., and Kelly, J. Improving services to gay and lesbian clients. *Social Work,* 1982, vol. 27, pp. 178–183.
4. White, T. A. Attitudes of psychiatric nurses toward same sex orientations. *Nursing Research,* 1979, vol. 28, pp. 276–281.
5. Dritz, S. K. Medical aspects of homosexuality. *New England Journal of Medicine,* 1980, vol. 302, pp. 463–464.
6. Dardick, L., and Grady, K. E. Openness between gay persons and health professionals. *Annals of Internal Medicine*, 1980, vol. 93, pp. 115–119.
7. McGhee, R. D., and Owen, W. F. Medical aspects of homosexuality. *New England Journal of Medicine,* 1980, vol. 303, pp. 50–51.
8. Johnson, S. R., Guenther, S. M., Laube, D. W., and Keettel, W. C. Factors influencing lesbian gynecologic care: A preliminary study. *American Journal of Obstetrics and Gynecology,* 1981, vol. 140, pp. 20–25.
9. Lawrence, J. C. Homosexuals, hospitalization, and the nurse. *Nursing Forum,* 1975, vol. 14, pp. 305–317.
10. Bell, A. P., and Weinberg, M. S. *Homosexualities: A Study of Diversity Among Men and Women.* New York: Simon & Schuster, 1978.
11. Council on Scientific Affairs. Health care needs of a homosexual population. *Journal of the American Medical Association,* 1982, vol. 248, pp. 736–739.
12. MacCulloch, M. J., and Waddington, J. L. Neuroendocrine mechanisms and the aetiology of male and female homosexuality. *British Journal of Psychiatry,* 1981, vol. 139, pp. 341–345.
13. Sigusch, V., Schorsch, E., Dannecker, M., and

Schmidt, G. Official statement by the German Society for Sex Research (Deutsche Gesellschaft für Sexualforschung e. V.) on the research of Prof. Dr. Günter Dörner on the subject of homosexuality. *Archives of Sexual Behavior*, 1982, vol. 11, pp. 445–449.

14. Pillard, R. C., Poumadere, J., and Carretta, R. A. Is homosexuality familial? A review, some data, and a suggestion. *Archives of Sexual Behavior,* 1981, vol. 10, pp. 465–475.

15. Siegelman, M. Parental backgrounds of homosexual and heterosexual women: A cross-national replication. *Archives of Sexual Behavior*, 1981, vol. 10, pp. 371–378.

16. Richardson, D. Lesbian identities. *In* Hart, J., and Richardson, D. *The Theory and Practice of Homosexuality*. London: Routledge & Kegan Paul, 1981.

17. Perkins, M. W. Female homosexuality and body build. *Archives of Sexual Behavior*, 1981, vol. 10, pp. 337–345.

18. Moses, A. E., and Hawkins, R. O. *Counseling Lesbian Women and Gay Men: a Life-Issues Approach*. St. Louis: C. V. Mosby, 1982.

19. Krieger, S. Lesbian identity and community: Recent social science literature. *Signs: Journal of Women in Culture and Society*, 1982, vol. 8, pp. 91–108.

20. Owen, W. F. The clinical approach to the homosexual patient. *Annals of Internal Medicine*, 1980, vol. 93, pp. 90–92.

21. Woodman, N. J., and Lenna, H. R. *Counseling with Gay Men and Women*. San Francisco: Jossey-Bass, 1980.

22. Krestan, J., and Bepko, C. S. The problem of fusion in the lesbian relationship. *Family Process*, 1980, vol. 19, pp. 277–289.

7

CHILDBEARING: ITS DILEMMAS

SHARON RISING

Sharon Rising writes of the dilemmas of childbearing. After an introduction to the issues, the decision for pregnancy is examined, followed by the choices for childbirth. The family unit, including the siblings, is reviewed. Finally, the preparation for parenting, including the necessary substantive areas for coverage, is delineated.

"Who controls a woman's body: Doctors? Lovers? Drugs? Women?" Thus reads the provocative cover of a recent addition to the growing library of books about issues of women. This book, *Vaginal Politics*, seeks to raise women's consciousness about what is possible in health care, for it is only through consumer pressure that our illness-oriented medical care system will change its focus to that of health/wellness care, treating "patients" as people and not as conditions.[1]

Perhaps in no area of human need has there been such exploitation as in the needs of women regarding their femaleness: childbearing, abortion, contraception and sterilization, rape, and gynecologic problems necessitating surgery and causing disfigurement. Women have not had the benefit of even basic information on which to base crucial decisions about their own lives or, if such knowledge was present, have had to struggle against great odds to find responsiveness in the system. There is no question that the rising tide of consumerism is a threat to the male-dominated medical care system. It is precisely this surge of activism that makes women and women's

health issues such an exciting avenue for exploration.

A chapter dealing with childbearing concerns could be endless. But the discussion in this chapter is confined primarily to an overview of the most pressing concerns surrounding childbearing, placed in a decision-making theoretic model. This is followed by an in-depth exploration of an area that has received little attention in our care systems: the preparation of parents for parenthood.

THE ISSUE

Is childbearing a crisis? How often this has been claimed—and yet studies demonstrate varied results. There are many definitions of crisis; for example, a turning point with potential for growth, a state of disease, or a state when usual behavioral patterns are inadequate and new ones are called for. The decisions surrounding childbearing certainly fall within these definitions for most women/couples. Within a family, the state of organization of the family unit at the time of the crisis is crucial. How severe or sustained that emotional disruption is for the woman and her family depends on many variables: Does she want to be pregnant? Now? Is there enough money? Now? Is there a support system? Does that system (father/couple) want to be preg-

Parts of this chapter have been revised from Rising, S. S. Preparation for Parenthood. *In* Sciarra, J. J. *Gynecology and Obstetrics.* Hagerstown, Maryland: Harper and Row, 1978.

67

nant? Now? If not, is abortion a viable option? Is adoption?

These issues probably come together most forcefully for caregivers in the pregnancy counseling situation. It is here that one sees intense joy, intense grief, and extreme ambivalence. "A baby, yes; now, no" is the ambivalence expressed by many women who struggle with issues of their autonomy, need for control, and emergence of personal essence, for having a baby is a lifetime decision, one that demands ongoing energy and investment. It is not a decision that can or should be made lightly. Whelan's book, *A Baby . . . Maybe*, clearly describes the conflicts inherent in making that decision.[2]

Women's "Coming Out"

The deluge of books directed toward and written by women is astounding. Women welcome the insights gained by sharing in them and feel the anger engendered by the truths expounded in them. Female nurses share in the corporate embarrassment over the inadequate, degrading system in which most women receive their medical care. As caregivers they also worry about the pressures that will be placed on the system of which they are a part by the response of consumers to the latest revelations. Being women and health care providers at times places them at opposite ends of the pole. That creative tension can lead to many new insights in both spheres.

The women's movement has helped women feel their personal power. As the initial surges of freedom have passed, some of the either/or dichotomy has also faded. It is now possible to talk of motherhood *and* career, marriage *and* freedom. A book entitled *Living with Contradictions: A Married Feminist* explores some of the discrepancies that are possible and resolvable for today's feminist. McBride states, "Press the button and I feel guilty about anything."[3] There is a constant pull in two directions: toward tradition and toward feminist ideology. Today's woman must learn to live with contradictions.

Coming to terms with self is essential if one is to survive healthily today. Part of that process is the recognition of one's self-worth as a person—apart from titles, occupation, or roles. It is in this context that the recognition of personal power has such meaning. As a woman comes to respect herself, she can also respect others in a way that is most powerful to the interpersonal relationship. Carl Rogers talks

of how issues are confronted openly, children are reared with respect, and each partner has freedom to pursue a life direction, make career choices, and engage in life's activities in his/her own way.[4] The emphasis for women on assertiveness has been a strong force for encouraging women to feel their power and to successfully negotiate their many relationships. Healthy avenues for the expression of anger have also demonstrated to women the validity of their anger and the ability of their significant people to respond meaningfully to that expression.

WHY THE CHANGE

One of the most monumental advances in recent years has been the development of "effective" contraception. As recently as the early 1960s some states still had not made the dispensing of birth control methods legal. As long as a woman had no control over her fertility she really had little control over the direction of her life. Even though there still is no ideal method of birth control, women do have the option of using methods with high reliability. In reviewing the field of birth control it is puzzling why more advances haven't been made in controlling male fertility. A strong hunch is that part of the reason must be due to the predominance of men in medical research leadership positions.

Women must deal with their anger over the "dumping" of responsibility for birth control. It is the woman who has had to deal with the side effects of the pill and intrauterine devices. It is the woman, primarily, who has had to deal with the emotions surrounding sterilization and abortion. It is no wonder that an increasing number of women are returning to the earlier methods of birth control: foam and condom and diaphragm, as well as the evolving natural family planning methods. And women are electing these methods partly because of the joint responsibility required.

Society and Change

Several social changes have given each woman "more options, more chance for dignity, more possibility of discovering her own self-worth."[5] Rogers has outlined the following changes:[6]

1. Greatly improved methods of contraception. As discussed above, this has had enormous impact. Years ago wives were expenda-

ble because there seemed to be no other alternative; death often came at an earlier age, the result of repeated childbearing.

2. Lengthened life span of men and women. This longer expectancy gives new significance to relationships. More effort is needed to keep pace with the ever-changing elements that affect relationships.

3. Increasing social acceptance of divorce. The increased liberalization of attitudes means that women do not necessarily have to feel bound to an undesirable marriage.

4. Family mobility. With the transiency of the family increasing, there tends to be less contact with an extended family.

5. Availability and acceptance of women working outside the home. This factor has made women more independent and has increased the potential for contact with other men.

6. Increased sexual freedom. More women are sexually experienced before entering a marriage contract. This can have a profound effect on the marriage itself.

One thing is certain. With this amount of change occurring within society, new patterns must be developed for dealing with the process of living in today's world. Old patterns aren't adequate; there are few prototypes. A woman's mother has lived a generation removed—perhaps completely removed—from the perplexing issues facing today's young woman. Only with great difficulty are values claimed and goals established.

DECISIONS

How often have we heard, "Just tell me what to do and I'll do it"? Why is it so difficult to make decisions? Clearly, the more that is at stake, the more difficult it is to make the decision. Considering the magnitude of the decisions surrounding childbearing, it is understandable that enormous ambivalence and indecision are present. It is a truism that no woman really decides to get pregnant; it just happens.

How does one make "good" decisions? There is no absolute answer, but guidelines have been developed. Janis and Mann have listed seven criteria to help ensure high-quality decisions:[7]

The decision maker, to the best of his/her ability:

1. Thoroughly canvasses a wide range of alternative courses of action.

2. Surveys the full range of objectives to be fulfilled and the values implicated by the choice.

3. Carefully weighs possible positive and negative consequences that could flow from each alternative.

4. Searches for new information relevant to further evaluation of alternatives.

5. Takes into account new information received about alternatives.

6. Re-examines positive and negative consequences of all known alternatives before making a final choice.

7. Makes detailed provisions for implementing the chosen course.

There is likely to be intense conflict whenever one must make a decision of great magnitude in the face of uncertainties. The decision is likely to be postponed. The person may experience hesitation, vacillation, and signs of acute stress, which may include apprehension, a desire to escape, and self-blame for allowing such a predicament to occur. Usually the intensity of symptoms experienced depends on the perceived magnitude of losses anticipated from the choice made. In general, it is felt that a moderate amount of stress actually leads to better decision making than either mild or severe stress. Some stress is needed to prod the person into thoughtful decision making, but too much stress may lead to panic.

When a person is faced with a decisional conflict, one with simultaneous opposing tendencies to accept or reject a given course of action, the consequence of each alternative course can be divided into four main categories:[8] (1) utilitarian gains and losses for self, (2) utilitarian gains and losses for significant others, (3) self-approval or disapproval, and (4) approval or disapproval from significant others. A very helpful tool, the balance sheet grid, has been developed by Janis and Mann to aid this process. A modification of this grid is shown in Figure 7.1.[9]

Identifying as many alternatives as possible and then carefully analyzing each, such as is required by this type of grid, will help ensure that a thoughtful decision is made. The clearer one is about the problem area the clearer the many alternatives will be. The more alternatives outlined, the less chance that the person will feel boxed in with no choices available. Probably one of our most serious problems with living today is that we fail to realize all the alternatives that are available. How often have we said, "She just seems to have her blinders on"?

TYPES OF ANTICIPATION	ALTERNATIVE COURSES OF ACTION			
Examples from Conflict with Pregnancy	Alternate 1: Continue with Pregnancy + −		Alternate 2: Terminate Pregnancy + −	
A. Gains or losses for self 1. Career 2. Income 3. Effect on health 4. Age				
B. Gains or losses for significant others 1. Prestige 2. Income 3. Family stability				
C. Self-approval or disapproval 1. Moral considerations 2. Body image, sexuality 3. Goals, aspirations 4. Self-esteem 5. Growth potential				
D. Social approval or disapproval 1. From significant other 2. From extended family 3. From close friends 4. National expectations				

Figure 7.1. Balance sheet grid for conceptualizing decisional conflict. (Adapted from Janis, I., and Mann, L. *Decision Making.* New York: Free Press, 1977.)

To further elaborate on the example used in the grid, it may be helpful to consider some of the material in Gail Sheehy's book, *Passages*.[10] Many of the conflicts in section A of the grid, "Gains and losses for self," are present in the state she describes as the Catch-30 transition. She sees that point (the transition from the 20s to the 30s) as a time of great change, turmoil, and crisis. Many who thought they knew what they wanted in their 20s find themselves tearing that up and striking out into new territory. Suddenly, they want to get married or want a child, or, if they have those, they are questioning both. Some literature has been exploring the postponement of childbearing until careers are established, the increasing number of couples who have one child or no children, the many older women who decide to be solo parents, and the large number of teenage parents who are electing to keep their children. Liberalization of the abortion option has also changed the alternative column for many women.

Sheehy also describes five life patterns of women, which have roots in history:[11]

Caregiver: woman who marries early in her 20s or before and at that time sees herself only in a domestic role.

Either-or: woman in her 20s who feels required to choose between children and love or work and accomplishment. There are two types:

Nurturer who defers achievement: postpones career but intends to pick it up later;

Achiever who defers nurturing: postpones motherhood and perhaps marriage until professional preparation is completed.

Integrator: woman who tries to combine marriage, career, and motherhood all in her 20s.

Never-married: these women include para-nurturers and office wives.

Transient: women who wander sexually, occupationally, and geographically.

There is no question that a woman's basic choices when she is in her late teens and 20s have a profound effect on her subsequent decisions regarding herself, her childbearing, and her relationships.

Decision for Pregnancy

Why do people actually decide to have babies? Many don't know, often because there really was no decision. "If you start believing that normal women have babies because they love children, you may be knee-deep in guilt before the doctor confirms you are pregnant."[12]

Many women and couples find that the satisfaction in their marriage or significant relationship is far from that romantically envisioned. They have grown farther apart and experienced communication that has become routine and shallow. Some of these couples decide that a child will fill the gap. This solution may work well for these couples throughout the childrearing years, but the crisis returns when the last child leaves home. The divorce rate among middle-aged and older couples is startling and undoubtedly is related to unresolved problems in the early relationship of the couple. Ironically, studies show that marital satisfaction is at a high before the advent of the first child, when it falls dramatically and doesn't again peak until the children have left home and married.[13]

Some women struggle with a sense of worthlessness and a lack of self-confidence. For so many years the stereotype for success included marriage and children; it was the "thing" for a woman to do. With the growing strength of the women's movement, this image has been seriously questioned. Such stereotypes are so ingrained in most individuals that they are largely unaware of their biases. Motherhood has been a sure way to say to the world, "I can produce; I am fertile; I can do what I was made to do." Children are a credential. Much of the identity of a woman with this bias is gained through identifying with her offspring. This often leads to an unhealthy relationship between mother and child, most aptly characterized by the hovering, oversolicitous mother whose children, in turn, tend to become demanding and unlikeable.

Many couples now postpone pregnancy until their relationship has matured. This provides time for husband and wife to become established in their respective careers. As the couples mature, their ability to provide a stable home increases. Many couples elect to live together for various periods before entering into a formal arrangement. There is little evidence in the literature as to the influence that the latter life style has on the ability to parent. It seems only fair to say that the more stable the relationship, the more problems and concerns the couple has had time to work out, and the more established each partner is in terms of her/his own identity, the greater the readiness of the couple to assume the tasks of parenting.

There is a well-recognized trend toward smaller families. This shift is partly in response to world overpopulation and the raising of the national and international consciousness. A decrease in population is seen as essential for survival. Also, there seems to be a change in the orientation toward family. Previously, the family was the focus for activity of its members. Children were essential for basic tasks necessary to keep the family alive. Transportation was not rapid, convenient, or readily available, and the family members relied on each other for entertainment and enrichment. Roles were clearly defined and family oriented.

Improvements in technology have led very quickly to changes in life style and to a shift in the original roles and family patterns. Making a living is considerably easier today, and there is more leisure time and money. The telephone, automobile, radio, and television promote instant communication. The movement toward urban areas has had an impact on the closeness of the family. Members have become more aware of their wants and needs, as individuals increasingly seek outside sources for gratification. A new loneliness and alienation have developed; some members have begun to look to nonfamily groups for significant relationships to fulfill basic needs.

The Human Potential Movement is extremely popular because it responds to a demonstrated need for personal growth. Glasser has described the phenomenon in terms of a major societal shift from a "civilized society" to an "identity society."[14] He sees the civilized society, existent since 10,000 B.C., as oriented toward power and security and directed by outside influences. The identity society is inwardly directed and focused on love and a sense of worth. It is more individual oriented than family oriented.

This change has led couples to re-evaluate the pattern of large families and has encouraged many to consider having no children or having only one or two. Studies show that children in smaller families tend to be more intelligent than those in large families. The ability of the parents to continue to develop their own relationship is enhanced by the fewer demands of the smaller family circle.

Many couples choose to have children because they genuinely enjoy them and want to share in their development and growth. These couples see their children as contributing to their increased appreciation of life and its wonder. They covet the privilege of sharing values and life experiences with the children. Children complete their family unit. These couples have a mature relationship and are ready to extend their personal and dual boundaries.

The Solo Parent

Many unmarried, or solo, parents struggle with parenthood. One group that continues to receive considerable attention is the adolescent pregnant girl. In 1981 there were 28,000 pregnancies in girls under 15 years of age. Of these pregnancies, 36 per cent became live births, 53 per cent were aborted, and 11 per cent ended as fetal deaths. In girls 15 to 19 years old, there were 1,103,000 pregnancies, of which 48 per cent became live births, 39 per cent were aborted, and 13 per cent ended as fetal deaths. The incidence of live births in the 10 to 14 year age group is 1.1/1000; in the 15 to 19 year age group it is 51.7/1000. Most of these pregnancies were unplanned and many of the babies unwanted. The economic demands made upon the family and the State are considerable and the disruption to the teenager's life long-lasting. Although the pregnancy and birth rates for this group have stabilized, the incidence is still a major concern.

Most younger teenagers live as part of their own nuclear family, and the baby becomes another member of that unit. When that happens, often the family becomes the parent, with responsibility for child care shared by many. It is not unusual for the grandmother to become the "mother" and raise the child as her own. Many times, though, the girl is looking for someone who will be special to her, who will provide her with the love that she has missed for herself. That parenting situation becomes even more difficult when if she is to do well at parenting she finds that she cannot "hang out" with her friends as before; this may result in considerable social isolation and depression.

The prevention of unwanted teenage pregnancy presents a challenge for our education system. It is clear that the pattern of having sex, becoming pregnant, and then considering contraceptive use is still prevalent. It is very difficult to get teenagers to plan ahead for contraceptive needs as they live almost completely in the present with little thought for the future.

Many single women are becoming parents either through their own pregnancy or by adoption. These women tend to be in their 20s and early 30s, secure in a career but wanting the experience of rearing a child. They may live in a commune to give the child exposure to men. Another special group consists of parents (or parents-to-be) who are separated, divorced, or widowed. This is a traumatic situation, especially when it occurs during pregnancy or the early postpartum period. In such cases, the relationship with the new child may be severely impaired. Solo parent groups have been formed in an attempt to give special support to those in this situation.

There is a definite difference in needs between a group of solo parents and a group of married couples. It is probably best to have single parents share together as a group to facilitate meeting their particular needs. One such group spent almost 2 hours dealing with concerns relating to their own mothers. Other concerns include dealing with society, ensuring income adequacy for basic needs, and providing positive male influence in childrearing. Group experience may be especially important for these women to give a support base and assist them in developing an assertive manner to deal with the complexities of their life.

PARENTS-TO-BE

Much of this chapter has dealt specifically with the concerns of women surrounding their own femaleness. It would be possible to discuss parenting simply in light of the woman herself, but that would be talking about a situation that is less than ideal for both the mother and the children in the family. Therefore, in the following sections, pregnancy is discussed in terms of the parents. If one of the parents is absent, the adjustments within the childbearing-childrearing experience are often much more acute, and the need for a firm support base is even more imperative.

When pregnancy occurs, parents are faced with many decisions; probably the most crucial are the steps that they must take to move themselves toward parenthood. Unfortunately, most parents have had little prior preparation for the kinds of responsibilities they must undertake when they become parents.

They may begin by reviewing their own experiences as a child with parents, including what they liked and what they wish to avoid repeating. This information should be shared because the parents often come from different backgrounds. They may consider their experiences of child care, e.g., caring for younger siblings, babysitting, or caring for children of relatives and friends. They should consider their ability to relate to children and their experience with neonates. Since infants tend to be sheltered, most people have had little experience in caring for them. If at all possible during this preparatory time, parents should have some contact with infants, preferably newborn. This will help put into perspective their images of the kind of child they will be bringing home from the hospital. If they are imagining the 6 month old Gerber baby, they may be very disappointed with their new offspring.

Together they may read some books on care of infants and share their attitudes on it. If they can begin to agree on what aspects are most important, they will begin to feel united in their movement toward parenthood. Some couples even get an animal on which to test their emotions and discipline techniques. A dog, especially, will help the parents learn some of the responsibility that comes with caring for another living being.

Perhaps the most important thing for a couple to do during pregnancy is to reassess their relationship as a couple. They should affirm activities that are important to them and that they enjoy doing together. These should be planned into their "parent schedule." They should also consider activities that are crucial to their survival as individuals. There must be continued provision for these activities in their new schedule. Contracting with each other for specific aspects of their day-to-day life may help them retain their individual identities and their relationship as a couple. Adjustments will have to be made, but they will be less threatening if provisions have been made to retain the most important aspects of the parents' individual and shared lives.

It is especially important for the woman to reaffirm her self-worth and to recognize her needs as legitimate. Otherwise, she may find herself in the trap of always responding to everyone else and neglecting her own wants and needs. After the baby comes, her wants and needs may be difficult to sort out as she responds to the many demands of her baby and family.

During this time the couple may begin looking for other couples who are also experiencing pregnancy. At one time, communities were relatively insulated from the rest of the world, and women and men shared ideas in a personal, helping way. Today we have mass media communication with essentially nonpersonal input. Also, the ease of travel and the move-ment to urban areas have contributed to a lack of community milieu for many young couples.

Alienation and lack of support can be rather frightening for a couple working through changing goals, new roles, and anxiety about labor, delivery, and parenthood. They have no background against which they can compare their dreams and fantasies and no objective sounding board.

Choices for Childbirth

How much choice should a woman/family have regarding the conduct of the childbearing experience? The demands of families on the health care system have created considerable conflict with systems and providers. Some have steadfastly refused to alter common practices; others have examined the need for "routine" procedures and have made considerable change both in environment and in practice.

Development of Alternative Birth Centers (ABCs) started in the 1970s as an in-hospital response to more homelike birth. In this more relaxed atmosphere women and families can feel a greater sense of participation and freedom in their birth experience. Across the country free-standing birth centers also have been proliferating. These centers, often staffed by nurse-midwives, perhaps provide the maximum freedom to families at low obstetric risk while providing reasonable safeguards for mother and baby. A recent study explored differences in women freely choosing in-hospital or out-of-hospital (including home) birth sites. One finding was that women who choose to deliver their babies out of the hospital tended to have a greater need for control of their own health and environment than did those choosing the hospital.[16] "Wherever rigorous scientific data to support an issue of policy or procedure are unavailable or at best controversial, then rigid application of that policy or procedure seems indefensible."[17] Within the sphere of childbearing, few practices could withstand such scrutiny.

Ironically, just when it seemed that these alternatives were strongly in place within the health care system, a major threat that threatens extinction has developed. The skyrocketing cost of malpractice insurance and the refusal of most insurance companies to insure alternative centers and certified nurse-midwives has resulted in the closing of many birth centers and has severely altered the freedom of practice of nurse-midwives. The threat to the entire profession of nurse-midwifery is clearly stated in this excerpt which appeared in the Washington Post, September 10, 1985, signed by the country's major nursing groups:

"We appeal for your urgent attention to the special plight of a vitally important segment of this country's nursing profession—and the tens of thousands of mothers and babies throughout this country who depend on them. . . .

Despite a low incidence of malpractice claims, insurance companies have made an arbitrary decision to cancel policies for nurse-midwives, refused to renew existing policies and refused to issue new policies. Professional nurse-midwives cannot practice without basic malpractice insurance. They are being denied their right to work."

This appeal, made to the members of Congress, is urgent. Given the data that have emerged on the safety and satisfaction of alternative maternity care, and its cost-effectiveness, a solution must be found. If one is not, the delivery of maternity care will become progressively more technical as care providers cover their concern for malpractice claims by using diagnostic tests and intervention procedures more frequently.

PARENTING PREPARATION

There is no question of the value of the programs presenting childbirth preparation. These programs are couple oriented and usually consist of about six sessions devoted to discussion and exercising. The topics discussed include conception and the menstrual cycle, physiologic and psychologic changes during pregnancy, stages of labor, analgesia and anesthesia, and delivery techniques. Some programs include material on breast preparation and feeding. The exercises emphasize relaxation with specific concentration techniques, as well as various types of abdominal and chest breathing.

These classes fill a void in helping couples prepare for childbirth but give them little help in adjusting to and caring for their child. Most hospitals have a series of demonstrations designed to help mothers with bathing and feeding infants as well as with birth control. Frequently, fathers are not present, and no special effort is made to include them. Follow-up studies indicate that these efforts seem to have little effect on the mother's ability to cope at home. What, then, needs to be done?

A Comprehensive Program

Most couples who are expecting are beset with many questions relating to the conduct of pregnancy, to concerns about parenthood, and

to their relationship as a couple. A formal parent preparation program starts with opportunities for group contact in both the first and second trimesters. Early in the program the parents's primary focus is not labor and delivery; this freedom provides an ideal atmosphere for promoting group cohesion and discussing issues of parenthood. Some of these issues are ambivalence of pregnancy, adjusting career to motherhood, changing sexual feelings, the couple's binding into the pregnancy, and anxieties about competence as a parent.

These groups should be small (four to six couples) and should be relatively unstructured to allow for a sharing of joys and concerns by the group members. The leader should be viewed as a facilitator rather than as a lecturer or teacher. Occasionally, resource people in family life education might be used to advantage. Phone numbers may be exchanged to facilitate continuing informal contact by group members. These contacts may help establish the couple's support base, which will be invaluable during the early stages of childrearing. Parenthood is much more difficult when faced alone.

The third trimester is usually the period for intense concentration on preparation for labor and delivery. Attendance at some formal series of classes should be strongly encouraged. Besides presenting information and providing an opportunity for learning relaxation and breathing methods, these classes should emphasize the couple's innate resources for dealing with labor, delivery, and early parenting. A couple should also be helped to develop realistic expectations for their birth experience, for subsequent satisfaction depends greatly on how closely these expectations were met.

Sibling Preparation

The preparation of older children for the arrival of a sibling is also an issue for many families. Some children are participating in the actual birth experience, others in the immediate postpartum bonding time. All siblings need to adjust and respond to the new child.

A variety of experiences can be planned to help the child feel included in the childbearing process. Attendance at prenatal visits can be encouraged with opportunity given for the child to listen to fetal heart tones, to palpate the enlarging uterus, and to ask questions. Many books prepared for children are available to assist the child with understanding the complex of feelings he or she may be having. Dolls may also assist the professional, parent, and child with comprehension of the birth process and early child care. Through repeated play with these dolls the child can become familiar with the birth process. Tours of the birth place are important for visualization and role playing. Movies, slides, and video tapes all help the child have a greater appreciation for the beauty and intensity of the whole event.

If the family is planning for the child to attend the birth, additional formal and informal preparation is needed. This should cover such areas as sounds, smells, episiotomy, blood, placenta, appearance of the newborn infant, and potential problems. A caring, prepared adult should always be present with and for the child.

THE NEW FAMILY UNIT

One day, with the onset of labor, the anticipation of having a new child clearly becomes reality. Besides feeling the concern for safety that they have related to labor, the couple realize that the reality of the newborn infant is soon to be on them. As the mother goes through labor she is also laboring psychologically to achieve a proper relationship with a new, nonparasitic person. It is not a simple jump from being pregnant, to having delivered, to needing to start nurturing a new being. In fact, if labor progresses too rapidly the mother may find that she has not done the necessary psychologic work of labor prior to delivery and may have to take considerable time after delivery to work through the process of delivering.

If it is a first child, the couple have not had to widen their circle to consider another dependent being. They still may be trying to determine who they are as a couple. The younger they are, the more probable it is that they are still working through self-identity. If this is their second or later pregnancy, they may be coping with such questions as, "Can we afford another?" "Do we have enough love, enough time, and enough of ourselves to give?" "Have we prepared our children adequately?" Feelings of confidence and self-doubt, anxiety, and excited anticipation race through them at the time of birth.

Integration within a family involves an understanding and a melding of all characteristics into a whole—perhaps not always a harmonious whole but one that is unique. Each member contributes unique characteristics to the larger unit, i.e., the family image. There is a certain openness during the first hour or two after delivery that may never occur again during the postpartum period. The mother tends to be very alert and almost oversensitive, and the baby, if she/he is not medicated, is usually crying and sucking in response to stimuli. This is a crucial time for all members of the triad to begin to get familiar with each other. Barring any unusual problems the baby should be kept with the parents, if they desire, and should be kept warm, preferably under the covers next to the mother's body. There the child is more likely to be content and to enjoy a continuation of the contact stimulation felt in utero.[18]

Siblings

As the couples have focused more on claiming childbirth as "their" experience, many have expressed a desire to have older siblings present during or immediately following the birth. This desire is motivated by several concerns: inclusion of the child as part of the total family unit, understanding of and knowledge for the child about birth, desire of child(ren) to participate, and congruence with family life style. Some birthing units have made an attempt to respond to this need by loosening policies, restructuring physical space, and developing educational programs. One such program provides parents with at least two opportunities for group discussion focused on ways to include children in the childbearing experience, parents' reasons for wanting their child to share the birth experience, and possible responses of the child to the birth experience.[19]

More research is needed to evaluate the effect on a sibling of being present at birth; in the meantime, families in increasing numbers are seeking facilities that will respond to this need. A recent study examined the impact on parents of having siblings present at birth. Three recurrent themes were reported by the 32 parents: (1) The family would choose again to have their children present at birth, (2) their presence added to a feeling of family unity, (3) their presence was viewed as a small part of the larger positive feelings about the birth experience.[19a] It can be hypothesized that the more included a sibling feels in the childbearing process, the less difficult it will be to accept a new child into the family. It also follows that the family itself should experience greater ease in redefining its image.

The Baby Is Born

A variety of behaviors is displayed by couples during these first few minutes. It is important that they have time with each other and the child. Claiming behavior is common to all animals and is essential if subsequent attachment is to occur. This early encounter forms the basis for their subsequent interactions and is critical in setting the tone. A father who is encouraged and becomes involved at this point is much less likely to feel like an outsider than a father who is excluded from any meaningful participation with his wife and new child.

During this early postpartum period, it is crucial that the couple identify their needs as clearly as possible. Studies have shown that a mother is not really ready to care for her infant until her needs for restoration have been met. The mother and father must be clearly attuned to the needs of each other or these needs will be overlooked in trying to meet the demands of their infant. One good practice is to go out together as a couple, perhaps for a meal, before leaving the hospital. If the couple has left the birthing place early, a delightful substitute might be for another couple to come over and assume the responsibilities for child care, thus freeing the new parents to enjoy some time alone. Support from professionals adds legitimacy to their needs as individuals and as a couple.

Postpartum Period

The first few weeks at home with the new baby are critical. The mother is tired and probably overwhelmed with her new responsibilities. If she is breastfeeding, she may wonder whether the baby is getting enough milk. What can be done if the baby has cried for half an hour and she has tried everything to quiet the child, or when she has been up for the fifth time in the night and may be tempted to abandon the demanding infant? When the father goes back to work, the mother often feels trapped at home and tries to rationalize her feelings of ambivalence. She may be experiencing an abrupt change from a very active work or career life to a life of domesticity. She may miss her old contacts and her old sense of achievement and may begin to wonder why she decided to have a child. She must be helped to see her achievement in her new mothering role.

When siblings are present in the family, the mother's adjustment is compounded by the need to respond to the varied demands presented by older children. These children often revert to more infantile behavior, which may intensify the mother's guilt at having to divide the time she has available. One recent study demonstrated that 92 percent of the children showed an increase of at least one problem after their mother's hospitalization.[20] Negative behaviors are frustrating to all in the family and are especially difficult to respond to when they occur at important interaction times with the baby, such as nursing. It is also much harder for a mother to take short daytime naps as she may use times when the baby is asleep to have quality time with her other children. The father often is a critical force in providing additional parenting time.

The mother must receive positive, nuturing input during this period to be able to give to the new baby and to her family. She may feel that everything is going out of her: the baby, the placenta, the lochial flow, her breast milk, her tears. She must have replacement of that output through love, care, affirmation, understanding, and encouragement. Physically and psychologically her body is experiencing emormous changes. There is no organ that even begins to match the outstanding involutional feat of the uterus, which shrinks 1000 grams in a period of only 6 weeks.

Support Group Concept

Human beings are social beings. Much of their lifetime is spent in interaction. One of the primary reasons for marriage and family life is to provide an opportunity for close sharing and support. However, neither a husband nor a wife can totally meet the needs of the other. Contact with a larger group is vital to a couple's relationship and to the health of each individual.

Gendlin has made some predictions relating to continued development of interaction. He believes that individals must be encouraged to focus on their own experience as the most honest, valid way of coping with life. He believes that in the future, children will be taught in school how to listen and to share meaningfully with each other. Ordinary people must be taught how to provide a therapeutic process for each other. He sees the need for social programs that build opportunity for intimate human interaction. In addition, he believes that one cannot effectively deal with only one part of a person; he or she is a total being that needs to be viewed in the entire life situation.[21]

A support group concept is employed at the University of Minnesota. A group of couples whose babies are due within the same month meets together weekly to share feelings and concerns about childbearing and parenthood.

The groups are formed 4 to 6 weeks before due dates; ideally, they will have met together occasionally since the first trimester.

These weekly meetings provide couples with an organized opportunity to discuss questions with a professional and also to gain considerable support from other group members struggling with similar concerns. Topics usually explored include dreams, concerns about death, continuance of the relationship of the couple, separation from the baby, coping with grandparents, division of household/baby responsibilities, resumption of career by the mother, and managing early labor. As soon as some couples become parents, they give a full report to the group; some have given reports on the same day as delivery. Besides giving the waiting couples firsthand data with which to compare their images, this approach gives the couple whose baby has arrived an opportunity to begin analyzing their own experience, which is essential to their successful progression as parents.

As couples in the group move beyond the childbearing event, the concerns begin to center on early childrearing, breast and bottle feeding, handling of crying, getting out of the house, and coping with fatigue. Babies are brought to the group sessions, and couples have an opportunity to watch each other handle crying infants and perform feeding and cleansing routines. It seems especially helpful to fathers to watch other fathers engaged in these activities. New parents of the group also have the satisfaction of seeing their own baby claimed by a larger community; this is a very important affirmation.

Participation in support groups should continue for at least 2 months after delivery. Many studies show that the new family is more crisis prone during these early months. It is wise to have co-group leadership that includes someone knowledgeable in childrearing. In our institution, leadership is usually shared by a nurse-midwife and a pediatric nurse practitioner, both of whom have had special preparation in group facilitation. Experienced parents can also add an important dimension to these groups.

A study was done of couples' perceptions of the support received while participating in one of these groups. These data included a listing of the following components of support: the opportunity to share experiences with group members, receiving assistance and information from group members, receiving positive feedback and pleasant attitudes and feelings, and-

sharing problems and feelings with other group members.[22]

A formal format for early childrearing classes could include a variety of topics dealing with caretaking activities of the neonate, mother-father relationship issues, changing roles, babysitters, and infant stimulation. Several excellent media resources are available that could supplement content presentation.

ACHIEVING PERSPECTIVE

Is the advent of the first child really a crisis for the family? Studies vary in their findings but clearly show that it is a crisis for many families. Le Masters interviewed 46 married, middle-class, well-educated couples. Eighty-three percent of the couples indicated "extensive" or "severe" crisis in adjusting to the first child. Among these couples, 92 percent of the pregnancies were either "planned" or "desired." One of the strongest findings was that these couples seemed to have completely romanticized pregnancy.[23]

In another study conducted by Dyer, couples indicating "extensive" and "severe" crisis totaled 53 percent, but a definite correlation was found with strength of family organization. Mothers and fathers were asked about their experiences, problems, and reactions in adjusting to their first child. Mothers responded as follows:[24]

Tiredness and exhaustion	87%
Loss of sleep	87%
Feelings of neglecting husband	67%
Feelings of inadequacy	58%
Inability to keep up with housework	35%
Difficulty in adjusting to being tied down at home and curtailing outside activities	35%

Fathers reported as follows:

Loss of sleep	50%
Adjustment to new responsibilities and routines	50%
Upset schedules and daily routines	50%
Ignorance of great amount of time and work required	—
Financial worries	—

Tremendous adjustments must be made by new parents; it is hoped that an increasing number will have the opportunity for more extensive preparation for their new role.

Recently, a workshop entitled "Parenthood: Full or Flat" was held. The response to the

Dimension	TIME SPENT (%)		WAY TIME SPENT (%)			EVALUATION	
	Now	Desired	Alone	With Significant Other	With Friends	Feels Okay	Needs Change
Sexual							
Intellectual							
Emotional							
Social							
Cultural							
Spiritual							
Recreational							
Vocational							
Family							

(Total time available in a week: 100 hours)

Figure 7.2. Dimensions of intimacy. (Adapted from Clinebell, H., and Clinebell, C. *The Intimate Marriage*. New York: Harper and Row, 1970.)

title was interesting. Did it mean pregnant and then delivered? Did it mean a house full of children and then an empty nest with all having left home? It could have meant either, but the focus was on how to make parenting a full, enriching experience rather than a flat, depressing one. Part of the key probably is to make good prepregnancy counseling available to couples who want to better understand the meaning of parenthood for them. This seems to be one of the best ways out of the loneliness and alienation that is felt by much of our society. Our sense of ourselves is best experienced through meaningful relationships with others: "We cannot be living, amusing, exciting, generous, forgiving, in isolation. Only the potential exists until there is someone present to be loved, to be amused, to be excited, to be grateful, to be forgiven. It is the response which this intimate other makes to us that validates our self-image."[25]

One tool that has been used to help individuals and couples focus on their needs for intimacy has the structure shown in Figure 7.2.

Included in the tool are dimensions of life in which each of us experiences interest and need. In some we may desire more intimacy than in others. Each person is encouraged to think about his/her needs in each area and to mark the approximate percentage of time currently spent in each area and the percentage of time desired. The next step focuses on how the person would like to spend that time—that is, alone, with significant others, or with friends. An additional step looks at whether the person judges the dimension overall to "feel okay" or whether it "needs work." This

exercise should help individuals and couples sort out where they are and where they would like to go.

Another mechanism is for the significant unit to participate periodically in enrichment groups: marriage, family, sex-related, sexuality. These programs are oriented toward "growth rather than problems . . . development rather than symptom relief."[27] These groups have a preventive approach and seek to stimulate insight and communication.

CONCLUSION

The factors to weigh, the decisions to make, and the dilemmas to resolve all contribute to the complexity and stress of the childbearing issue for women today. There are many, and they are difficult to resolve. Our changing society has provided a dynamic climate in which to live. But the pace is almost breathtaking. When is there time to engage in thoughtful decision making? Who has time to listen and reflect? Where are those caring people who are needed for the support base so essential for survival today?

It is not only possible but important for self-fulfillment to approach living intentionally by taking control of life rather than letting it be in control. This intentionality has several characteristics:

1. Valuing yourself, developing self-esteem through quality interpersonal relationships, acknowledging differing wants and needs
2. Taking charge of your own destiny
3. Consciously balancing expectations of society with your own wants, needs, and values

4. Deciding your future by setting goals, setting strategy, looking ahead, and being accountable

5. Acting in a proactive, rather than reactive, fashion

6. Constantly reflecting on your experience, and repeating the cycle

As women become clearer about their needs and are therefore better able to articulate them, there may be a surprising response from other women and from men. Slowly there is a response building to some of these needs: daycare facilities, pregnancy benefits, part-time benefits, the Equal Rights Amendment, and equal pay for equal work. As women find other opportunities both available and satisfying there may not be as great a need to have a baby because it is "the thing to do" or "the only way to achieve some status." And for those women who do decide to have children, it need not be such a stressful experience; in fact, it can be an exciting and rewarding one.

References

1. Frankfort, Ellen. *Vaginal Politics*. New York: Bantam Books, 1972.
2. Whelan, E. M. *A Baby . . . Maybe*. New York: Bobbs-Merrill Company, 1975.
3. McBride, A. B. *Living with Contradictions: A Married Feminist*. New York: Harper and Row, 1976.
4. Rogers, Carl. *On Personal Power*. New York: Delacorte Press, 1977.
5. Rogers, Carl, ibid., p. 45.
6. Rogers, Carl, ibid., pp. 43–44.
7. Janis, J., and Mann, L. *Decision Making*. New York: Free Press, 1977.
8. Janis, J., and Mann, L., ibid., p. 137.
9. Janis, J., and Mann, L., ibid., p. 138.
10. Sheehy, Gail. *Passages*. New York: E. P. Dutton & Company, 1974.
11. Sheehy, Gail, ibid., p. 242.
12. McBride, A. B. *The Growth and Development of Mothers*. New York: Harper and Row, 1973.
13. Campbell, A. American way of mating: Marriage si, children only maybe. *Psychology Today*, May 1975, pp. 37–43.
14. Glasser, W. *The Identity Society*. New York: Harper and Row, 1972.
15. Birth Rate for Teens Soaring, Alarming. Minneapolis Tribune Section B, September 25, 1977, p. 3.
16. Fullerton, Judith. The choice of in-hospital or alternative birth environment as related to the concept of control. *Journal of Nurse-Midwifery*, vol. 27, March/April 1982, pp. 17–22.
17. Fullerton, Judith, ibid., p. 22.
18. Rising, S. S. Fourth stage of labor: Family integration. *American Journal of Nursing*, May 1974, pp. 870–874.
19. Daniels, Mary. The birth experience for the sibling. *Journal of Nurse-Midwifery*, vol. 28, Sept./Oct. 1983, pp. 15–22.
19a. Krutsky, Christina. Siblings at birth: Impact on parents. *Journal of Nurse-Widwifery*, vol. 30, Sept./Oct. 1985, p. 269.
20. Trause, Mary, et al. Separation for childbirth: The effect on the sibling. *Child Psychiatry and Human Development*, vol. 12, Fall 1981, pp. 32–39.
21. Gendlin, E. T. A short summary and some long predictions. *In* Hart, J. T., and Tomlinson, J. M. (eds.). *New Directions in Client-Centered Therapy*. Boston: Houghton-Mifflin, 1970.
22. Lindquist, K., and Meyer, M. Childbearing and child-rearing support group: Verbal interaction and support. Plan B Paper, University of Minnesota, 1976.
23. Le Masters, E. E. Parenthood as crisis. *In* Parad, H. J. (ed.). *Crisis Intervention*. New York: Family Service Association of America, 1965, pp. 111–117.
24. Dyer, E. Parenthood as crisis: A re-study. *In* Parad, H. J. (ed.). *Crisis Intervention*. New York: Family Service Association of America, 1965, pp. 312–323.
25. Fullerton, G. P. *Survival in Marriage*. New York: Holt, Rinehart and Winston, 1972.
26. Clinebell H., and Clinebell, C. *The Intimate Marriage*. New York: Harper and Row, 1970.
27. Fowler, R,, and Schultz, D. Total family enrichment: A systems approach. *Theological Markings 5*, Winter 1975, pp. 31–37.

COMMUNICATION PATTERNS OF WOMEN AND NURSES

MARIE LELAND MENIKHEIM
MIRIAM WATKINS MEYERS

This chapter by Marie Menikheim and Miriam Meyers begins with identification of the societal status and communication patterns and then proceeds to identify the communication patterns of men and women in stress and conflict. The chapter closes with suggestions for change in communication patterns.

INFLUENCE OF SOCIETAL STATUS ON COMMUNICATION PATTERNS

Positions that individuals occupy in society are sociologically defined as social statuses. Status provides a basis for social identity. Each status has rights, obligations, and prestige, which constitute a social role. A social role is the pattern of behaviors expected with a particular status position in society.[1]

A social role is attached to sex status, just as roles are attached to all positions in society. Sex status is considered an "ascribed status," along with race and age.[2] This type of status is assigned at birth and is independent of skill, effort, and ability. Nonetheless, virtually every society has formed a complex set of explicit and implicit rules for proper behavior based on sex differences. Different cultural expectations for male and female social roles are taught and reinforced from birth.

This socialization determines in large part identity development and sex concept. In general, socialization is considered training for a social environment or culture.[3] Brim more specifically defines socialization as "the process by which individuals acquire the knowledge, skills and dispositions that enable them to participate as more or less effective members of groups and society."[4]

Socialization is a reciprocal process. Culture provides the framework of societal standards. As the individual learns and demonstrates appropriate behaviors consistent with societal standards, the framework is strengthened. The individual, in turn, is rewarded for behavior that conforms to these societal standards.

Infants are given behavioral reinforcement consistently for appropriate behavior. Parents treat infant boys and girls differently as they talk to them, play with them, and handle them. Youngsters observe their parents and other adults, imagining themselves in the role of the adult. Children learn to differentiate between men and women and identify a sex role preference. Schooling, peer groups, and various media further influence sex role formation. Children then begin to live out sex role behavior, ultimately internalizing it.

The sex status ascribed to men continues to be superior to the sex status ascribed to women in American society. Men and masculine characteristics are more highly valued. Even as young children, boys prefer their social role to that of girls. Some girls wish they were boys.[5]

Culturally determined social roles based on unequal sex status determine in large part the interaction patterns between men and women in American society. The value system and behavior are interactive. Communication patterns reflect this paternalistic orientation with its authority/subordinate parameters.

Communication patterns also reflect sex role stereotypes, i.e., consensual beliefs about the different characteristics of men and women. Broverman et al. found that stereotypes continue to be persistent and pervasive in American society. Female traits are regarded as less socially desirable than male traits and less mentally healthy.[6] Table 8.1 identifies current stereotypic behaviors based on sex role as described by Broverman et al.[7] and Bardwick and Donavan.[8]

Despite the apparently higher value placed on maleness, American society proclaims equality for both sexes. Consequently, there is conflict between the ideal of sexual equality and the reality of sexual equality. Although men and women are told they are equals, the American system does not provide equal reinforcement or support for women's advancement. The values and norms revolving about the social role related to sex status for women are contradictory and ambiguous. Behaviors appropriate to the feminine stereotype may be incompatible with behaviors appropriate to equality.

Communication patterns between men and women reflect this conflict in roles. As the inconsistencies in role increase, communication patterns reflect the stress of the role conflict.

Individuals occupy several statuses in society at one time. Thus far, this chapter has discussed sex status, an ascribed status in American society. Individuals also occupy statuses that are classified as achieved. "Achieved statuses" are not assigned at birth; they are chosen and earned. Special educational preparation may be necessary for their attainment. The statuses of wife, mother, and nurse are achieved. As the statuses occupied by a person multiply, the roles associated with them often contradict each other. Communication patterns of women that conflict between ascribed (sex) and achieved (wife, mother, and nurse) roles are uncertain and often unclear. The communication style is futher influenced by this additional conflict.

Communication patterns are further affected by the institutional inconsistencies relative to equality. In American society attributes associated with leadership in organizations are considered masculine. Attributes associated with most professional roles are also considered masculine. The behaviors associated with the role of a professional woman and those appropriate to the social role of the female in society can be mutually exclusive, further complicating woman's concept of herself.

The further women move from stereotypical behaviors associated with sex status, the more conflict occurs in their communication patterns with others.

SEX-RELATED COMMUNICATION PATTERNS

Patterns that reflect male and female roles have been found in language. The linguist assumes that there is a system in the language and that data gathered from it can be analyzed and described. Though linguists (and other communication researchers) vary in how they view the implications of their findings about language, many subscribe to the views of Sapir and Whorf, whose widely discussed linguistic relativity theory argues that structure not only reflects culture but shapes reality by predisposing language users to think in habitual patterns.[9]

The English language has been said to reinforce male dominance and female subordination. In a classic work, Otto Jespersen described English as the "most positively and expressly masculine" of languages.[10]

The Bible regards Eve as merely an offshoot from Adam's rib—and English follows suit by the use of many Adam's rib words. The scientific name for both sexes of our species is the word for only one of them, *Homo,* "man" in Latin; our species is also referred to as *human* (derived from Homo) or *mankind,* two other words which similarly serve to make women invisible. The average person is always

Table 8.1. **Stereotypical Characteristics of Men and Women**

Men	Women
independent	dependent, passive, fragile
aggressive	nonaggressive
competitive	noncompetitive
task-oriented	interpersonally oriented
outwardly oriented	inner-oriented
assertive	passive
self-disciplined	other-disciplined
stoic	empathic
objective	subjective
innovative	conforming
analytic-minded	intuitive
unsentimental	sensitive

(Adapted from Broverman, I. K., et al. Sex-role stereotypes: A current appraisal. *Journal of Social Issues,* vol. 28, 1972, pp. 59–78; and Bardwick, T., and Donavan, G. Ambivalence: The socialization of women. *In* Gornick, V., and Moran, B. K. (eds). *Women in Sexist Society.* New York: Basic Books, 1971, pp. 225–241.)

masculine (as in "the man in the street") and so is the hypothetical person in riddles and in examination questions (If a man can walk ten miles in seven minutes, how many miles can he walk in twelve minutes?).[11]

Male identity is considered the norm. It is men, until recently, who virtually always retained their name in marriage. It is men who represent the nation, the race. Consider "Four score and seven years ago our *fathers* brought forth upon this continent a new nation, conceived in liberty and dedicated to the proposition that all *men* are created equal" (italics added). Some analysts have found that such masculine forms, while purportedly inclusive of all human beings, are interpreted by both speaker and addressee as referring to males only.[12]

Miller and Swift found words associated with masculinity and femininity reflecting the stereotypic bias.[13] *Sissy*, from the word *sister*, indicates timidity, whereas *buddy*, from *brother*, indicates friendship or closeness. Lakoff noted, in comparing word pairs such as *bachelor:spinster* and *master:mistress*, that the feminine member carries negative connotations.[14] Furthermore, male identity is associated with high-ranking job categories. Though the masculine forms *he, his,* and *him* have been prescribed as "generic" pronouns, research has shown that the personal pronoun *he* is applied to physicians and lawyers, whereas *she* is applied to elementary school teachers, nurses, and secretaries.[15] This linguistic sexism permeates everyday activity, influencing the thought and communication patterns of even small children.

In addition to patterns within the language itself, researchers have investigated patterns of sex-linked language *use*. We know that people hold strong opinions about the language of men and women. Kramer's study of young people in Illinois showed that they believe women are friendlier, gentler, more emotional, more grammatically correct, and more enthusiastic than men when they speak, whereas men are believed to be louder, more forceful, dominating, boastful, authoritarian, blunt, and straight to the point as speakers. Kramer summarized their view of women's speech as "kind, correct, but unimportant."[16] Edelsky has shown, furthermore, that a language/sex of speaker stereotype is firmly established in children by the time they reach sixth grade.[17] Chaika argues that the crucial difference in such perceptions of women's and men's speech is one of *potency*.[18]

It is surprising that scholars have been among those offering assertions about female speech with little evidence to support them. Jespersen alleged that women talk more, and faster, than men.[19] More recently, Lakoff set off a flurry of research by claiming that women use "empty adjectives" (such as *divine, charming*), use tag questions that tend to weaken their own authority ("That was a good meeting, wasn't it?"), use question intonation on statements, are more concerned about politeness than about content, and "hedge" when they speak.[20] Few of Lakoff's claims have been corroborated by the research they sparked. Indeed, superior/subordinate status (or "power") has been found to be more important a determinant of so-called "women's language" than sex.[21]

Differences in female and male communication, which have been substantiated and which have bearing on this discussion, are that men interrupt women overwhelmingly more than women interrupt men;[22] that women ask more questions and introduce more topics than men whereas men make statements and introduce the topics that get discussed;[23] and that women speak a more socially "correct" variety of language than men of their social group.[24] Some investigators have found that women use tag questions on statements about their own ideas and feelings, robbing their speech of confidence and power.[25] With regard to topics of conversation, men show greater interest in action, movement, and doing, whereas women focus more on feelings and expressions.[26] Baird found that studies of sex differences in verbal interaction patterns in groups (1950–1975) generated results that parallel sex role expectations;[27] Table 8.2 illustrates identified differences in interaction patterns.

Table 8.2. **Differences in Interaction Patterns Between Men and Women in Group Communication**

Men	Women
initiate interaction	respond to interaction
give more information	express warmth, helpfulness
are task/goal oriented	are socially oriented
use more words	participate less as men talk
talk more often	more
interrupt more often	withdraw from unpleasant interaction
demonstrate positive attitudes	communicate negative attitudes
are objective	are opinionated

(Adapted from Baird, J. E. Sex differences in group communication: A review of relevant research. *Quarterly Journal of Speech*, vol. 62, April 1976, pp. 179–192.)

This chapter has focused thus far on communication patterns of women in relation to men as determined by position in society (status) and socialization into role. The marginality of women is reflected in the dominant "maleness" of the language. The subordination of women to men is further exemplified in society's expectations of the ways in which women should speak and the ways in which women are spoken to. One of the most consistent findings produced by studies of sex differences in communication is that women tend to conform more to group norms than do men.[28] Frost reported that female college students try to avoid confrontation in conflict situations, whereas male college students try to assert themselves. Women's conformity is maximized in mixed groups, in which they often express concern about disagreements and wish to maintain good personal relationships.[29] As women conform to fulfill societal role expectations, their behavior is reinforced and societal values are strengthened.

COMMUNICATION PATTERNS INDICATING STRESS AND CONFLICT

Many women today are dissatisfied with their sex status in society. The implicit programming of sex stereotypic roles through socialization is being questioned. The conservative model of sex role evolution, which adheres rigidly to male dominance based on survival needs, is being disputed. Cross-cultural studies indicate that a variety of sex roles is appropriate, thereby challenging basic assumptions about what is "right" and "natural" for men and women in American society. Maccoby and Jacklen indicate that many of the popular beliefs about the psychologic characteristics of the two sexes have little or no basis in fact.[30]

New, alternative models have been proposed that focus on differential access of men and women to scarce resources and commodities as determinants of sex role. Men have greater access to means of production, ownership, and control.[31]

Many women wish to change the social role associated with their sex status in society. There is, however, great pressure on women from society to conform to the norms. As differences in values and beliefs are expressed, conflict results. A conflict exists whenever incompatible activities occur together.[32] Communication patterns in conflict often represent exaggerated forms of day-to-day communication styles. Women under stress may respond to conflict helplessly. Out of fear of the au-

thority figure, a woman may hesitate and respond apologetically for her position. She may express behaviors considered "childlike." These behaviors, which may include pouting and crying, may have been dependent responses to conflict during childhood.

The polarized response of power is also seen. As women learn that control is established through authoritarian means, they may unconsciously copy this behavior during "conflict." Aggressiveness is also seen in women acting out in rage against society. Aggression may be indirect or passive. Women respond to conflict with confusing communication. There are incongruences between verbal and nonverbal patterns. Women may use qualifying statements such as those beginning with "yes, but" or "it depends." Women who are unable to express anger in conflict may feel guilt. Women who are dissatisfied may suppress their anger, misplacing it and thereby punishing themselves.[33]

NURSING AS AN OCCUPATIONAL ROLE REFLECTING FEMALE SEX STATUS AND COMMUNICATION STYLE

Nursing is said to be a profession that supports the sex status of women in American society. Nursing has come to be viewed as an extension of the sex role. Mauksch studied personality traits common to nurses before, during, and after educational preparation.[34] Generally, the nurse was found to be an individual who genuinely wants to help people, who is very conscious of what others think of her, and who is compliant. The nurse is fearful of making mistakes. This fear manifests itself in what Mauksch describes as "blame avoidance." Blame avoidance is characterized by a fear of being wrong which is so strong that the person can *never* be responsible for a wrong act; the individual *always* has to be right. There is an extreme desire to be safe and correct.

The authority/subordinate relationship between physicians and nurses reinforces the male/female societal role. Society sees the physician role as most important. The doctor's influence, even control, can be seen in the Nightingale Pledge and the Nurse Practice Act. Duberman discusses nursing as a sex-stereotyped occupation along with elementary school teaching, social work, and librarianship.[35] Like men and women, occupations hold status, and nursing has consistently been labeled as inferior to medicine.

Some studies indicated means by which

these status inequalities are communicated. Goffmann discusses interaction rituals associated with status. "Doctors had the right to saunter into the nurses' station, lounge on the station's dispensing counter, and engage in joking with other nurses. Other ranks participated in this informal interaction with doctors, but only doctors had initiated it."[36] Between persons of equal status, interactions are guided by symmetric familiarity. Some evidence indicates that conversational interaction between male and female doctors, for example, shows a more symmetric pattern.[37] In interactions occurring between persons of unequal status such as doctors and nurses, on the other hand, the relations are asymmetric.

Acquiescence with paternalism, self-sacrifice, and self-dedication are qualities Leininger identifies with nursing. Traditionally, nurses have been socialized to be quiet and humble in the presence of father-like authority figures, and their behavior revealed signs of respect, attention, and reverence to them.[38]

The phrase "doctor's orders" says a great deal about the type of communication patterns that exist. Consider the following anecdote in which a nurse noted that a male physician prescribed Librium for a patient. After thanking the doctor for the drug orders, the nurse commented, "Oh Doctor, I forgot to tell you that the night nurse reported that Mrs. M. was nauseated after each Librium. Did you want to write a new order?"

"Yes thanks, Trudy, I did want to change the order."[39]

This doctor-nurse game situation reflects how a nurse can indirectly demonstrate knowledge without threatening the physician's authority. According to Hoekelman, the most important rule of the game is that open disagreement between the players must be avoided at all costs.[40] How distant are these communication patterns from those of the wife who informs her husband of the need to buy a washer for the sink after identifying a dripping faucet or of the secretary who validates with her boss that contracts are to be countersigned? The nurse protects the physician as the wife cares for her husband and as the secretary cares for her boss.

Nurses also relate to nursing leaders as authorities. Historically, a nurse responded to a nurse educator, nurse supervisor, or nurse director as she did to a physician/administrator. Seldom did a nurse question the decision of a nurse leader since the leader has been perceived as possessing great intelligence and knowledge.

This model of authority continues as Yura, Ozimek, and Walsh identify the strong authoritarianism that characterizes nursing service today: "Authoritarianism is a vestige of the developments of nursing from the military hospital model. . . . Militarism is a curse upon nursing that endures."[41]

This authoritarian frame is also visible in communication patterns among nurses. The behaviors that relate to the need to be correct in situations are often present in conflict situations. For example, often a great deal of time is spent by nurse faculty members in criticizing and fault finding, even scapegoating, among themselves. In attempting to do the best for clients, patients, and students in communities, hospitals, and colleges, nurses often negate one another and themselves.

Finally, patterns of communication between nurses and patients reflect this authority/subordinate role. The care recipient has been a passive, dependent model. It has been relatively easy for nurses, having been conditioned as women, to relate to that passive model and to discourage independence and autonomy in clients.[42] The nurse often evades direct questions from the patient. There is often a compulsory pretense regarding the patient's condition. This communication style indirectly negates the nurse's understanding of the patient's condition from the patient's perspective. It encourages the patient to seek answers from the doctor. Like the tag-question discussed earlier, it negates commitment on the part of the speaker, in this case the nurse. This can have a profound effect on the patient as well as the nurse. In a recent study,[43] 261 medical-surgical patients ranked 49 events related to the experience of hospitalization from most to least stressful. Important stressful events as expressed by the patients were related to a lack of communication of information by the nurse or a lack of communication in a meaningful way.[44]

Just as women in American society are questioning their position in the culture, so nurses are questioning the highly authoritarian behavior of physicians and nurses in the leadership positions of their profession. Conflicts are coming into being as the concepts of authority are challenged. Nurses may be inclined to respond to conflicts either submissively or aggressively, unless they know how to respond more appropriately.

ALTERNATIVE COMMUNICATION PATTERNS: STRATEGIES FOR CHANGE

A need exists for women to recognize that a constraining image has been accepted and internalized in learning to be women in our society. Once this is recognized, old roles can be unlearned and new roles accepted. As the underlying assumptions that influence sex role behavior continue to be exposed as myths rather than realities, the social role can be identified. Relearning will gradually occur. Attitudes will slowly change.

A communication pattern that reflects such a change is the movement from the statement "There is nothing to be done about the situation" to the question: "What can be done about the situation?" The question is then rephrased as a statement: "This is what can be done about the situation."

The process of developing new communication patterns can be awkward, even painful. Old ways are predictable and comfortable to everyone. Motivation for change develops within oneself. Although the steps to change may appear complex and strange, they may not be as difficult as they seem.

Change can be as simple as a practical relaxation exercise. For example, once an individual recognizes feeling tense in a communication and begins to feel helpless, the person can consciously tell herself or himself to relax, take a deep breath and hold it for 5 seconds, and then let the breath out slowly. As the muscles are relaxed the breath is released deliberately. Conversation can be continued. Nine times out of ten no one even notices the silence or if they do they will more than likely attribute it to interest in the conversation.

Since the 1970s the need for changes in communication patterns has been reinforced by consciousness-raising groups. These groups help women increase their awareness of their sex role in society. What is unconscious becomes conscious as common experiences are shared. This new insight often causes emotional responses in the member. Feelings of anger, frustration, sadness, fear, and even rage are not uncommon. Once the person recognizes the discrepancy between the real and the assumptive world there is strong incentive to change.

Many present psychosocial theories encourage relearning of communication patterns. Approaches toward more egalitarian communication patterns are presented within these frameworks. The human potential movement shifts emphasis from continuous criticism of self to recognition of personal strengths and development of individual potential. The concept of personal power and its impact on making choices and responsible decisions is also stressed by Rogers.[45] He asserts that there is a natural tendency toward complete development in human beings, an underlying flow of movement toward a constructive fulfillment of their inherent possibilities. Facilitating self-ownership by the client, placing the locus of decision-making on the client, and placing responsibility for the effects of these decisions on the client form the politics of Rogers' client-centered approach.[46] Rather than focusing on what one should have and blaming others for what one does not have, emphasis is placed on assessing one's position and then taking responsibility for changing it.

The values clarification approach encourages individuals to personally and consciously choose beliefs and establish certain behavioral patterns to act on these beliefs.[47] Assertiveness training focuses on speaking for oneself, taking responsibility for one's actions. It fosters the emergence of new communication styles based on honest, direct, open communication.[48]

Transactional analysis emphasizes equality-oriented communication patterns (transactions). The parent/childlike nature of most learned human interaction is identified, and adult/adult (egalitarian) patterns are encouraged.[49] Behavior modification addresses specific patterns of communication, reinforcing appropriate patterns and extinguishing patterns seen as negative to individual development.[50]

Once a woman realizes the authoritarian/subordinate nature of language and has learned methods by which a more equal communication pattern can be established, she is able to act on her new beliefs and practice a new communication style. The communication style, if egalitarian, will conflict within the esablished norms of almost every group with which the woman has contact. Equal communication patterns create imbalance in aggressive/submissive language styles.

An egalitarian communication style redefines external and internal expectations of a relationship. It facilitates a collegial, cooperative perspective. Communication becomes more direct and lateral rather than vertical, as prevails in authority/subordinate relationships. As the communication style is practiced consistently, the imbalance creates uneasiness and stress. Equal communication patterns challenge the powerful position in authority/subordinate relationships. No person, group, or institution gives up power easily. Much work and struggle are involved in this type of pervasive change. A sociologist has identified major changes in life that affect large areas of the assumptive world as *"psychosocial* transitions."[51] Such transitions are seen as turning points for better or worse in psychosocial adjustment.

There is great pressure to accept and submit to societal norms of communication once an individual identifies the consequences of a true commitment to an egalitarian communication style. To make a satifactory adjustment, an individual must give up one view of herself and her assumptive world and acquire another. Parkes states that avoidance and depression are the two most common alternatives to the acceptance of reality.[52] It is interesting to consider how common are these behaviors among many women in society today.

Communication in conflict situations is particularly difficult for women. It has also been found to be difficult for nurses as a group. Kramer encourages a reorientation of nurses toward conflict, advocating the learning of appropriate skills for the management of constructive conflict.[53]

Acting out these new communication patterns can be a great challenge; research indicates that conflict, if faced reasonably, contributes to rather than detracts from growth.[54] Potential is enhanced for all relationships as the dyad-group-institution is broadened to include the feminine perspective. Though not the same as the masculine perspective, it is not less than or more than the male contribution; it is a different contribution.

The cry within the sciences to open up what one can see by admitting as data that which one feels, to place emphasis on the whole of the experience instead of the measurable parts, is a rejection of the limitations of a scientific, masculine reality and an acceptance of the need for the addition of the holistic feminine. In addition to knowing, it is necessary to feel—to know love and tenderness and fire and rage and passion.[55]

As attitudes change, the caring orientation of nursing will be seen as equal to the cure orientation of medicine. Nursing is different than, rather than less than, medicine. As personal characteristics are accepted in communication, the affective orientation of women

will be reinforced. Conflict patterns will move from competitive situations to cooperative ones. The indirect communications system described by Stein as the doctor-nurse game will become more open and direct.[56] This collaborative approach is prevalent in true interdisciplinary functioning in rehabilitative centers today. The "win-lose" orientation of the authority-subordinate relationship can be changed to a "win-win" situation if all members' perspectives are taken seriously.

References

1. Stoll, C. S. *Female and Male.* Dubuque, Iowa: W. M. C. Brown, 1974.
2. Stoll, C. S., ibid.
3. *Webster's 7th New Collegiate Dictionary,* under the word "Socialization."
4. Brim, Jr., O. G. Socialization through the life cycle. *In* Brim, Jr., O. G., and Wheeler, S. (eds.). *Socialization After Childhood.* New York: John Wiley and Sons, 1966.
5. Lynn, David B. The process of learning parental and sex role identification. *Journal of Marriage and the Family,* vol. 28, 1966, pp. 446–470.
6. Broverman, I. K., et al. Sex-role stereotypes: A current appraisal. *Journal of Social Issues,* vol. 28, 1972, pp. 59–78.
7. Broverman, I. K., et al., ibid.
8. Bardwick, T., and Donavan, E. Ambivalence: The socialization of women. *In* Gornick, V., and Moran, B. K. (eds.). *Women in Sexist Society.* New York: Basic Books, 1971, pp. 225–241.
9. Sapir, E., and Whorf, B. L. Language and thinking. *In* Laird, Charlton, and Gorell, R. M. (eds.). *Reading About Language.* New York: Harcourt, Brace, Jovanovich, 1970, pp. 18–20.
10. Jespersen, Otto. *The Growth and Structure of the English Language.* New York: D. Appleton, 1923.
11. Farb, Peter. *Word Play.* New York: Alfred A. Knopf, 1975, p. 160.
12. Blaubergs, Maija S. The nurse was a doctor. Paper presented to the Southeastern Conference on Linguistics, October, 1975.
13. Miller, C., and Swift, K. One small step for mankind. *New York Times Magazine,* April 16, 1972.
14. Lakoff, Robin. *Language and Woman's Place.* New York: Harper and Row, 1975, pp. 28–33.
15. Martyna, Wendy. What does "he" mean? Use of the generic masculine. *Journal of Communication,* vol. 28, 1978, pp. 131–138.
16. Kramer, Cheris. Female and male perception of female and male speech. *Language and Speech,* vol. 20, 1978, pp. 151–161.
17. Edelsky, Carole. Acquisition of communicative competence: Learning what it means to talk like a lady. *In* Ervin-Tripp, S., and Mitchell-Kernan, C. (eds.). *Child Discourse.* New York: Academic Press, 1977, p. 225–243.
18. Chaika, Elaine. *Language: The Social Mirror.* Rowley, Mass.: Newbury House, 1982, p. 204.
19. Jespersen, Otto. *Language: Its Nature, Development and Origin.* New York: W. W. Norton, 1964, pp. 252–253.

20. Lakoff, R. op. cit.
21. Crosby, F., and Nyquist, L. The female register: An empirical study of Lakoff's hypothesis. *Language and Society*, vol. 6, 1977, pp. 163–189, and Erickson, B., Lind, E. A., Johnson, B. C., and O'Barr, W. M. Speech style and impression formation in a court setting: The effect of "power" and "powerless" speech. *Journal of Experimental Social Psychology*, vol. 14, 1978, pp. 266–279.
22. Zimmerman, Don H., and West, C. Sex roles, interruptions, and silences in conversation. *In* Thorne, B., and Henley, N. (eds.). *Language and Sex: Difference and Dominance*. Rowley, Mass.: Newbury House, 1975, pp. 105–129.
23. Fishman, Pamela. Interaction: The work women do. *In* Thorne, B., Kramerae, C., and Henley, N. (eds.). *Language, Gender and Society*. Rowley, Mass.: Newbury House, 1973, pp. 89–101.
24. Trudgill, Peter. Language and sex. *In Sociolinguistics: An Introduction*. New York: Penguin Books, 1974, pp. 91–101.
25. Chaika, Elaine. *Language: The Social Mirror*. Rowley, Mass.: Newbury House, 1982, p. 214, and Nelson, Bruce: The tag question: Women and men use them differently, don't they? Unpublished paper, 1983.
26. Barrch, N. Sex-typed language: The production of grammatical cases. *Acta Sociologia*, vol. 14, Winter, 1971, pp. 24–42.
27. Baird, J. E. Sex differences in group communication: A review of relevant research. *Quarterly Journal of Speech*, vol. 62, April, 1976, pp. 179–192.
28. Baird, J. E., ibid.
29. Frost, J. H. The influence of female and male communication styles on conflict strategies: Problem areas. Paper presented at the International Communication Association Convention, Berlin, West Germany, 1977.
30. Maccoby, E. E., and Jacklin, C. N. *The Psychology of Sex Differences*. Stanford, Cal.: Stanford University Press, 1974.
31. Caine, C. A. H., and Caine, T. A. The evolution of male dominance. Paper submitted to the Department of Women's Studies, University of Minnesota, January 6, 1976.
32. Deutsch, M. Conflicts: Productive and destructive. *Journal of Social Issues*, vol. 25, 1969, pp. 7–43.
33. Madow, Leo. *Anger*. New York: Charles Scribner's Sons, 1972, p. 6.
34. Mauksch, H. O. The Nurse: A Study in Self and Role Perception. Dissertation, University of Chicago, 1966.
35. Duberman, Lucile. *Gender and Sex in Society*. New York: Praeger Publishers, 1975.
36. Goffmann, Erving. *Interaction Ritual*. New York: Anchor Books, 1967, pp. 47–95.
37. Sauer, Sue. Interruptive behavior in cross-sex physician conversations. Unpublished paper, Metropolitan State University, 1983.
38. Leininger, Madeline. *Nursing and Anthropology: Two Worlds to Blend*. New York: John Wiley and Sons, 1970, p. 67.
39. Lewis, F. The nurse as lackey: A sociological perspective. *Supervisor Nurse*, April, 1976, pp. 24–27.
40. Hoekelman, R. A. Nurse-physician relationships. *American Journal of Nursing*, July, 1975, p. 1151.
41. Yura, Helen, Ozimek, Dorothy, and Walsh, Mary B. *Nursing Leadership: Theory and Process*. New York: Appleton-Century-Crofts, 1976.
42. Heide, W. S. Nursing and Women's Liberation: A parallel. *American Journal of Nursing*, May, 1973, p. 826.
43. Valicer, B. S., and Bohannon, M. W. A hospital stress rating scale. *Nursing Research*, vol. 24, September/October, 1975, pp. 352–359.
44. Valicer, B. S., and Bohannon, M. W., ibid.
45. Rogers, C. *On Personal Power, Inner Strength and Its Revolutionary Impact*. New York: Delacorte Press, 1977.
46. Rogers, C., ibid., p. 14.
47. Simon, S. B., Howe, L. W., and Kirschenbaum, H. *Values Clarification*. New York: Hart Publishing Company, 1972.
48. Alberti, R. E., and Emmons, M. L. *Your Perfect Right: A Guide to Assertive Behavior*. St. Luis Obispo, Cal.: Impact, 1970.
49. Harris, T. A. *I'm OK, You're OK*. New York: Avon Books, 1967.
50. Sherman, A. R. *Behavior Modification Theory and Practice*. Monterey, Cal.: Brooks Kole, 1973.
51. Parkes, C. M. Psycho-social transitions. *Social Science and Medicine*, vol. 5, 1971, pp. 101–115.
52. Parkes, C. M., ibid., p. 110.
53. Kramer, M. S. Conflict: The cutting edge of growth. *Journal of Nursing Administration*, October, 1976, pp. 19–25.
54. Nye, R. D. *Conflict Among Humans*. New York: Springer Verlag, 1973.
55. Bardwick, J. Androgyny and humanistic goals, or goodbye cardboard people. *In* McBee, M. L., and Blake, K. A. (eds.). *The American Female: Who Will She Be*. Beverly Hills, Cal.: Glencoe Press, 1974, p. 63.
56. Stein, Leonard J. Male and female: The doctor-nurse game. *Archives of General Psychiatry*, June, 1967, pp. 699–703.

DEPENDENCY IN WOMEN

ELIZABETH A. PETERSON
DIANE KJERVIK

This chapter by Beth Peterson and Diane Kjervik starts with three brief case studies of dependent women, followed by a review of the literature regarding dependency. The assessment of necessary dependency interventions is then described for the reader.

Midge LaPorte is a 25 year old woman who comes to the clinic for immunization for her four children. She is unemployed and divorced and is living in a large rented house. She receives monthly welfare checks. She is a high school graduate and has worked as a legal secretary. She is eligible for energy assistance and food stamps but has not applied for them. When she is questioned about that, she responds, "I know I should, but I hate going down there. Couldn't someone here help me with that?" She has had considerable interpersonal difficulties with neighbors. Initially she had good relationships with them, but later they seemed to have withdrawn from her. She explains this by saying, "I can't understand them. They said they'd help me keep up my yard and take care of the kids. Now when I really need them, where are they?"

She has had a series of relationships with men, all of which have been unsatisfying to her. She talks about wanting to meet the "right man," her need for a companion, and her dislike of being alone.

Sue Callahan is a 32 year old woman who is a newly diagnosed diabetic patient. She is a college graduate who is working as a sales clerk in a clothing store. She is unmarried and lives with several other women in an apartment. She is hospitalized for regulation of insulin and for learning her medical care. For 3 days the nurses assigned to Sue have been encouraging her to self-administer her insulin.

Each day Sue responds, "Oh, would you do it for me? I just don't feel up to it. Besides, Sarah, the other nurse, said that she'd help me any time I wanted it." Later she became angry with her sister and brother-in-law after he declined to take her car to the repair shop for repairs that he had suggested were needed 6 months ago.

Christine Davis is a 56 year old woman. She is married and the mother of two children, both of whom are out of the home. She is a college graduate and worked for 3 years as an elementary school teacher, but has not worked since her children were born. Four weeks ago she had a cholecystectomy. Her recovery was slowed by a wound infection. She has been home for 5 days. Her incision still drains, and she needs to change the dressing several times a day. When the hospital staff showed her how to change her dressings, she insisted that her husband be present. "You better explain all of this to my husband. He knows how to do things better than I." At home she has expressed concern about being left home alone and has asked her daughter to spend the day with her. When the nurse visits her at home, she commonly asks, "Do you think that I should take a bath today? Will you give me my pills so I'm sure that I take the right ones?"

Midge LaPorte, Sue Callahan, and Christine Davis have at least three things in common. They are women, they are recipients of nursing care, and they exhibit behaviors that reflect dependence. Dependency is not a foreign concept, either to lay people or to professionals. Yet, when it comes to defining dependency, most people have a hard time. In much of Western society, we applaud independence and decry dependence. At the same time, most of us acknowledge that we are dependent on such people as farmers, postal workers, car mechanics, central supply workers, drug companies, families, friends. Immediately we realize that all dependence is not bad. It is crucial for survival and necessary for rich, meaningful relationships. yet sometimes dependence gets in the way of growth and maturity. The three women described earlier exhibit that kind of dependency, and it is that kind of dependency we need to be concerned with in nursing practice. The dependence that stems from mutuality and strength needs to be separated from the kind that inhibits growth and maturity. The easiest way to do that is to give the first a different name. i.e., interdependence. When interdependence is seen in clients and families, it is a strength and should be promoted and encouraged.

This leaves us with the task of defining and describing dependence. Webster's dictionary defines dependence as the "state of being contingent upon or influenced or determined by something else."[1] According to Tavris and Offir, "Dependence is the need for other people. The independent person copes with life's big and little frustrations in an active, vigorous manner, exercising personal initiative. The dependent person stands there, suffering the slings and arrows of outrageous fortune, hoping that help will arrive quickly."[2] Julia Sherman further describes dependency by saying, "A passive dependent attitude is apt to evoke anxiety, since the individual feels helpless and vulnerable, unable to act. Moreover, a dependent person, provoked to justifiable anger, may conceal his anger for fear of antagonizing the person upon whom he is dependent."[3]

Combining the ideas from these authors, dependency can be defined as (1) the inability or failure to exercise personal initiative in dealing with circumstances of life, (2) the expectation that someone or something else can and should provide that initiative, and (3) the need to rely upon the approval of valued others in order to maintain a sense of personal well-being.

What The Experts Say

Psychosocial literature is filled with references to dependency, often in relationship to women. Much of the early literature that describes dependency was written by Freud. "Regardless of the form in which it is present, a psychoanalytic theory makes the critical assumption that a pre-determined relationship exists between the nature of genital differences and the psychological characteristics of males and females. Freud assumed that there are sex-typed differences in aggressiveness, dependency, jealousy, and passivity, differences which represent an inevitable emotional response to unconscious fears and impulses about genital differences."[4]

Karen Horney provides another psychoanalytic approach. She discusses dependency in relationship to a number of commonly accepted female traits.[5]

In particular one must consider the fact that when some . . . elements [such as blocking of outlets for sexuality, estimation of woman as being inferior, economic dependence of women on men] are present in the culture-complex, there may appear fixed ideologies concerning the "nature" of women; such as doctrines that woman is innately weak, emotional, enjoys dependence, is limited in capabilities for independent work and autonomous thinking . . . The influence that these ideologies exert on women is materially strengthened by the fact that women presenting the specified traits are more frequently chosen by men . . . qualities like emotional dependence on the other sex, absorption in "love." Inhibition of expansive, autonomous development, etc. are regarded as quite desirable in women but are treated with opprobrium and ridicule when found in men.[5]

According to Erik Erikson, autonomy and initiative occur early in the developmental sequence. If an individual does not develop autonomy, shame and doubt will develop instead. "For if denied the gradual and well-guided experience of the autonomy of free choice, the child will turn against himself all his urge to discriminate and to manipulate. He will overmanipulate himself, he will develop a precocious conscience."[6] Later, if the young child does not develop initiative, guilt will develop instead. "Initiative adds to autonomy the quality of undertaking, planning and attacking a task for the sake of being active and on the move . . . The danger in this stage is a sense of guilt over the goals contemplated and the acts initiated in one's exuberant enjoyment of new locomotor and mental power. . . . "[7] The lack of developing a sense of autonomy or of initiative may influence or at least be related to the development of dependence in which the person lacks the inability to exercise personal initiative in dealing with his or her circumstances of life.

It is important to note that Erikson makes no distinction between the development of males and females, either in terms of the cultural context or in terms of the sex-typed differences that are rooted in psychoanalytic thought. According to Sanguilano, this oversight may be problematic, especially in understanding female development.[8]

Like most theoretical constructs it has its shortcomings. One of them is the area of predictability. Predictability has always been the hornet's nest of social scientists, and well it should be. Has anyone known a woman's life that was predictable? There are a myriad of influences that shape a life; the social climate and expectations; the personal psychological response to those expectations—which makes every woman unique; and the values and meanings, at first borrowed, later personally derived.

Paradoxically, however, not only do the stage theories fall short on the issue of predictability, but they also fall short on the flip side—that question of unpredictability. The view of adulthood as a series of orderly, predictable, linear progressions—steps that are age-specific—makes little room for the impact of those "unexpected" critical events that have changed the focus and direction of women's lives.

Contemporary theorists are still struggling to explain the seemingly higher incidence of dependency in women. Although most of them reject the biologic determinism of Freud, they offer a number of explanations as to its origin.

Jean Baker Miller provides a view of society in which men are the dominants and women are the subordinates.[9] According to her,

Dominant groups usually define one or more acceptable roles for the subordinate. Acceptable roles typically involve providing services that no dominant group wants to perform for itself. Functions that a dominant group prefers to perform, on the other hand, are carefully guarded and closed to subordinates . . . Subordinates are usually said to be unable to perform the preferred roles.

Consequently, according to Miller, women have been relegated nurturing tasks and emotional, nonactive behaviors, which, in fact, are less valued by dominant men. This frees men to avoid dealing with the tasks and behaviors which they do not value.[10]

. . . if the members of the dominant group—that is, men—claim they do not have feelings of insecurity [etc], subordinates (women) cannot challenge their claim. Furthermore, it is women's responsibility to supply the needs of the dominant group so that its members can continue to deny these feelings.

If women have become the repository for emotions, weaknesses, fears, and defenselessness, they are by necessity dependent upon (strong) males for protection.

To further complicate matters, not only is it important to the dominants to get rid of their seemingly "negative" tasks and behaviors by attributing them to the subordinates but also doing so accentuates their seemingly "positive" tasks and behaviors. This frees men to tell themselves that they are strong, independent, rational beings who are not subject to "raging hormones" or unpredictable mood swings. Consequently, women beginning to question the tasks and behaviors traditionally assigned to them not only affects men but also becomes extremely disconcerting to men's understanding of who they are.

Although the previous discussion helps explain why men would encourage or reinforce dependency in women, it certainly does not explain why women would accept dependency. Jean Baker Miller provides some insight into this subject.[11]

If subordinates do not accept their place as inferior or secondary, they will initiate open conflict. That is, if women assume that their own needs have equal validity and proceed to explore and state them openly, they will be seen as creating conflict and must bear the psychological burden of rejecting men's images of true "womanhood."

The conflict has the potential of pulling apart a woman. She may be forced to decide between personal growth or development of an intimate relationship with a man.

According to the author of a popular contemporary book, women have been socialized for dependent roles and actually choose them. "We've been encouraged to avoid anything that scares us, taught from the time we are very young to do only those things which allow us to feel comfortable and secure. In fact we are not trained for freedom at all, but for its categorical opposite—dependency."[12] She suggests that ". . . personal, psychological dependency—the deep wish to be taken care of by others—is the chief force holding women down today. I call this 'The Cinderella Complex'—a network of largely repressed attitudes and fears that keeps women in a kind of half-life, retreating from the full use of their minds and creativity. Like Cinderella, women today are still waiting for something external to transform their lives."[13]

One of the greatest difficulties in examining what writers currently have to say about dependency in women is that there are a number of other phenomena that may or may not occur in conjunction with dependency. These include a higher incidence of fears in general, an external locus of control, learned helplessness, less valued sex-role characteristics, and decreased achievement motivation. Research from each of these areas may help illuminate the context in which dependency occurs.

A study by Alan Krasnoff compared the self-attribution of fear between women and men. His findings showed that "to the extent that men or women endorse adjectives that represent feminine sex-role orientations or stereotypes, the greater is the likelihood that these people will attribute more fear to themselves."[14]

Julian Potter has summarized and duplicated a number of experiments dealing with the difference in subjects' behavior when they perceive reinforcement as contingent upon their behavior versus chance or experimental control.[15] In summarizing the research, he asserts:

A series of studies provides strong support for the hypothesis that the individual who has a strong belief that he can control his own destiny is likely to (a) be more alert to those aspects of the environment which provide useful information for his future behavior, (b) take steps to improve his environmental condition, (c) place greater value on skill and achievement reinforcements and be generally more concerned with his ability, particularly his failures, and (d) be resistive to subtle attempts to influence him.

Some of the research by Martin Seligman and others regarding learned helplessness is also relevant. According to Seligman, an organism learns to be helpless when it is repeatedly exposed to stress conditions in which no behavior in which the organism engages reduces stress.[16] If, as the other studies seem to suggest, women are socialized to be more passive and dependent, they may never develop the necessary skills to take initiative in life situations. As a result, none of their "learned" coping skills reduce their stress or change their life situations. This could naturally lead them to the conclusion that they are unable to change anything and that they must find themselves someone else who can change something.

The studies done by Broverman, which have now almost become classics, discuss sex roles. College students were asked to rate the typical adult female and male according to a list of adjectives. The results indicated that the traits attributed to men by both sexes were the most socially desirable. Furthermore, the women described themselves as high on feminine traits which were not socially desirable, and low on masculine but socially desirable traits such as being independent, objective, logical, direct, self-conscious, and ambitious.[17]

Ellen Lenney examined the issue on self-confidence in relationship to women's achievement motivation.[18] She had her subjects complete several lists and then estimate their own score, the score of the average undergraduate, the average male undergraduate, or the average female undergraduate. Her findings showed that:

Women did not compare their own work less favorably than men to that of their peers in either the verbal section, an ability area in which women typically perform better than men, or in the interpersonal perceptiveness section, an ability area closer to the stereotype of feminine than of masculine skills. Thus, in neither of the more female-oriented sections was there any evidence that women had less self-confidence than men.
. . . Women's self-confidence was lower than men's in both the spatial-mechanical section and the creativity section. These results indicate that while women may express low self-confidence in more ability areas than men, this tendency is actually quite discriminative.
. . . Women's self-confidence was more dependent than men's upon the specific peer to whom they compared themselves. In sharp contrast to men's independence from these social comparison cues, women's evaluation of the relative quality of their own work depended greatly upon the specific individual to whom they compared themselves.

A number of studies look at dependency behavior in young children (both boys and girls) and also examine attitudes and behaviors of parents that may influence the development of dependency behaviors. Goldberg and Lewis made the following discovery:[19]

Thirty-two boys and girls, aged 12 months, were observed at home with their mothers. They found that mothers of girls looked at and talked to their children more but that boys got more touching and cuddling. When the observation was repeated six months later, it was found that girls received more attention and physical contact. Then at age twenty-three months the children were observed playing with toys with their mothers. They observed that boys were less reluctant to leave their mothers, returned less often, wandered farther away, and stayed away longer. Later a fence was placed in the middle of the room. They found that the boys were more likely to attack the fence and try to get around it, while the girls cried.

Lois Hoffman summarizes the work of several different investigators and suggests that parents may respond differently toward their daughter's independent and dependent behavior.[20]

Parents begin independence training earlier for boys than for girls and emphasize it more. Asked at what age parents should let children use scissors without supervision, cross the street, tie one's shoes, play away from home without first telling the parents, and take a bus ride, parents of girls invariably set a later age than parents of boys (Collard). In addition, parents allow boys free access to a wider area of the community (Saegert and Hart).

Julia Sherman describes some works dealing with older children.[21]

Among . . . children during the grade school years, there are consistent reports that girls receive more love and nurturance than boys (Bronfenbrenner, Droppelman, and Schaefer). During grade school years, a boy who is still behaving in a dependent manner would be expected to encounter increasing censure from parents, especially fathers, and from peers as well. In the fifth and sixth grades, a sample of girls with a high need for approval were among the most popular, while boys with a high need for approval were among the least popular (Tulkin, Muller, and Conn). It seems likely that if a boy does not "naturally" come to show independent behavior, various environmental pressures will be applied to achieve that end. If a girl shows excessive dependent behavior, her father is less likely to help her develop independence, and if her mother becomes annoyed with her dependency it may only increase.

Mabel Cohen carried out an exploratory and descriptive study of 50 pregnant women and their husbands.[22] She had weekly interviews with these women from the third or fourth month of pregnancy through the first 3 months postpartum. In summarizing her findings, she reports:

We found the problem of dependency to be intimately related to questions of masculine and feminine identity. . . Part of the mythology of the sexes is that the man is independent and the woman dependent, but this is only a myth. The man's dependency needs are largely cloaked beneath the masculine image, while those of the woman are more in the open, and indeed are exaggerated by the popular stereotype of femininity.

A study by Peterson and Kjervik questions the notion of whether women are more dependent than men.[23] A questionnaire designed to measure dependency was distributed to 150 college students. They were asked to rate themselves according to a number of different statements dealing with dependency, such as relationships with others, perceived ability in making life decisions, and sense of personal adequacy. The scores between men and women were very similar (X = 71.6 in females, and X = 71.2 in males). The standard deviation for female scores was greater than for male scores (S.D. = 8.3 for women and 6.9 for men), suggesting that some women may be more dependent than their male counterparts, but the study certainly casts doubt upon the notion that women as a group are more dependent than men as a group.

After review of the literature, one must conclude that dependence is a pervasive and complex issue that requires skillful and directed assessment and intervention.

Assessment of Dependence

Assessment of dependence involves a thorough assessment of all aspects of a person: physical, psychosocial, and spiritual, since dependence can be manifested in all those areas. The physical manifestations of dependence include such things as making requests for assistance in an activity when no physical limitations prevent a person from carrying out the activity without assistance. In the hospital, these requests may be overt—"Will you do my Clinitest for me? I'm just too tired"—or they may be much more covert and often manipulative—"I feel so secure when you empty my colostomy bag. Then I know it's done right." Another physical manifestation of dependency is the desire for closeness. Again, this can be manifested overtly. "Please sit by my bed and talk to me," or by the familiar grasping of the hand and not letting go. Covert indications involve frequent use of the call light or many seemingly unnecessary requests. According to Jasmin and Trygstad, "Persons who are excessively dependent . . . may substitute substances or objects when others refuse to fulfill their excessive needs."[24] Thus, addictive behaviors such as smoking, use of alcohol, and compulsive eating, may also be manifestations of dependence.

Psychosocial manifestations of dependence are varied. Dependent individuals may request a great deal of affirmation and acknowledgement. They may ask for it—"How did I do?"—or they may complain bitterly to others about the lack of support and encouragement. They may also express self-deprecating ideas, such as "I'll never learn how to do this," or "This is beyond me. I've never been good at this." Whatever their behavior, one of the following emotions usually underlies the manifestations:

anger, anxiety, depression, or fear of being abandoned.

Spiritual manifestations of dependence are even more varied and complex. For purposes of this discussion the term spiritual is used synonomously with what are commonly referred to as existential questions: what is the nature of personhood, what is one's purpose in life, how does one deal with finiteness, limitations, and imperfections. Dependent individuals may exhibit magical thinking in relationship to God or some other supernatural force. They may also look for miraculous solutions to their problems and may gravitate to messianic figures who offer advice and assistance. In understanding spiritual manifestations of dependency, it is important to realize that the significant concept is not a belief in the supernatural or the expectation of something positive happening in the face of difficult circumstances. Rather, it is the abdication of personal responsibility, the failure to act, the belief that one's actions would be impotent, and the expectation that finding a solution to one's difficulties is the sole responsibility of some great supernatural force or being.

Intervention in Dependency

One of the most ironic outcomes of dealing with dependent women is promoting further dependency, but this time on the helper. This danger is especially great in nurse-client relationships since the individuals are often in a dependent position because of their health-related needs. Probably one of the greatest nursing challenges is to avoid promoting dependence in clients who need a great deal of assistance in carrying out all or some of their activities of daily living. To avoid that, a nurse must first take a long look at his or her motives and behaviors. For instance, the nurse who gains deep personal satisfaction from "taking care" of others or the nurse who is so busy that he or she does things for clients rather than taking the time to assist the clients to do them may find that he or she is inadvertently encouraging dependence. Consequently, self-assessment is the first and maybe the most important step in intervention.

The goal of intervention with dependent women is for them to assume responsibility for their own life situation. This does not preclude their asking others for help or support, but it does mean that they do not look to other people to act while they remain inert. To promote this goal, the nurse must assist the woman in problem solving, in dealing with

strong emotions, and in working through issues of the nurse-client relationship.

Dependent women are often caught in a web of relationships that serve to promote further dependence. This is why problem solving is so crucial. For many women economic dependence is a major contributor to their inertia. "If I leave my husband, how will I support myself? Even though he beats me, I know that he'll pay the rent." Another factor is their inability or unfamiliarity in dealing with the person or persons upon whom they are dependent. "I could never tell my boyfriend how I'm feeling. He might get mad," or "I couldn't ask my boss for a raise. What would he think?" Anticipatory problem-solving techniques, such as role playing, assertiveness training, and providing group support, can all be valuable in assisting the women to accept responsibility for her life, while also providing information, feedback, and support from others.

Strong emotions almost always surface as women begin to deal with dependence. Anxiety about one's limitations, fear of abandonment, and anger are some of the most common. Most dependent women truly believe that they are inadequate to deal with their life situation. Consequently, the suggestion or expectation that they should is frightening. It is so frightening that it may paralyze them if it is done in pieces too large. Dealing with life must be broken down into smaller, achievable tasks; for example, calling the clinic to make an appointment, or asking a friend for a ride. Successful experiences are crucial, so the tasks need to be achievable. Positive reinforcement for the successes is also an important way of reinforcing the benefits of actively dealing with life.

Many dependent women also fear that any change in their attitude or behavior will result in the loss of the relationship with the person upon whom they are dependent. This fear of abandonment can be debilitating and is a challenge for nursing intervention. Assisting the woman in asking and answering the very painful question, "What would happen if I were all alone?" may serve to help the woman discover personal resources. It is important to understand that the purpose of this question is not to encourage problem-solving, although it may do that, but rather to encourage a woman to describe and explore the depth of her feelings about changing her dependent behavior.

As a women begins to face her dependency, she will almost always feel anger. The anger will probably be very frightening for the woman and maybe for the nurse. The nurse can assist the woman to deal with her anger by allowing her to express her feelings and by later helping her decide how best to act upon those feelings.

Several issues in the relationship between a nurse and a dependent woman are also important to consider. Working through these issues is a crucial aspect of intervention. Manipulation is a common behavior in an individual who perceives herself as dependent. Manipulation involves an attempt by the woman to get the nurse to meet her needs. It is especially detrimental in the relationship with a dependent woman because it serves to reinforce her belief in her own dependence and in her inability to meet her own needs. Manipulative behavior is usually aimed at making the nurse feel strong, competent, or needed. Intervention for manipulative behavior consists of providing firm, consistent responses to the behavior. When the client in good physical condition says, "Will you please give me a bath today? I feel so tired. That's one thing I like about you here. All of you are so good to me when I don't feel well," the nurse might respond, "You sound tired, but I'm concerned that your staying in bed might actually make you weaker. If you'd like to rest now, I'll come back later and you can take a tub bath or shower then." It is crucial that all the nursing staff are also aware of and abide by that same approach, since it is highly probable that the client will make the same request of every other staff person who comes her way. It may even be embellished with, "You are the only nurse who really cares about me. I'm glad when you're here because you give such good care." Again, a firm, specific response is crucial. Unfortunately, there is also the possibility that the woman may travel from one health care provider to the next using that same approach. Currently, little can be done to work with manipulation happening that way since one has little or no control over what happens in other agencies.

Because dependent women are convinced that they need help from other more powerful people, initiating action can be very frightening for them. Consequently, to do so they need a great deal of support from someone with whom they feel comfortable. The nurse-client relationship can provide them with needed support and encouragement. Sometimes providing that support is agonizing because the woman seems so fearful and hesitant. However, providing positive reinforcement, even for small tasks, such as making a phone call or filling out a form, may help make the next phone call easier and less complicated. As important as providing encouragement is assisting the woman to find positive reinforcement in taking the action rather than in receiving praise from someone else. Thus, the nurse always must have the goal that the client will not need him or her to provide reinforcement but will be able to find it within herself.

In addition to providing support, setting limits and maintaining separateness is also critical. "I'm sorry that I can't take you to the doctor. I have several other home visits that I must make today." This approach is very important because it contradicts the notion that the woman is dependent and therefore unable to act and that the helper is strong and able to do anything. Telling a client, "I have 15 minutes to spend with you. How would you like to spend that time?" is much more therapeutic for the dependent client than to cancel all other responsibilities and spend great amounts of time trying to meet her needs.

CASE STUDY

Earlier in the chapter we were introduced to Midge LaPorte. The brief assessment data provided suggests that she is exhibiting dependent behavior. As she enters the examining room, she announces, "I'm glad to see you again. You're so good to me. Those other nurses don't ever listen to me. You understand how awful life has been for me. I don't think I can do all the things those other nurses expect me to do."

Fortunately, the clinic nurse realized that Midge's concerns were too great to be handled in one visit, so she used the office visit to deal with the health care needs of the children. She then referred Midge to the mental health nursing specialist. Although she made the referral, she didn't give away her role with Midge. Instead, the two nurses developed a care plan which they communicated to the rest of the staff. The clinic nurses worked primarily with problem solving, dealing with manipulation, providing encouragement, and limit setting. As noted earlier, Midge was eligible for food stamps and some other assistance programs, about which she had done nothing. The clinic nurses began to ask her what she felt she needed to do about the shortage of food at her house. After a while she started talking about applying for some assistance. When she brought up the subject, the nurse responded, "Do you know how to do that?" When Midge responded, "No, what should I do?" the nurse asked, "Would you like to talk to someone who could give you the right forms to fill out?" Eventually Midge applied for food stamps. Each action step was acknowledged and supported by the nursing staff, but Midge was the one taking action.

The clinical specialist dealt primarily with her relationship with others and her anger. Midge often talked about her feelings toward men. She had been involved in a number of abusive relationships and explained that, to her, it was better than being alone. Her fear of aloneness and abandonment was explored and contrasted with the way in which she was providing for herself and her children. Gradually she was able to acknowledge that she was able to provide for herself and her family, and that most of the abusive men made minimal contributions to their well-being. Midge later began to talk about what she wanted in relationships and slowly became more selective in the men that she related to.

As Midge continued with the clinical specialist, she did experience a great deal of anger: at her parents, at her male friends, at her ex-husband, at society, at the therapist, and at the clinic staff. She was very fearful of her anger and expressed concern that she couldn't control it once she let it out. The clinical specialist worked with her in learning how to express anger in a way that was not destructive to herself or to others and in accepting anger as a normal human response. One day at the clinic a physician gave her a prescription for one of her children without telling her the purpose or action of the drug. She became angry and felt herself losing control, but then was able to regain control and responded, "I need to know what this medication is for before I give it to my child. If you're unable to tell me about it, please find someone who will."

Midge made slow but steady progress. She began to take the initiative in dealing with her situation. She learned to ask for help in specific, concrete ways: "Could you take care of my children on Tuesday afternoon while I go grocery shopping?", and she began expressing pleasure in taking responsibility for herself. She still expressed the desire for someone to take care of her but was able to laugh about it and acknowledge that it was not realistic or healthy.

Dependence in women is not inevitable or intractable, even within the context of the nurse-client relationship, but it is a challenge and prevention requires astute nursing care. On the other hand, working with a woman to assist her in taking or maintaining responsibility for her own life can be one of the most rewarding aspects of nursing and may represent one of our most important responsibilities.

References

1. *Webster's New World Dictionary of the American Language.* college edition. Cleveland: World Publishing, 1959, pp. 393–394.
2. Tavris, Carol, and Offir, Carole. *The Longest War: Sex Differences in Perspective.* New York: Harcourt, Brace, Jovanovich, 1977, p. 50.
3. Sherman, Julia, *On the Psychology of Women.* Springfield, Ill.: Charles C Thomas, 1971, p. 38.
4. Ullian, Dorothy. The development of conceptions of masculinity and femininity. *In* Lloyd, Barbara, and Archer, John (eds.). *Exploring Sex Differences.* London: Academic Press, 1976, p. 26.
5. Horney, Karen. *Feminine Psychology.* New York: Norton, 1977, p. 231.
6. Erikson, Erik. *Childhood and Society.* New York: Norton, 1963, p. 252.
7. Erikson, Erik, ibid., p. 255.
8. Sanguilano, Iris. *In Her Time.* New York: Morrow Quill, 1980, p. 20.
9. Miller, Jean Baker. *Toward a New Psychology of Women.* Boston: Beacon Press, 1976, p. 67.
10. Miller, Jean Baker, ibid., p. 34.
11. Miller, Jean Baker, ibid., p. 17.
12. Dowling, Collette. *The Cinderella Complex.* New York: Summit Books, 1981, p. 15.
13. Dowling, Collette, ibid., p. 31.
14. Krasnoff, Alan G. The sex differences in self-assessed fears. *Sex Roles: A Journal of Research,* vol. 7, January, 1981, p. 22.
15. Potter, Julian B. Generalized expectances for internal versus external control of reinforcement. *Psychological Monographs: General and Applied,* vol. 80, 1966, p. 25.
16. Seligman, Martin. Fall into helplessness. *Psychology Today,* June, 1973, p. 43.
17. Broverman, I. K., et al. Sex-role stereotypes and clinical judgments of mental health. *Journal of Consulting and Clinical Psychology,* vol. 34, 1970, p. 18.
18. Lenney, Ellen. What's good for the gander isn't always good for the goose: Sex differences in self confidence as a function of ability area and comparison with others. *Sex Roles: A Journal of Research,* vol. 7, September, 1981, p. 921.
19. Goldberg, Susan, and Lewis, Michael. Play behavior in the year-old infant: Early sex difference. *Child Development,* 1969, p. 21.
20. Hoffman, Lois Waldis. Early childhood experiences and women's achievement motives. *Journal of Social Issues,* vol. 28, 1972, p. 142.
21. Sherman, Julia, op. cit., p. 32.
22. Cohen, Mabel. Personal identity and sexual identity. *Psychiatry,* vol. 29, 1966, p. 89.
23. Peterson, Elizabeth, and Kjervik, Diane. *A Comparison of the Incidence of Dependency in College Age Males and Females.* Unpublished Plan B project, University of Minnesota School of Nursing, p. 17.
24. Jasmin, Sylvia, and Trygstad, Louise. *Behavioral Concepts and the Nursing Process.* St. Louis: Mosby, 1979, p. 110.

10

WOMEN AND CHEMICALS

MARJORIE JAMIESON
CATHERINE SCHABOT

This chapter by Marjorie Jamieson and
Catherine Schabot on women and chemical
abuse begins with information regarding the
disease of alcoholism. The chapter proceeds
with the impact of female life changes and its
relationship to the unique characteristics of
alcohol and other drugs. The chapter
concludes with a major section on
interventions and treatments.

THE STIGMA

Nice women are not alcoholics. Alcoholics
are not nice women. Therefore, I (or my wife,
my aunt, my mom) am (is) not an alcoholic.

We know that "boys will be boys," and that
a stressful job and financial responsibilities of
supporting a wife and children afford legitimate reasons for drinking—for a man. Drinking is a sign of masculinity; the amount of
booze a man can hold indicates his manhood.

We're amused at the behavior of a drunken
man, but we turn in disgust from a drunken
woman. We see a "fallen" woman who hangs
out in bars and sleeps around, or a hopeless
housewife who neglects her husband and kids
and generally disgraces womanhood.

A double standard? Yes.

Although studies suggest that chemical dependency (including alcoholism, a dependency
on the chemical, alcohol) is shared equally
among men and women, known chemically
dependent females range from 25 to 35 per
cent, a figure that is growing.[1-3] This is partly
true because female alcoholics and their families keep the alcoholic woman a secret.

I telephoned my dad the day I was admitted to
an alcohol treatment center. He told me not to tell
anyone, that he'd come and get me, and things

would straighten out at home. After all I'd left
home too early (I was 22!) etc., etc.*

We are motivated to protect our women so
that drinking is concealed and the illness of
chemical dependency is disguised. We cannot
tolerate a "failed mother," a "bad wife," or a
"drunk sister." Consequently, society helps
women drink longer and thereby progress to
advanced stages of alcohol or drug dependency
before detection. The alcoholic woman shares
society's opinion of herself and has more
shame than the alcoholic man. She therefore
drinks in secret and resists treatment. We go
to such extremes that a diagnosis of mental
illness is preferred to a diagnosis of alcoholism.

I wanted to be crazy.

When I went into treatment for my chemical
dependency, my sister came to "prove" that I was
not an alcoholic but needed psychiatric help.

Twice when I was on a psych ward because of
my depression my entire family visited and supported me. But when I was in an alcoholic treatment center they never acknowledged I was in treatment
nor did they visit me.

---

*All quotes in this chapter are from nurses who have
been through treatment for chemical dependency; they
were dependent on alcohol, other drugs, or both.

My mother talks about my "poor" aunt who is having a "nervous breakdown"! I know she is an alcoholic.

Society's protective attitude toward this woman is demonstrated in many ways. Physicians prescribe "a small glass of wine before bed." Women quit their jobs when they no longer can function.

For almost ten years I worked as a night nurse. During that time I was using "speed" and "downers" to different degrees. Whenever things became unmanageable or I felt someone might be catching on, I'd take a leave of absence.

Police officers drive drunk women home instead of giving them DWIs (Driving While Intoxicated) tests; husbands send their wives to a psychiatrist and obtain household help; and children call Mom "sick," while the oldest daughter takes on Mom's role.

Society is protecting the mother who drinks after Dad and the kids leave each morning, but who also manages to get the beds made and supper started before they come home. Society is ignoring the alcoholic professional woman who functions at work but whose company is a bottle or pill on weekends and evenings because she does not fit into the couple configuration of society.

The chemically dependent woman may be managing a home and family and is probably working outside her home too. Life appears normal, even though it is not as simple and orderly as it could be. The housewife hides her wine in the bleach bottle, while the professional pops valium with her coffee or sits in the bathroom cubicle as she has a drink. Most are "respectable" women who are socially integrated; those suspect are, ironically, protected by society.

My job was very important to me. I expended lots of time and energy being a good nurse—and covering up and denying my alcoholism. When I was in treatment my supervisor visited me and told me I had never stopped functioning as a nurse. What she didn't know was that I was functioning but not living.

A chemically dependent woman could be any woman involved in any role, living in any community, at any age, within any income level. Her dependency is unrelated to her religion, education, ethnicity, or intelligence quotient. She becomes chemically dependent because of the inter-relationship of the drug she chooses, whether alcohol, tranquilizers, marijuana, or others, and how she views herself as she perceives and relates to her world.

Because of the nature of these drugs, the central nervous system is affected. One can predict how each drug affects the central nervous system and the behaviors that will result, until eventually her emotions and behavior are controlled by the drug.

THE DISEASE

In 1956, the American Medical Association officially recognized alcoholism as a disease, with specific, well-defined and described physical, emotional, and psychologic problems. It is a chronic, progressive, incurable biochemical process.

The suggestion that genetic factors are important in the development of chemical dependency is becoming more credible as evidence accumulates; genetics are more important than any other factor. Arguments weighing the blame of chemical dependency on environment or inheritance have been interminable, but no one can argue with the fact that 85 to 88 per cent of alcoholics have a family history of alcoholism. Surveys of twins from alcoholic familes who have been adopted separately indicate that, although their different adoptive parents did not have drinking problems, both twins became alcoholic.[2, 4, 5] People are born predisposed to chemical dependency; the abnormal brain chemistry functions well until the first drink of alcohol.

There is a difference between how a social drinker and how an alcoholic metabolizes alcohol, with consequent predictable pathophysiology. When alcohol is broken down in the body of a social drinker, the end products are carbon dioxide and water. In an alcoholic, tetrahydroisoquinaline (THIQ), which is extremely addictive, is manufactured. When THIQ is injected into animals with an inherited aversion to alcohol, they will seek alcohol and choose it over water.[6]

Like diabetes, the disease of chemical dependency can be treated, but it cannot be cured. The drug chosen by the chemically dependent person *always* affects the central nervous system by altering the mood with behavioral results. The type of behavior can be predicted when the drug of choice is known. Depressants (alcohol, barbiturates, minor tranquilizers, sedatives, opiates, cannabis) affect the cerebral cortex, the center of intellect and emotions where awareness of reality is achieved. Stimulants and hallucinogens (amphetamines, PCP, preludin, mescaline) affect the limbic system (a section of the midbrain), which controls the affective (emotional) nature of sensory sensations, whether pleasant or painful, depressing or exciting. All psychotropic drugs produce both acute effects that are reversible, as well as chronic organic changes.[7] The chronic damage is limited to the midbrain (conducting impulses between "lower" and "higher" brain centers), whereas toxic levels affect the medulla (controlling visceral functions such as temperature), with death as a possible consequence. These drugs affect the cerebral cortex first, then the limbic system, and finally the medulla. Most drug-dependent people use enough drug(s) to alter the functioning of the limbic system so that their basic mood is changed, as is their emotional response to reality.

Of every 36 alcoholics, 96 per cent will die of alcoholism though the death certificates will name many other causes. Alcoholics are treated for all sorts of diseases, often with other drugs, which compounds the problem. They've been diagnosed as mentally ill or have been admitted to hospitals for pancreatitis, stomach ulcers, and so on. Of the 36 alcoholics, 3 per cent will recover; 1 per cent will become custodial in a nursing home or mental institution.[8]

FEMALE LIFE CHANGES

The way a woman copes with stress from infancy determines whether she will become dependent. As a child, adolescent, or adult, her coping skills and ability to deal with life's vicissitudes in her world of events and personal relationships are both rational and emotional. Reality includes pain, frustration, anger, anxiety, and unfulfilled needs. If parents have removed pain, solved problems, and protected her, she will be incapable of dealing rationally and emotionally with reality in a healthy way when confronted with conflict and anxiety.[2]

A teenager does not see drugs as a future problem as she experiments with pot and alcohol and discovers "euphoria" or "peace" while coping with the normal stress of adolescence. The maturation level of the adolescent causes her to seek instant gratification; the future is an hour away. Drugs work, for emotional pain is instantly alleviated. Therefore, she abdicates her chances of learning to manage frustration, rejection by a boyfriend, or tense situations at home.

When drugs are used to cope with reality by dulling the perception of stress, chemical dependency is a possible consequence primarily because of the physiologic affects. Alcohol is frequently the drug first used to relieve anxiety.[2]

Whether physical or psychic dependence or both, a woman's "need" is satisfied by the ingestion of a chemical. She wants the feeling that is a result of the chemical action in her body. The effects shield her from reality.

I soon learned that if I drank enough fast enough I could escape from reality. It was an "out" for me. I didn't drink to get high. I didn't like hang-overs, but I liked the feelings I got from alcohol.

Different decades within the life of a woman tend to have the same emotional and psychologic stress and exigencies of living. As an adolescent, she copes with her changing body and separation from home. During her 20s, she searches for intimacy and commitment while balancing the concomitant loyalty to a career. During her 30s, she realizes that her girlhood dreams have not been realized, that a toll has been extracted for her mistakes, and that she's ended up on the short end. In her 40s and 50s, she's lost her identity in her home and children, and suddenly she's old and unattractive.[3]

If it's okay for boys to be boys at whatever age, what happens when a teenaged girl drinks, even if her peers don't? Adolescent boys prove their masculinity by drinking, and parents will excuse a son's DWI as part of growing up. Although teenaged girls may not want to prove themselves adults, new role expectations suggest they can do anything boys can do. One author states that alcohol use among girls equals that of boys.[9]

I led a very sheltered life. I wasn't pretty, I thought I was fat, I didn't know how to flirt or act on a date.

I remember my first drink at a party when I was a high school senior. Suddenly I wasn't shy or clumsy, I could "put on the make" with a guy. I could even dance—provided I had a drink first!

I discovered that night that alcohol was the key to [overcoming] my total lack of self worth in relationships with my peers.

The stress of being a teenager requires a heightened ability to manage conflicts with parental values, decisions about sexual activity, frustrations and pressures of peers, and choices of college and career. Chemical dependency is a potential hazard if the adolescent experiments with alcohol and other drugs and discovers a relief from emotional trauma. When chemicals "solve" problems, constructive coping mechanisms are not developed. At the exact point of chemical dependency, the teenager stops growing emotionally. There-fore, a 20-year-old who became addicted at age 13 behaves like a 13 year-old and must make up "lost time" during and after treatment.

Teenagers dream, and the American dream includes the right to be free from pain, to be happy and fulfilled. Chemicals will provide this . . . for the moment. Even the average American adult believes that any discomfort can be eradicated with a chemical to provide instant relief. We are a nation that consumes tranquilizers at a rate of 120 million prescriptions a year.[10]

Changes in mood that correspond to hormonal shifts during menses are currently accepted as fact. The way in which a woman copes with the stress of these mood swings may lead to the use of alcohol. In a 1971 study by Belfer and associates, of 34 alcoholic women who related drinking to their menstrual cycle, 20 indicated that their drinking began or increased premenstrually.[11] Of the alcoholic women surveyed in this study, 67 per cent of the menstruating women linked their drinking to their menstrual cycle. Other studies point to specific physiologic trauma ranging from infertility to menopause.[2]

Hippocrates blamed premenstrual tension on poisonous blood.[12] The etiology is still uncertain, although water retention due to hormone imbalances seems important. Alcohol as a diuretic relieves symptoms associated with water retention: bloating, headache, irritability. Women learn that alcohol relieves cramps. Older nurses remember intravenous feedings of alcohol used to prevent a uterus from contracting during premature labor!

Mothers and well-meaning physicians give medication to teenaged girls to relieve premenstrual tension and menstrual cramping. Women describe the feeling of tension as irritability, depression, sensitivity, anxiety, and insecurity. When some cannot face these feelings with equanimity, they moderate their feelings with alcohol to alleviate the symptoms.

I drank much heavier during my period to relieve my feelings and the cramps. I have a natural "high" at the end of my period. So I drank then to get a "super high." Now, after treatment it helps to know when my period is coming so I can obtain emotional support, do exercises for the cramps, and enjoy the natural high afterwards!

As far back as 1937, a physician stated, "excessive drinking is more intimately associated with a definite life situation in females than in males." He suggested a relationship in women among premenstrual tension, cramping, and the use of alcohol. Postpartum depression and difficulty with menopause were also postulated.[13]

Because documentation does show a correlation between alcoholism and obstetric-gynecologic problems, the issue appears to be whether alcohol contributes to or is a consequence of these problems. It is clear from the literature that two research tracks have been followed. One studies the relationship between sex hormones and alcohol metabolism; the other is the inter-relationship of mood, hormonal changes, and patterns of alcohol use. Alcoholism in women is a product of our culture, but it is also because of the physiologic and endocrinologic reactions of women to alcohol, which are different from those of men.

Little research has addressed endocrine functions related to alcohol consumption, whereas numerous studies have documented the feminization of the male alcoholic as well as impotence and sterility. Alcohol-related endocrinologic dysfunction in females suggests clinical implications similar to testicular failure in men, such as ovarian failure and cessation of menstruation.[14]

An experiment conducted with female subjects indicates that sex hormone levels may be related to behavioral effects of alcohol. The females studied became more intoxicated than males with equivalent amounts of alcohol, especially if the alcohol was given premenstrually.[15]

Until the late 1960s, a wife expected to be "happy and fulfilled" in a well-polished house with several "lovely" children, chicken and apple pie on Sunday, and a contented husband who adored her. Reality hit abruptly when the kids went to school and hubby slopped in front of the T.V. every evening. Her enthusiam for daily living evaporated, because she had seen others only in relation to herself. She became bored, discontented, and felt like a dud.

I grew up thinking a woman's mission was to help a man. I had to be a lady, and being a person was to be female, cute, sexy. I knew that when the right man came into my life he would make me whole and everything would be alright. My ultimate dream was happiness with a husband, children, my home. But it didn't solve my problems and fix me for life. Now that I'm divorced my family still inquires, "Are you *really* happy as a single person?"

She not only felt unfulfilled; she believed she was a failure! Because she was a good wife, the woman's social life revolved around her husband's colleagues and friends, and she transferred with him from job to job. In the drinking atmosphere of her husband's social life, she felt less lonesome and ill-at-ease when she had a drink, which was also expected of her.

I felt more and more lifeless. I felt totally worthless to anyone and decided my family would be better without me. I reasoned that my husband was still young and could marry again and that because my children were very small they would adjust.

Her chemical dependency may have begun with a doctor's prescription for emotional discomfort such as anxiety, a sense of inadequacy, or loneliness—all normal emotions. The natural disinclination for scrubbing dirty saucepans or for worrying over a sick baby was cured by medicine in lieu of healthy coping mechanisms. Her physician knew her complaints did not have an organic basis, but the patient demanded to be well. The physician was probably unaware that she was an incipient alcoholic and enabled her disease to progress by adding another chemical. Physicians have treated female alcoholics much as they have male alcoholics, except for prescribing more combinations of drugs such as Antabuse, tranquilizers, and antidepressants.[3] Additionally, a woman who already has problems knows exactly what symptoms and signs to bring to her doctor's attention. She calls for help, as her family enables her to do, by protecting her problem, and her doctor helps mask the problem with pills. Later, she tells her family that the doctor suggested she's overworked, needs more rest, or has a case of "nerves."

A similar scenario is enacted with her clergyman, who agrees to counsel her and her husband concerning their "communication" problems. The pastor understands that she's overworked, is constantly giving of herself, and deserves a husband who is a better communicator. Other professionals are just as blind. Lawyers feel sorry for women, and judges give lenient sentences for alcohol-related offenses.

After her recovery and return to work, a nurse remarked:

I was astonished at the ignorance of doctors and nurses; obvious alcoholics did not have this disease mentioned anywhere on their chart. One was in a coma and dying—yet no one spoke about the disease of alcoholism which was killing him.

I've noticed in nursing journals where articles and studies deal with obvious alcohol problems—even cirrhosis of the liver—but the alcoholism is ignored.

Both role changes (e.g., the "empty nest syndrome") and physiologic changes in middle age send the middle-aged woman to the doctor or the bottle, or both. This woman has received her basic identity through her husband and her children. She's no longer needed. She feels empty; each day is a drag. She's lonely; the house is so quiet. Her pride has been in being a wife, mother, housekeeper, and hostess. She has little to offer in an inter-relationship with her husband. She suspects or accuses him of being interested in more vital women. And he may be! Either way, she feels innocent, a victim of circumstances, which makes her very resentful. Aha! Her age is to blame.

Because age serves as a rationale for stress, and for using drugs, menopause adds credence to the woman's argument. In addition, studies suggest that hormone changes during menopause may affect the pattern of alcohol use. Data collected from alcoholic women pinpoint menopause as the onset of their problem drinking.[15, 16] A British journal indicates that women are significantly older than men when their regular drinking begins. In addition, they have been drinking for a shorter period of time.[3] The hormonal imbalance during menopause may be a risk factor in the pathogenesis of cirrhosis of the liver, which occurs more frequently in alcoholic women than in alcoholic men.[2]

UNIQUE CHARACTERISTICS

Alcohol

Alcoholism, by its very nature, contributes to stress in a woman's life. Whether stress precipitated the alcoholism or alcoholism created the stress is a moot question. Studies debate both.

Stress escalates as a woman spends more time and energy hiding her disease. The more drink or medication she takes, the less she sees of what is actually happening and the more vehemently she denies her illness. There follows a merry-go-round of self-denial, family denial, society's denial, and perhaps denial by professionals to whom she goes for help. She's terrified that people will discover her problem and that her husband will divorce her (90 per cent of husbands leave their chemically dependent wives, whereas 10 per cent of wives leave their chemically dependent husbands[17]) or that her boss will fire her (if she were a man, her boss would arrange treatment).

A phenomenon labeled "telescoping" suggests that once women become heavy drinkers, the course of alcoholism is swift and grave. Theories blame women's extended period of secret drinking and their apparent ability to absorb alcohol faster and to reach higher peak blood alcohol levels than men.[1, 2]

Drugs

More women than men consume psychotropic drugs.[18, 19] When an annual physical exam indicates emotional stress, a physician typically prescribes a medication or refers the woman to a psychologist or psychiatrist.[7]

I went to a psychiatrist for one year. I thought I was mentally ill but he said I just drank too much. And he thought it was funny! He wanted to talk about dreams—and I don't dream!

Men consult a physician for physical problems. Women usually go to physicians when they are healthy. They go for birth control, abortion, prenatal care, childbirth, breast exams, and pap smears. They are also the ones who take children to the doctor for routine check-ups, immunizations, school physicals, and summer camp health records.

Women go to physicians more often, are admitted more frequently to hospitals, have more surgery, consume more medications, and are committed to mental hospitals more often than men. This dependence on doctors has created a situation in which healthy American women are given medications and even surgery that are not medically justified.[10]

Women often describe their signs and symptoms in emotional terms. When physicians find no physical pathophysiology, the physician, who has been taught in medical school that women's problems are usually emotional, prescribes pharmaceuticals.

I was so tired. I went to my doctor who prescribed an amphetamine to get me going each morning, a tranquilizer to get me through the day, and a sedative so I could sleep at night. I never told him—nor did he ask—that I was drinking.

Prescriptions against "migraine," "diet," "insomnia," "nerves," "exhaustion," and "loss of energy" give the woman an excuse to use these drugs, and she can "blame" her doctor when convenient. Concomitantly, drug companies bias advertisements of psychotropics toward females. Liquor advertisements are also targeted at the female market.

A wide variety of chemicals, ranging from uppers (amphetamines, speed) to downers (Valium, sedatives, alcohol), produce central nervous system effects ranging from stimulation to depression. Drugs with alcohol are a combination becoming more widespread among women. People who have developed a tolerance to alcohol usually have a cross tolerance to other chemicals that are sedative in nature. The interaction of alcohol with psychotropic drugs is not well understood by physicians. The effect of taking two chemicals may be more pronounced than a larger dose of one chemical; women do overdose unintentionally.

Without variance, statistics show that the pattern of stress factors and the way women cope with them are of consequence; they are very different from the stress factors of men.[8] In women, a specific traumatic event more probably precipitates drinking, even without a history of alcohol abuse, than it does in men. The crises cited include infidelity, desertion, divorce, postpartum depression, a child leaving home, a death of a member of the family, and a wide range of physical problems.[2, 8] As mentioned earlier, female alcoholics are more frequently divorced than are male alcoholics; they are also more often widowed.[3] Psychologist Joan Curlee[19] discovered that in a sample of 200 people undergoing treatment of alcoholism, one third of the women and only one twenty-fifth of the men could specify a particular traumatic event that triggered their alcoholism. Almost all traumatic events articulated by the women revolved around their perceived "lower status" as wives and mothers.[8]

Women who have entered treatment institutions have had poorer physical health, a lower satisfaction with self, and fewer resources for support.[3]

Alcoholics have the same percentage of mental illnessess and emotional problems as other people, and this clouds the issue. Recovering from chemical dependency does not mean recovery from physical disease or mental disorders. A diagnosis of chemical dependency is difficult even without the complications of physical or psychologic diseases or both.[7]

Women are more vulnerable to depression than men; and more women have a primary diagnosis of depression, with alcoholism as a secondary diagnosis. Approximately 25 per cent of alcoholic women are primary depressives, a rate that is four to eight times higher than the 3 to 5 per cent rate in the general population.[20] A metaphor may facilitate the understanding of someone who starts drinking and who has a primary diagnosis of depression, and ends up an alcoholic. She drops a match in a building, a small fire starts (marital unhappiness, a child dying). While the woman addresses this fire, the rest of the building has caught fire (alcoholism), and it's burning down. While alleviating or curing the depression, the woman has become an alcoholic.[21]

Because affective behavior in alcoholism and depression are similar, it may be necessary for a woman to be free of alcohol to make an accurate determination of her disease.

WOMEN IN THE 1980s

Contributing to the etiology of alcoholism are the disparate social roles of men and women, which produce very divergent types of psychologic tensions and life problems; culturally defined behaviors demanded of women are extremely important.[8]

"You've come a long way, baby" epitomizes the liberated females of the 1980s. More women meet their male colleagues in bars, compete with men on their turf, and accept drinking as part of their role. More women are having a drink before dinner to relax after a hard day. Some "drink like a man." Some order "men's" drinks—and make their orders directly to the wine steward instead of to their escorts, as was "proper" until recently.

Perhaps the liberated female of the 1980s is not liberated. Because of social transition, the movement toward independence, autonomy, and self-realization is accompanied by the stress of coping with older role expectations and the new self. Stress is heightened as women struggle to construct new lives in a social environment that sometimes expects old roles and sometimes expects a new, autonomous role. The highest number of female alcoholics are women who are married and work away from their homes.[8] A dual identity including living up to others' expectations is confusing, to say the least. Consider the female executive who comes home to a husband relaxing with the paper while he waits for her to prepare dinner; or to a child who expects a caring listener; or to guests who expect graciousness, poise, and stimulating conversation. This is to say nothing of the alive, exciting sexual partner she is expected to be later that evening.

I was married and had three children in 3½ years. In addition to the diapers, bottles and runny noses I worked full-time. My husband came home from work and sat in front of the T.V. drinking beer. I waited on him hand and foot but resented every minute of it.

This woman has no extended family for support when daily life gets to be too much. Mother and grandmother aren't around to help out for a day or two, so that she can catch up. In days gone by, women were expected to be "more emotional" and "delicate," and it was accepted practice to go to bed for several days when under stress. Who knows how many tranquilizers and drinks are taken to ward off what was previously taken care of by a day or two in bed?

PATHOPHYSIOLOGY

It is extremely important to remember that, although alcohol is a sedative and depresses the function of the brain cells, in small doses (only one or two drinks) it stimulates the appetite, reduces anxiety, and increases self-confidence. A person does not feel depressed, because the drug reduces inhibitions and allows for good feelings.[7] Because anxiety is lessened and confidence is up, the drinker does not perceive alcohol as a sedative. Before drowsiness is noted, the brain function changes, producing relaxation, talkativeness, and friendliness—but also produces changes with regard to reflexes and judgement.

Voluminous literature[2, 9, 17, 22–27] delineates the effects of chemicals on virtually every system in the body. Alcohol impedes blood flow to the heart, causes loss of body heat because of the dilation of blood vessels in the skin, depresses the formation of various blood cells, lowers resistance to infection, precipitates bleeding/clotting problems, raises the blood pressure, destroys muscle cells with consequent weakness, causes the head of the femur (hip bone) to become necrotic, leaches calcium from bones, and inflames the kidney. People who are chemically dependent have a higher incidence of diabetes, hypertension, and emphysema. As alcoholism progresses, other diseases progress as well.[7] Psychologic phenomena, such as stress, speed up the emptying time of food in the stomach, and consequently the rate of absorption of alcohol is increased. For men and women, there are differential health risks. Morbidity in females appears to be accelerated. Anemias are more prevalent in women alcoholics. A shorter heavy drinking history before the initial occurrence of most diseases is found in women.

Blood levels of alcohol depend on a person's size, for the effect of alcohol depends on how much is concentrated in the blood. Women are usually smaller than men, have less blood, and therefore can expect higher blood levels from the same-sized drink than man can expect. In addition, the greater amount of muscle (not fat) the lower the blood level of alcohol, because muscle fibers assimilate alcohol.

High blood pressure and cancer, especially breast cancer, seem to have special relevance when related to alcohol abuse. Interestingly, stress appears significant in the development of high blood pressure, breast cancer, and correlations with alcoholism. Records of menstrual irregularities in chronic alcoholic women go back to 1813.[2]

The pathophysiologic effects of chemicals present a consequence for the innocent—from the person driving a car on the same highway to the fetus growing in an alcoholic mother's uterus.

Small amounts of alcohol cause the eyes to accommodate to bright light in about double the time, and they remain in such a state for up to six hours. Visual acuity is then impaired, with resultant inability to follow a moving object. Consequently, only large objects are recognized and small things, such as a child, are not identified. Large amounts of alcohol cause double vision. Reaction time is protracted and coordination impaired.

FETAL ALCOHOL SYNDROME

The past five years have produced information about the fetal alcohol syndrome, a set of signs and symptoms that characterize a baby born of an alcoholic mother.

Greek and Roman mythology refer to what we now know as fetal alcohol syndrome. Bridal couples in Carthage were not allowed to drink wine on their wedding night, to prevent defective babies from being conceived.[28]

A report in 1834 describes infants born to alcoholic mothers with "a starved, shrivelled and imperfect look."[2] Up to the present, studies on both animals and humans document a definite pattern of fetal malformation resulting from maternal alcoholism.[25, 29–32] Most profound are characteristic facial features, small stature, and mental deficiency. There has been no indication that children have caught up in growth or performance later in life; some effects may appear only when the child is older.[2, 28]

What has been termed the "placental barrier" appears not to be a barrier to alcohol; alcohol enters the fetal blood stream and gains access to the fetal tissues, including the brain tissue, at about the same level as it enters the mother's. Even the baby's breath after birth and the amniotic fluid may have an alcoholic odor.[30] Alcohol itself is toxic, but the products of alcohol breakdown in the body also affect the fetus.[32] Evidence does not conclude whether the problem is from the alcohol, its metabolites, or both.

The newborn fetus can be physically addicted; within hours after birth, alcohol withdrawal, including delirium tremens and convulsions, occurs with severity that depends on the amount and duration of the mother's drinking. Treatment may be delayed if the physician is unaware of the mother's alcohol intake, for he or she may suspect various other diagnoses. Different degrees of fetal liver damage may occur, owing to heavy alcohol exposure. It is clearly possible that less severely affected children may be born of women who drink less than the alcoholic.[30] Poor food intake and hyperactivity of the newborn child may be subtle disturbances that interfere with infant-mother bonding and were caused by alcohol consumption during pregnancy. In this case, the mother may question her adequacy as a mother and then turn to the bottle for solace.[2] In addition, alcohol is secreted in the breast milk of nursing mothers.[32]

The National Institute of Neurological Diseases and Stroke completed a study of 55,000 pregnancies in 1973. Women who were alcoholic during their pregnancies delivered babies with fetal alcohol syndrome at a rate of 32 out of 100. Perinatal mortality was 17 per cent, and 44 per cent of the babies were mentally retarded. Women who consume about four drinks daily risk a 10 per cent chance of giving birth to a child with fetal alcohol syndrome; more than four increases the chances to between 19 and 74 per cent.[31, 33]

The first three months of pregnancy, the time when some women do not realize they are pregnant, appear to be most critical. High blood levels of alcohol during this trimester may place the fetal developing cells and tissues at great risk. A fetus cannot, even for an hour or so, tolerate a toxic chemical environment.[34] Even the mother's getting drunk at a party only once may coincide with the critical moment when the roof of the mouth is being formed and, as a result of the alcohol, the child may be born with a cleft palate. One physician goes far enough to suggest that ". . . ideally such women should be encouraged and assisted in exercising effective birth control until such time as they can discontinue the alcohol intake. If pregnancy should occur in such a woman, she should be offered the alternative of terminating the pregnancy."[30] The Surgeon General advises women to abstain even when considering pregnancy, and to be aware of the amount of alcohol in foods and medication.[35] Obviously, a safe level of alcohol consumption during pregnancy is zero. Fetal alcohol syndrome is 100 per cent preventable.

INTERVENTION AND TREATMENT

Given that alcohol presents a problem for women in our society, how can such a hopeless situation as an alcoholic woman be changed? How does the chemically dependent woman receive help? Unfortunately for many, the agony for the entire family continues. The family has already pleaded, manipulated, bargained, prayed, reasoned, and threatened. It is hoped that someone will intervene—a family member who will finally let out the secret; an employer who gives an alternative of treatment or termination; or a physician, clergyman, or counselor who becomes suspicious.

Intervention is the process used when people who are important to the chemically dependent person, with the help of professionals, present data about behavior and chemical use that forces the woman to look at herself, assessing the woman for chemical dependency, and persuading her to enter treatment if drug-dependence is determined. Vernon E. Johnson, in *I'll Quit Tomorrow,* spells out the specific steps.[36] Dr. George Mann, in *Recovery of Reality,* writes about the treatment process.[7]

If up to 64 per cent of all hospital admissions are related to alcohol consumption[37] and if more women than men are hospitalized, nurses need to ask about patients' alcohol intake just as they ask about allergies when doing a nursing assessment. Often a clinic, public health, or home health nurse is the first to become aware of problems. Women, more than men, during their early alcoholism report searching for a change of mood, and talk about finding bruises and injuries that they have no knowledge of incurring. Women with alcoholic problems report more gynecologic and obstetric problems than the general population. A higher incidence of jaundice and ascites among women is known, and one study suggests that physical illness secondary to alcoholism is more common among women than among men.[38]

Nurses are doing a patient a favor by documenting the possibility of alcoholism, for an alcoholic requires different anesthetics, special postoperative management, and medications, to prevent withdrawal symptoms and delirium tremens. This is especially important for patients with early symptoms of alcoholism: frequent gastrointestinal problems, sleep disturbances, liver or pancreatic disease, frequent respiratory disease, or emotional problems. The admitting diagnosis can range from gastritis to depression, or from hypertension to liver disease. Often, the physical signs and symptoms of alcoholism are treated without reference to this primary disease. A potential diagnosis of alcoholism or a subterfuged diagnosis from physicians needs to be communicated by nurses to their peers, so that disruptive behavior, elevated vital signs, diaphoresis, or even delirium tremens are not a surprise, and so that appropriate nursing intervention can augment the medical management. Even a nonalcoholic patient who drinks regularly can experience some agitation because alcohol is not available during hospitalization.

A nonjudgmental inquiry seeking only information with direct, factual questions often provides a picture, even when the alcoholic denies any problem. Questions need to focus on what, where, and when drinking is done; not on why it is done. Specific assessment strategies for nurses can be found in an *American Journal of Nursing* article.[39]

Nurses need to be aware of chemical abuse among their colleagues. High-stress working conditions, readily available drugs, and easily obtained prescriptions from physician friends contribute to the misuse of chemicals for nurses. Some nurses, although keenly aware of the potential for drug abuse, may not associate the use of alcohol as a drug with its insidious potential for addiction. Confronting colleagues about drug and alcohol abuse and supporting them in a recovery program, rather than protecting and covering for them, for fear of their losing jobs and licenses, ultimately restores health and sanity. The American Nurses' Association House of Delegates' position statement of 1982 about alcohol and drug abuse by nurses clearly supports this type of caring.

The chemically dependent woman has unique needs both during and after treatment. Usually, she will need treatment for depression or for polydrug use, or both. Very real concerns associated with her role also need attention.

My stress over the care of the kids while I was in treatment made it difficult to concentrate on my recovery. I felt guilty because I believed I was neglecting them. These worries, plus financial concerns, limited my choices for aftercare treatment following discharge.

A white-knuckled, teeth-gritting sobriety is very lonely and often leads to relapse. The woman will always be recovering because of the chronic nature of her disease, and she'll initially require the support and care that can be given only by other women who are confident and assertive about being female and who can be role models for parenting and who can help her to capitalize on her vocational skills. An Alcoholics Anonymous (A.A.) group for women, or a group suited to specific areas (e.g., a group for recovering nurses), may be vital at first.

I used to, while drinking, get good feelings having a man on my arm. I felt complete when he made love to me. I didn't realize that I was prostituting my personhood. A woman's AA helped reinforce that at first. Now I'm in a mixed group where I'm a person who is an alcoholic before I'm a woman. I am now proud of being a woman, a woman who has a job and am whole without my husband.

The label and stigma of alcoholism follows a recovered alcoholic woman. The perception of society continues after a woman's rehabilitation. She is punished and discriminated against in a variety of ways, from employment to insurance coverage. She wonders if it is safe to risk telling of her history, and she and those close to her are tempted to use terms such as "problem" and "little illness" and to provide rationales for abstinence to "allergies," "stomach problems," and "nerves."

After treatment I became employed at a different hospital. I didn't tell people about my alcoholism because I suspected it would jeopardize my professional future. I was glad I hadn't for the nurses talked about alcoholics with derogation and contempt.

I was open about my alcoholism but I felt like a prime suspect. After six weeks I was accused of drinking on the job and was asked to resign. They even complained to the State Board of Nursing. Consequently I had to hire a lawyer and was given a 2 year conditional license.

Recovered male alcoholics have a double standard, too. The loneliness of being an odd one in a predominantly male A.A. is very real.

Eleven years ago after I'd completed treatment for alcoholism, I felt like a tramp in A.A. The innuendoes and offers of the men in the group indicated their judgment of me as a bar hop and prostitute.

The men in my A.A. group had no problem with my use of tranquilizers. But my drinking was another matter!

Changes of attitudes are indicated, though.

Four years ago when I joined A.A. I was put on a pedestal and considered very courageous.

A chemically dependent woman cannot depend solely on others for sobriety. The miracle of recovery is made up of the combination of a program for increasing inner strength and peace, and of sharing experiences, strengths, and hopes with other recovering people.[7]

The stresses I live with are the same as the stresses I had before. I just cope with them differently now.

I socialize with living things and am having fun in sobriety.

I need to verbalize about my stress; that takes the power out of it. My sponsor and AA friends are marvelous listeners.

One nurse, recovering for almost 15 years, exclaims,

I did it—with the help of others—but I did it!!

It is obvious that the most thoughtful writing and the most current research efforts must culminate in a statement that more information is required before any valid conclusions based on solid data about female chemical dependency can be made. All that has been accepted as fact is being questioned and re-examined. We know how much we do not know.

References

1. Estes, Nada, Smith-Dijulio, and Heinemann, M. *Nursing Diagnosis of the Alcoholic Person.* St. Louis: C. V. Mosby, 1980.
2. Mendelson, Jack, and Mellow, Nancy (eds). *The Diagnosis and Treatment of Alcoholism.* New York: McGraw-Hill, 1979.
3. Smart, Reginald G. Female and male alcoholics in treatment: Characteristics at intake and recovery rates. *British Journal of Addiction,* Vol. 74, 1979, pp. 275–281.
4. Goodwin, D. W., Schulsinger, R., et al. Drinking problems in adopted and non-adopted sons of alcoholics. *Archives of General Psychiatry,* vol. 32, 1974, pp. 164–169.
5. Kinney, Jean, and Leaton, Gwen. *Loosening the Grip.* St. Louis: C. V. Mosby, 1978.
6. Ohlms, David. *Disease Concept of Alcoholism*: A Basic Lecture for Alcoholism Treatment. Detection, Prevention, and Public Education. Belleville, IL: Gary Whiteaker Co., 1981.
7. Mann, George. *Recovery of Reality.* New York: Harper and Row, 1979.
8. Sandmaier, Marian. *The Invisible Alcoholics.* New York: McGraw-Hill, 1980.
9. Oh, S. U. Chronic alcoholic myopathy. *Southern Medical Journal,* vol. 65, 1972, pp. 449–452.
10. Hughes, Richard, and Brewin, Robert. *The Tranquilizing of America.* New York and London: Harcourt, Brace, Jovanovich, 1979.
11. Belfer, J. L., Shader, R. L., Carroll, M., Harmatz, J. S. Alcoholism in women. *Archives of General Psychiatry,* 1971, pp. 540–544.
12. Podolsky, Edward. The woman alcoholic and premenstrual tensions. *Journal of the American Medical Women's Association,* vol. 18, pp. 816–818.
13. Wall, J. H. A study of alcoholism in women. *American Journal of Psychiatry,* vol. 93, 1937, pp. 943–952.
14. Ryback, Ralph. Chronic alcohol consumption and menstruation. *Journal of the American Medical Association,* vol. 238, 1977, p. 2143.
15. Jones, B. M., and Jones, M. K. Alcohol effects in women during the menstrual cycle. *Annals, New York Academy of Sciences,* vol. 273, 1976, pp. 576–587.

16. Belfer, J. L., and Shader, R. I. *Alcoholism Problems in Women and Children.* New York: Grune and Stratton, 1976.
17. Cowan, D. W., and Hines, J. D. Thrombocytopenia of severe alcoholism. *Annals of Internal Medicine,* vol. 74, 1971, pp. 37–43.
18. Cooperstock, R. Women and psychotropic drugs. *In* MacLennan, A. (ed.). *Women: Their Use of Alcohol and Other Legal Drugs.* Toronto: Addiction Research Foundation of Ontario, 1976.
19. Curlee, J. A. A comparison of male and female patients at an alcoholism treatment center. *Journal of Psychiatry,* vol. 129, 1972, p. 127.
20. Halsukami, Dorothy, and Pickins, Ray. *Depression and Alcoholism.* Center City, MN: Hazelden Literature, 1980, pp. 1–30.
21. Scarf, Maggie. *Unfinished Business, Pressure Points in the Lives of Women.* New York: Doubleday, 1980.
22. Beard, J. D., and Knott, D. H. Hematopoietic response to experimental chronic alcoholism. *American Journal of Medical Science,* vol. 252, 1966, pp. 518–525.
23. Guyton, Arthur. *Textbook of Medical Physiology.* Philadelphia: W. B. Saunders, 1985.
24. Hourihane, D. O. B. Suppression of erythropoiesis by alcohol. *British Medical Journal,* vol. 1, 1970, pp. 86–89.
25. McCurdy, P. R., et al. Abnormal bone marrow morphology in acute alcoholism. *New England Journal of Medicine,* vol. 2, 1957, pp. 236–240.
26. Shanoff, H. M. Alcoholic cardiomyopathy, an introductory review. *Canadian Medical Association Journal,* vol. 106, 1972, pp. 55–61.
27. Webb, W. R., et al. Ethyl alcohol and the cardiovascular system. *Journal of the American Medical Association,* vol. 191, March 1965, pp. 1055–1058.
28. Haggard, H. W., and Jellinek, E. M. *Alcohol Explored.* Garden City, NY, 1942.
29. Ferrier, P. E., Nicod, I., and Ferrier, S. Fetal alcohol syndrome. *Lancet,* vol. 2, 1973.
30. Hanson, J., et al. Fetal alcohol syndrome: Experience with forty-one patients. *Journal of the American Medical Association,* vol. 235, April 1976, pp. 1458–1460.
31. Jones, R., et al. Outcome in offspring of chronic alcoholic women. *Lancet,* vol. 1, 1974, pp. 1267–1270.
32. Waltman, R., and Iniquez, E. S. Placental transfer of ethahol and its elimination at term. *Obstetrics and Gynecology,* vol. 40, 1972, pp. 180–185.

33. Kaminski, M., et al. Consumption of alcohol among pregnant women and outcome of pregnancy. Transl. from *Paris Revue d'Epidémiologie et Santé Publique,* vol. 24, 1966, pp. 27–40.
34. Noble, E. P. National awareness of fetal alcohol syndrome sought. *NIAAA Information and Feature Service,* vol. 39, September 8, 1977.
35. U.S. Department of Health and Human Services. A Practical Guide for Ob/Gyn Physicians and Nurses. Alcohol, Drug Abuse and Mental Health Administration, National Institute on Alcohol Abuse and Alcoholism, Public Health Service, Pub. No. (ADM) 81–1163, 1981.
36. Johnson, Vernon. *I'll Quit Tomorrow.* New York: Harper and Row, 1973.
37. Stark, J. J., and Nichols, H. G. Alcohol-related admissions to a general hospital. *Alcohol Health and Research World,* vol. 1, 1977, pp. 11–14.
38. Estes, Nada, and Heinemann, M. *Alcoholism; Development, Consequences, and Intervention.* St. Louis, C. V. Mosby, 1982.
39. Weist, J. K., Lindeman, M. C., and Newton, M. Hospital dialogues. *American Journal of Nursing,* vol. 82, 1982, pp. 1874–1877.

General References

Goodwin, D. W., Schulsinger, R., et al. Alcoholism and depression in adopted-out daughters of alcoholics. *Archives of General Psychiatry,* vol. 34, 1974, pp. 751–755.

Jones, Kenneth L, and Smith, David W. Recognition of the fetal alcohol syndrome in early infancy. *Lancet,* vol. 2, 1973, pp. 999–1001.

Jones, K., Smith, D., et al. Patterns of malformation in offspring of chronic alcoholic mothers. *Lancet,* vol. 1, 1973, pp. 1267–1270.

Kaij, L., and Dock, J. Grandsons of alcoholics. *Archives of General Psychiatry,* vol. 32, 1975, pp. 1379–1381.

Kreisberg, R. A. Glucose-lactate inter-relations in men. *New England Journal of Medicine,* vol. 287, 1972, pp. 132–137.

Van Thiel, D. H. Testicular atrophy and other endocrine changes in alcoholic men. *Journal of Human Sexuality,* June 1976.

11

SEXISM AND ITS RESULTING EFFECT ON THE MENTAL HEALTH OF WOMEN

DIANE KJERVIK

Diane Kjervik's chapter on the role of sexism and its effect on women's mental health first addresses both the definition of sexism and its manifestations. A closer examination is given to women and mental health, which includes the undoing of sexism in mental health by the therapist and the role of feminist-oriented counseling. The chapter closes with implications for education and research.

The mental health of women has been jeopardized by the sexist orientation in our society, a society that has taught women to believe that they are inferior to men. Women are often able to overturn the effects of sexism, at least in part, and to become more assertive, autonomous individuals. Stages through which women pass in confronting sexism are discussed in this chapter, along with methods that therapists can use to facilitate this process.

SEXISM: DEFINITION AND MANIFESTATIONS

In order to understand the status of women in this society, the concept of *sexism* must be clarified. Sexism, according to Shortridge, is "a belief that the human sexes have a distinctive make-up that determines their respective lives, usually involving the idea that one sex is superior and has the right to rule the other."[1] Shortridge also includes the political and societal support of such an asserted right in her definition. This concept is similar to the concept of caste, according to which, by birthright, persons' roles within society are fixed. Sexism exists in educational, economic, religious, legal, and political arenas of this society. Less

apparent to the public is the sexism that exists in the health care field, specifically in the mental health care system.

Women are cast into societal roles at birth. Women, as a group (and there are always a few exceptions to the rule), are taught in school and in their families to be passive, nurturant, and expressive of emotion; whereas males are reinforced for aggressive, emotionless, and rational behavior. Girls learn to look to boys or men rather than to themselves for answers. They grow up being encouraged to marry a lawyer rather than to become a lawyer. We know about this sex role socialization process, and some of us know that women earn 57 per cent of what men earn, according to the government's latest figures. This percentage has been steadily declining since 1960, when women were earning 61 per cent of male salaries (median income for year-round, full-time workers).[2] As a sidelight, male nurses earn one-third higher salaries than female nurses on the average.[3] In that money is a kind of power, one can see that women are disadvantaged economically.

Also, in religious, legal, and political areas, women are under-represented in leadership roles. It is interesting that female achievement in occupational, economic, and educational realms between 1940 and 1965 declined to below the pre-1940 levels. Before 1940, women were not equally represented.[4] One could speculate that the declining status of women has been an impetus to the resurgence of the women's movement in the 1960s.

Despite the efforts of the women's movement, sexism holds fast in many facets of our society. Recent evidence points to a lack of progress for women in higher educational administration. Two surveys have found that colleges and universities have not achieved equality for women administrators, in either salaries or number of positions held; in fact, women were found to be grossly under-represented.[5]

The abortion rights of poor women are threatened by recent congressional action limiting federal funds to pay for abortions. The Supreme Court ruled in December 1976 that companies do not have to pay for pregnancy-related disability benefits (General Electric v. Gilbert), which meant that working women had to choose between their jobs and motherhood if they suffered disabilities such as severe varicose veins that prohibited walking following labor and delivery. This decision was changed by the Pregnancy Discrimination Act of 1978, which includes pregnancy discrimination as a form of sex-based discrimination. Pornographic images in magazines and movies increasingly eroticize violence against women.

On the other hand, progress toward equality continues in other places. Married couples, as of June 1977, may maintain individual credit accounts if they so choose. A recall election was held in Madison, Wisconsin, which resulted in the removal of a judge from office for ruling as "normal" the behavior of an adolescent boy who allegedly raped a 16-year-old girl. A nurse who was discharged from the Navy in 1967 because she was pregnant will be allowed reinstatement at her old rank and will receive 10 years of back pay.[6]

It is not the purpose of this chapter to examine why or how discrimination against women evolved but rather to focus on one way that sexism is maintained, that is, by beliefs about the mental health of males and females, respectively.

WOMEN AND MENTAL HEALTH

John Stuart Mill, the great 19th-century philosopher, acknowledged in his essay entitled "On the Subjection of Women" the impor-

tance of the subversion of the mind to the maintenance of the second-class status of women: "All men, except the most brutish, desire to have, in the women most nearly connected with them, not a forced slave but a willing one, not a slave merely, but a favourite [sic]. They have therefore put everything in practice to enslave their minds."[7] Mill goes on to say that the enslavement of a female's mind occurs as a result of males conveying to females that meekness, submissiveness, and resignation of their will into male hands is essential to sexual attractiveness.[8] Whenever one's identity is so wrapped up in one's sexual attractiveness, as in our society, this form of mental enslavement as described by Mill contributes to keeping women in a submissive, dependent position in relation to men.

Work done by a psychologist in Colorado, Anne Wilson Schaef, tends to support the idea that women need to seek male (specifically white male) approval. She relates this need for approval to the "original sin of being born female," which she believes every woman carries with her.[9] If males like what a woman does, she can eliminate some of the pain of this original sin that is inherently a part of her femaleness. Thus, a woman can save herself only by being saved by someone else!

Alexandra Symonds, a psychoanalyst, describes women who are very successful professionally yet have great dependency needs on the personal level. She notes the difficulty in working with these women because of their deep sense of inferiority and repulsion about their femaleness. These clients believe that they need a man so that they can value themselves.[10]

The effect of this need for validation from others is a tremendous lessening of a woman's self-esteem. In my practice as a psychotherapist, I find that often female patients do not have a negative or poor opinion of themselves; rather, they have no self-concept. When asked what they need or want, they answer that "my father wants me to be . . ." or "my sister thinks I am . . . ." They draw a blank on self-evaluations.

One of my clients stated that she felt unreal, not human. Part of this nonperson feeling she connected to the possibility of not having a male lover. On the other hand, she felt worthless when she cared for a man, as if her self was abnegated. This conflict manifested a very weak, if not absent, sense of self. Her relationships with females were no better. She distrusted other women and was jealous of any woman her male friend was near. She could not accept these jealous and nonperson feelings and, probably as a result of this, was extremely anxious and suffered from asthmatic attacks. Despite these limitations she was a successful artist. This client was much like Symonds' who displayed extreme dependency on the personal level. At one point, the client acknowledged her wish to be mothered and admitted that she clung to her "sick role" in an effort to maintain the therapy relationship. The deep dependency need is described by Horney as "having the center of gravity outside oneself."[11]

Another of my clients was trying to decide whether to stay in an unsatisfying relationship with a man. One of her primary wishes was to be taken care of by him, and her chief complaint was that he was too dependent on her. She put it this way: "If he needs me that much, he isn't a man." The belief that men and women have distinctly different psychologic needs and abilities led this client to a rigid way of viewing herself and her partner. Mental health is often seen as the ability to move flexibly from one stage of development to the next or from one role to another without major conflictual problems. This client's stereotyping held her to a rigid expectation of herself and her friend. It did not allow her to grow beyond the assigned behavior.

These women in therapy acted out, in a sense, attitudes toward females that are present in society. Studies have shown that negative opinions of females prevail generally in our society, among both women and men. Broverman and co-workers showed that, regardless of the respondent's age, sex, religion, educational level, or marital status, men and women were described differently—men having characteristics in the "competence" realm, and women having characteristics in the "warmth and expressiveness" realm.[12] Very significantly, the male characteristics were more often valued than the female characteristics. A recent study showed that sex-role stereotypes remain, although attitudes about desirable characteristics have changed during the 1970s.[13]

Statistics relating to psychiatric diagnosis, treatment, and prognosis reveal further differences based on sex. Women are more often treated for mental illness; Chesler's study showed that around 60 per cent of the total patient population was female.[14] Brandon found that women are more often admitted to psychiatric hospitals and once there stay longer than men.[15] Fabrikant found similar evidence when he looked at psychotherapy that therapists themselves had received: Female therapists had had more treatment than male therapists and spent more time in psychotherapy. Female patients were found to have been in therapy over twice as long as male patients.[16] Fabrikant's evidence was gathered from the patients' own reports and might have been influenced by the possibility that it is more acceptable for women to be in a sick role in society than it is for men.

Ineichen reports that women, more often than men, are afflicted with neuroses.[17] Seiden states that more women than men are judged to be clinically depressed.[18] Chesler discovered that females are more often labeled depressed, frigid, paranoid, neurotic, suicidal, and anxious. Men's symptoms are alcoholism, drug addiction, personality disorders, and brain diseases.[19] Think of why these diagnostic differences might exist. Notice that the symptoms attributed to women are considered more treatable than the male symptoms. Treatability means, of course, the opportunity to become dependent on a therapist. Since the vast majority of psychotherapists are male, this means another kind of dependence on males in a form different from dependence on a husband or a father.

A 1976 study showed that the use of mood-altering drugs is a major problem for the mental health of women. Women consume 70 per cent of prescribed tranquilizers and 72 per cent of prescribed antidepressants.[20] This again supports women in their passive patient roles. Thomas Szasz calls the conglomerate of female symptoms "dread of happiness" indicators—part of a slave psychology or, as I see it, the psychology of oppression.[21] A question that could be posed is: Do the symptoms really vary or are people placed in slots according to their sex?

Another 1976 study supports the latter contention by demonstrating that children were apt to be referred to mental health professionals when they demonstrated behavior inappropriate to their sex. That is, when boys were passive or girls were aggressive they were often judged to be in need of psychiatric help.[22]

The judgments in the Feinblatt study were made by graduate students in one of the mental health training programs. What becomes apparent, then, is the importance of the beliefs of the mental health professionals themselves in making supposedly objective decisions about diagnosis and treatment plans. A study conducted by Broverman and co-workers and published in 1970 showed that mental health professionals considered mental health to be a different phenomenon for men than for women. Mentally healthy men were considered the same as mentally healthy adults, but mentally healthy women were given a separate description. Mature, mentally healthy women were considered to be different from healthy men or adults by being "more submissive, less independent, less adventurous, more easily influenced, less aggressive, less competitive, more excitable in minor crises, having their feelings hurt more easily, being more emotional, more conceited about their appearance, less objective and disliking math and science."[23] The beliefs of these clinicians (psychiatrists, psychologists, and psychiatric social workers) were in agreement with generally held beliefs about the characteristics that are socially desirable for a man or woman. Also, there was no significant difference between male and female clinicians in holding these beliefs. The results of this study pointed to a double standard of mental health for men and women, whereby a woman might have to give up her femininity in order to be considered mentally healthy. One wonders then, what route a therapist will take in guiding her or his female client to mental health—a road to femininity or a road to adulthood? Psychotherapists are very influential, not only with individual clients but also in directing societal notions of mental health. The Broverman study indicates a subtle form of sexism being supported by mental health professionals.

The ramifications of this double standard of mental health are great. If women cannot achieve adulthood without losing their femininity, is it any wonder that our language reflects such a situation? For example, women of any age are referred to as "girls;" and, not surprisingly, masculine pronouns are used generically, to mean everyone. Occasionally, reference is made to an individual having to decide whether *he* will have an abortion.[24] Adult men typify normalcy—women are deviations from the norm—and our language reflects this. The problem with the use of "man" for everyone is that authors often switch from the generic to the specific in very confusing ways, especially if the reader is a woman. For example, Swami Ajaya in *Yoga Psychology* discussed the process of meditation by mentioning that people often try to find happiness in external objects, which only provide temporary solace—examples of external objects being a football game, an ice cream cone, or a girl. People are always stated to be "man,"

of course. Later he says that meditation leads to enriched relationships with other people: "Seeing people less as objects to satisfy your desires allows you to notice things about them which previously went unobserved." However, seeing women as objects seems to be something this swami continues to do after years of meditation.[25]

Is it surprising that women fear success so often, as Matina Horner's studies have found?[26] Studies conducted after Horner's showed that when women feared success it was because they feared social rejection, whereas when men feared success it was the value of success itself that the men questioned.[27] These studies indicating that women fear social rejection if they are successful tend to support Schaef's idea of the female need for approval, an approval that begins to seem impossible to find. Approval by men then loses its impact. It becomes meaningless in view of a double standard of mental health. If a woman is commended for aspects of her femininity, then her adulthood is challenged and vice versa. This kind of conflict could lead to emotional problems, and, with women who choose a contemporary sex role behavior, this is apparently what happens. Powell and Reznikoff found that women with contemporary sex role orientations have more symptoms of psychologic problems than those who are oriented to traditional roles. They speculated that the reason for this difference is a conflict between personal needs and cultural role expectations within the women with contemporary orientations.[28]

The double standard of mental health also affects treatment plans. A good example of this is in an article by Dr. J. Houck, entitled "The Intractable Female Patient."[29] Behavioral problems in this type of patient are depression, anxiety, and dependency needs. The treatment suggested is, among other things, that the patient's attention be firmly fixed on home, family, and adult obligations. The husband must also be worked with because "he is obliged to modify lifelong attitudes of passivity and diffidence and to assume a posture of strength and resolution—especially toward his wife."[30] She will resist, of course, and test the husband to see if he means it, "but she is often aware at last that she really hopes she will not win."[31] This physician has taken a prevalent societal attitude that women enjoy being pushed around and has manufactured a psychotherapeutic regimen based on it. Szasz possibly would refer to this as a victimization and dehumanization process that happens to persons who deviate from the norm.[32] It is doubtful that a man would be subjected to this kind of treatment since the diagnosis is in terms of female intractability.

A replication of the Broverman study published in 1975 showed that male counselors in training (not female trainees) held differential standards of mental health.[33] 1974 and 1977 studies showed that female therapists were more accepting of new roles for women than were male therapists.[34] The study by Brown and Hellinger in Canada included psychiatric nurses, although their educational backgrounds were not identified. Psychiatric nurses were the most accepting of new roles for women, but Brown and Hellinger were not certain whether this was because of their profession or the fact that most of the nurses were female.

A study that focused on assessments of mental health by psychiatric–mental health nurses prepared at the master's level showed less sex-role stereotyping than that found by Broverman in 1970. In fact, these nurses rated ideals of mental health higher for women than men on some traditionally male characteristics such as self-confidence and higher overall on both male and female valued qualities.[35] This was a primarily female clinician population, and some authors believe that female clinicians might hold less sexist attitudes than male therapists.[36] The Kjervik and Palta study indicates the possibility that a different kind of sex role stereotyping is occurring, that is, that in which women are expected to achieve higher levels of behavior than men in order to be considered "healthy" by clinicians. This could be indicative of attitude change, possibly a swing away from old sexist ideals to new beliefs.[37]

Expecting more from women could have the beneficial effect of the self-fulfilling prophecy: If you expect little, you often get little in return. Women so often look to external persons for encouragement or validation that, if they get this from a psychiatric nurse, they may respond favorably, by meeting higher standards. On the other hand, being expected to leave a comfortable status in a traditional female role for a more demanding role as combination career woman and homemaker might be a problem.

The research that has been presented indicates that a change in attitude with regard to women's roles in society is possibly occurring. Traits that have been labeled masculine such as aggressiveness and leadership are being seen more often as proper for women as well as for men. Traditional female qualities such as expression of tender feelings are becoming more acceptable for men. In this sense, a kind of androgyny is evolving, not in which men and women are the same any more than individual persons are carbon copies of one another, but in which men and women can choose from among a variety of behaviors and not feel compelled to act passively or aggressively if they do not want to.

This change has become apparent in our language. Politicians are now more careful to say "women" instead of "girls," and many curricula in the human service areas are substituting the concept of humankind or humanity for mankind. Simone de Beauvoir, in her book *The Second Sex,* talks about the "otherness" of the woman.[38] The man is the subject—he is the doer, whereas the women is the object—she has things done to her or watches the man being active. It is hoped that changing language usage will bring the woman into the subject category and out of her role as "the other." If our language acknowledges both female and male counterparts, women will learn to think of themselves as responsible, important adults.

As women have been considered "others" in society, so, too, have they been thought of as "others" in their roles as health caregivers. Anne Davis reported during the American Nurses' Association convention in June 1976 that female psychotherapists are stereotypically considered to be quiet, practical, nurturant earth mothers.[39] Chesler notes that there are many more male therapists than female therapists in the two leading mental health groups—psychiatry and psychology.[40] These evidences of sexism may be removed as the public and health caregivers learn that female clinicians often have attitudes that are less sexist than those of their male colleagues.

UNDOING THE SEXISM IN MENTAL HEALTH

The major aspects of the concept of mental health that have been alluded to thus far and that are pertinent to this section are the following: (1) a sense of self, (2) a sense of control or authority over one's own self, (3) communication of one's needs and desires to others, and (4) valuing oneself. Women have learned that others are more important than they are and that they exist to serve others rather than to develop themselves. This is detrimental to reaching a mentally healthy state. As one client said, "My happiness comes when others are happy." Pleasing herself, for herself only, did not occur to her. When I was a child I was told that pleasing myself was selfish and was to be avoided. Selfishness could be restated as self-assertiveness and then not seen in such a negative light. Total other-directedness leads to not knowing oneself. Men, by the way, suffer from the impact of sexism as well. They must affiliate with individuals on an unequal basis, that is, with women who cannot state a need or desire clearly and who thus look totally to men for support, thus placing a great burden on the men.

Four stages through which women pass in undoing their own sexist attitudes will now be discussed. These ideas are based on my work with clients and contact with other women who were at various stages and on my own growth and change as well.

Stage 1: Making Connections

This stage could be likened to a honeymoon; that is, one that is pleasant. The "ah ha" reaction is predominant, and the woman is delighted to see that things that made her feel uncomfortable in her past now make sense. She may have wondered why masculine pronouns are used for everyone, why female nudity and rape are more common than male nudity and rape, and why physicians are mostly male. Now these odd occurrences fall together and manifest a pattern. The woman also experiences a sense of diminished guilt, which is refreshing. Whereas she felt guilt for being uncomfortable about these things and receiving strange looks at parties for mentioning them, she can now comment on them and know that others (persons sympathetic to the women's movement) are on her side. The extent of her exposure to feminist ideas and feminist persons will determine the length of time spent in this and subsequent stages.

Stage 2: Anger

Because enlightenment alone does not remove the problem, the woman begins to be irritated. She thinks, "It makes so much sense. Why don't others want to change their behaviors? Anything this obvious should be easy to remedy. It's so logically wrong." She begins to show others the errors of their ways. She may give men dirty looks for opening doors for her or make sure that, when a man touches her, she touches him back (and in the same place) or insist that she be addressed as Ms. rather than Miss or Mrs. This is the time when she joins a consciousness-raising group, which serves to increase her anger and outrage as she listens to the numerous injustices suffered by her "sisters." She begins to experience the problem of sexism as overwhelming, and she

may at this point enter therapy (usually with a female therapist) to handle the growing anger. Some clients project fear onto the therapist, expressing their concern that the therapist might be overwhelmed by their anger.

Stage 3: Action

After the woman discovers that her anger can be expressed without destroying herself or others, she begins working (usually with a feminist group) to undo sexist practices. She attends lectures on legislative effectiveness and assertiveness and begins to practice these. She takes a less hostile approach than in the previous stage and therefore expects to be effective in changing others' behaviors. Change does not come as quickly as she expects, because her expectations continue to be based on what she now thinks is logically right and just treatment for women. Since sexism defies her newly acquired sense of right and wrong, her expectations are not met and she becomes hopeless and depressed.

Stage 4: Balance

As the woman shares her hopelessness with others in therapy or women's groups, she learns that these feelings have been experienced by others, and she learns that she can reach out for support from other women and receive it. This point is extremely important, because her previous socialization has taught her not to trust other women (they might take her man away from her). She learns the necessity of delaying gratification, because attitude change does not happen in a few weeks. However, she does not lose her commitment to the cause. Within women's groups she learns to work for small, objective changes, one at a time. I worked on an "action" with a local women's group to enable nurse-midwives to have their names on the birth certificates of the babies they delivered. I experienced a great sense of satisfaction when a favorable decision was made by the State Department of Health. The woman learns patience with others who are in previous stages or who have not even reached stage 1. Part of her patience comes from the realization that what is logical, right, and just will not happen right away because the feelings that support sexism (inferiority versus superiority) are not based on logic—*they just are.*

Therapist's Role in Undoing Sexism

When a woman has not reached the first stage of undoing her own sexist beliefs, the therapist may be faced with an extremely difficult task, that is, dealing with a woman who genuinely believes that she is inferior to men. An extreme example of a woman in this position is one who is being battered by her male companion. A less extreme example is the "happy homemaker" who probably would not come into therapy for herself but might appear because of her concern with another family member. The ethical question for the therapist is whether to begin pointing out the realities of sexism in order to foster the onset of stage 1.

In these cases, the therapist can question the happiness or satisfaction that is expressed by the woman. She may ask, "If you're so happy, what about these problems in your family?" Then if the patient retorts, "I just want to learn how to please my husband," the therapist can ask what she thinks pleases him. Often a double-binding situation is discovered in which the husband directs the wife to do her own thing, stand up to him, be intelligent, and express her desires. He also expects her to do what he tells her to do (for example, make his meals and clean the house). The treatment in this instance would be the same as dealing with any double-binding communication, that is, increasing the awareness of the dysfunctional pattern, or changing the relationship rules through the use of therapeutic double binds, or both.[41, 42]

Dealing with these women is similar to being faced with someone who denies the reality of a death. Change is needed, but the woman isn't ready for it. She would have to give up too much of herself. As in working with denial, the therapist would not hit the problem head on, thus reinforcing the defensiveness. Rather, it would be important to follow the immediate concerns of the woman and to role-model attention giving. Assuming that she will learn behavior displayed by the therapist, the woman will learn to attend more acutely to herself. Battered women may need direction (rather than support) such as, "No one deserves to be hit or pushed around."

The therapist's role is one of teaching new attitudes through role modeling. Respecting the woman (having an idea of what has led to her current behavior) while not agreeing with the values that she expresses is important for the therapist for use in dealing with the woman's other relationships (for example, with unruly children or a difficult husband). As in dealing with a suicidal patient, the therapist should show the woman alternative choices for action. Exaggeration of the existing situation can be used as a paradoxical strategy to change

the problematic behavior. Watzlawick might refer to this strategy as prescribing the symptom.[43] For instance, the therapist may direct the client to "elaborate on the feeling about yourself when you are waiting on your husband. What is that like for you?" She may discover that "waiting on" is not always fun and there is a tiny bit of resentment for the giving without receiving.

During stage 1, the woman probably will not seek out therapy for sexism-related concerns. The enlightenment is rewarding. When she becomes angry in stage 2, the feelings might become overwhelming so that rage needs to be expressed. Schaef provides a "rage room" where women can vent this anger by hitting or destroying items of their choice without having to clean up their messes.[44] It is useful not to allow the woman to vent all her anger, because anger is a form of energy that is basic to the action stage. During the third stage, the woman may want to develop assertiveness skills, which the therapist can facilitate. Along with assertiveness, the woman needs to learn more about what she wants and needs so that she knows what to assert. This builds her sense of self. When she becomes hopeless during stage 3, the therapist should provide a supportive atmosphere of listening and responding to the woman's concerns. Reminding her that change will take a long time will help her begin to put the desired changes in a reality-centered perspective. Helping her to see that being assertive about what she wants does not guarantee getting what she wants will again teach her the limitations of reality. This reality is the boundary between herself and others' selves. Again, this will help her develop her self-concept.

FEMINIST-ORIENTED COUNSELING

In the practice of psychotherapy, a new interest in feminist-oriented therapy has evolved. According to Williams, feminist therapy gears itself to the following goals:[45]

1. To support women who are struggling to become assertive
2. To increase women's sense of power, self-esteem, and autonomy
3. To help women lessen self-defeating feelings in roles they currently play
4. To help women see that they have choices in their patterns of living
5. To give women insights into the connection between their own behaviors and societal structures that nurture these behaviors
6. To acknowledge the therapist's sociali-

zation as a woman, which might lead to a kind of motherly "overprotectiveness"

These goals direct the therapist as well as the client. For example, goal 6 is the expectation that the therapist will be aware of her own conditioning within society, which affects her ongoing behavior in therapy. Reynolds discusses what she considers to be distinctive elements of the feminist perspective in counseling. One element is the assumption that all women are oppressed, and another is·that women are distinct human persons who are not extensions of other persons. To this end, the therapist must identify her own oppression and empathize with the oppression of her clients. Reynolds recommends that her patients attend consciousness-raising groups, women's support groups, or assertiveness training groups so that they will begin to believe that change can be made. She also recommends bibliotherapy with feminist-oriented books if the client enjoys reading.[46]

Both Reynolds and Williams emphasize the importance of the therapist's self-knowledge and appreciation of her own oppression. It is useful for the therapist to review her past in order to decipher any sexist messages that were taught her. One such message might be that girls should grow up to marry men who are stronger and more intelligent than they are. This overlooks several possibilities for a woman: that she may choose a man of equal intelligence or strength, that she may choose a female partner, or that she may choose no one at all, to mention a few. The therapist must examine her feelings about these various possibilities for lifestyles. Some therapists and educators have noticed a change in their attitudes toward their students and clients after they have begun to conceive of them as women rather than girls. Kronsky also believes that the feminist-oriented therapist should be aware of the subjective experience of being caught in a double-binding kind of situation in the male-dominated society. She concludes that in this sense, the feminist-oriented therapist may have to be a female.[47] Self-knowledge on the therapist's part, as this is shared with the client, gives her the message that it is valuable to know oneself and that it is acceptable to develop control over oneself. In this way, the therapist role models self-appreciation.

Williams discusses the value of role modeling expressions of anger with the depressed woman. The depressed woman often suppresses competitive urges and feels guilty about having these urges. She is basically angry about having to behave "nicely" toward persons who treat her shabbily, usually persons who are perceived as authority figures. The woman needs to learn that expressing angry feelings is acceptable. If the therapist expresses her own anger openly to the patient, the patient learns that it is acceptable for her to do the same. If the therapist does not role model this anger, the woman is reinforced in believing that she is bad or guilty for feeling hurt or anger, since the authority figure, in this case the therapist, apparently doesn't ever feel anger.[48]

Kronsky suggests that, if a woman is feeling guilty about overidentification with men in her life, a feminist-oriented therapist should attempt to remove the woman's guilt instead of emphasizing an interpretation such as penis envy. Identification with men could be considered normal in a male-dominated society in which men are able to be assertive. The woman in identifying with men is possibly in touch with her wish to become assertive.[49]

Although one of the goals of feminist-oriented therapy is to increase the woman's sense of power over her destiny, the therapist could possibly exacerbate the woman's feeling of inadequacy by reminding her of all the power that she has lying dormant. Schaef believes that, if the therapist tells the client how much power she has, it will reinforce society's message that she is too sick, bad, crazy, or stupid to have known this.[50] It seems that a better approach is to build on the woman's statement of concern in the here-and-now situation, as has been described previously.

IMPLICATIONS FOR EDUCATION AND RESEARCH

Educational programs should gear themselves not only to conscious manifestations of sexism, such as those found in textbooks, but also to less obvious forms, such as nonverbal expressions of approval given by teachers to students. In other words, negative attitudes about women should be explored in a discussion of students' feelings about the changing roles of women and men in society in conjunction with provision of facts about the status of women in society.

Research should focus on clinicians' attitudes toward female and male clients, effects of clinicians' attitudes on outcomes of therapy, the status of women's self-concepts, the public's understanding of sexism and its ramifications, and psychotherapeutic or educational practices that are effective in removing sexist attitudes. Both research and education are vital to changing the attitudes in our society from androcentric to androgynous.

CONCLUSION

It is apparent that legal, economic, religious, and health care positions will have to be changed in order to deal with the totality of sexism. Yet it is comforting to accept the system-theory principle that a change in part will effect a change in the whole. If a change can be made in society's view of the mentally healthy state of women, perhaps changes in other areas of society will follow.

References

1. Shortridge, K. Women as university nigger, *University of Michigan Daily Magazine,* April 12, 1970, pp. 4–5, 21.
2. U.S. Department of Commerce, Bureau of the Census. *A Statistical Portrait of Women in the U.S.* Washington, D.C.: U.S. Government Printing Office, April 1976.
3. Chapman, W. *Minneapolis Star,* February 26, 1974, p. 8B.
4. Knudsen, D. The declining status of women: Popular myths and the failure of functionalist thought. *Social Forces,* vol. 48, December 1969, pp. 183–193.
5. Women Administrators Found Unequal in Pay Status. *Chronicle of Higher Education,* vol. 14, June 1977, p. 8.
6. *Spokeswoman,* vol. 8, July 1977, pp. 7–8.
7. Mill, J.S. The subjection of women. *In* Rossi, A. (ed.). *Essays on Sex Equality.* Chicago: University of Chicago Press, 1970, p. 141.
8. Ibid., p. 142.
9. Schaef, Anne Wilson. *Women's Reality.* Minneapolis, MN: Winston Press, 1981, p. 24.
10. Symonds, Alexandra. Neurotic dependency in successful women. *Journal of American Academy of Psychoanalysis,* vol. 4, 1976, pp. 96–102.
11. Symonds, Alexandra. The liberated woman: Healthy and neurotic. *American Journal of Psychoanalysis,* vol. 34, 1974.
12. Broverman, I. et al. Sex-role stereotypes: A current appraisal. *Journal of Social Issues,* vol. 8, 1972, pp. 59–78.
13. Ruble, T. Sex stereotypes: Issues and Changes in the 1970s. *Sex Roles: A Journal of Research,* vol. 9, March 1983, pp. 397–402.
14. Chesler, Phyllis. *Women and Madness.* Garden City, NY: Doubleday and Co., 1972, p. 119.
15. Brandon, Sydney. Psychiatric illness in women. *Nursing Mirror,* vol. 134, January 1972, pp. 17–18.
16. Fabrikant, Benjamin. The psychotherapist and the female patient: Perceptions, misperceptions, and change. Franks, Violet, and Burtle, Vasanti (eds.), New York: Brunner-Mazel, 1974, pp. 94–96.
17. Ineichen, Bernard. Neurotic wives in a modern residential suburb: A modern residential profile. *Social Science and Medicine,* vol. 9, 1975, pp. 481–487.
18. Seiden, Anne M. Overview: Research on the psychology of women. II. Women in families, work and psychotherapy. *American Journal of Psychiatry,* vol. 113, October 1976, p. 1115.
19. Chesler, Phyllis, op. cit., p. 40.
20. *Spokeswoman,* p. 12
21. Chesler, Phyllis, op. cit., p. 40.
22. Feinblatt, J., and Gold, A. Sex Roles and the Psychiatric Referral Process. *Sex Roles: A Journal of Research,* vol. 2, June 1976, pp. 109–122.
23. Broverman, I. et al. Sex-role stereotypes and clinical judgments of mental health. *Journal of Consulting and Clinical Psychology,* vol. 34, 1970, pp. 1–7.
24. *Ms.,* vol. 3, February 1975, p. 93.
25. Swami Ajaya. *Yoga Psychology: A Guide to Practical Meditation,* 2 vols. Glenview, IL: Himalayan International Institute of Yoga Science and Philosophy of U.S.A., 1974, vol. 1, pp. 17–23.
26. Horner, M. Fail: Bright women. *Psychology Today,* vol. 3, November 1969, pp. 36–38.
27. Tresemer, D. Fear of success: Popular, but unproven. *Psychology Today,* vol. 7, March 1974, pp. 82–85; Kemper, S. Graven, Paludi, M. Fear of success revisited: Introducing an ambiguous cue. *Sex Roles: A Journal of Research,* vol. 9, August 1983, pp. 897–900.
28. Powell, Barbara and Reznikoff, M. Role conflict and symptoms of psychological distress in college educated women. *Journal of Consulting and Clinical Psychology,* vol. 44, 1976, pp. 473–479.
29. Houck, J. The intractable female patient. *American Journal of Psychiatry,* vol. 129, July 1972, p. 27.
30. Ibid., p. 30.
31. Ibid., p. 31.
32. Szasz, Thomas, quoted in Rosner, S. The rights of mental patients: The new Massachusetts law. *Mental Hygiene,* vol. 56, Winter 1972, pp. 117–119.
33. Feinblatt and Gold, op. cit., pp. 109–122.
34. Brown, D. R. and Hellinger, M. S. Therapists' attitudes toward women. *Social Work,* vol. 20, July 1975, pp. 266–270; Aslin, A. Feminist and community health center psychotherapists' expectations of mental health for women. *Sex Roles: A Journal of Research,* vol. 3, December 1977, pp. 537–543.
35. Kjervik, Diane, and Palta, Mari. Sex-role stereotyping in assessments of mental health made by psychiatric–mental health nurses. *Nursing Research,* vol. 27, May-June 1978, pp. 166–171.
36. American Psychological Association. *Report of the Task Force on Sex Bias and Sex-Role Stereotyping.* Washington, D.C., August 1975, p. 8.
37. Kjervik and Palta, op. cit.
38. de Beauvoir, Simone. *Le Deuxième Sexe.* Paris: Gallimard, 1949.
39. Davis, Anne. Issues in the mental health of women. Audiotape, American Nurses' Association Convention, Atlantic City, NJ, June, 1976. On-the-Spot Duplicators, Northridge, CA.
40. Chesler, Phyllis, op. cit., pp. 61–65.
41. Watzlawick, Paul. *An Anthology of Human Communication.* Palo Alto, CA: Science and Behavior Books, 1964, p. 48.
42. Watzlawick, Paul, Beavin, J. and Jackson, D. *Pragmatics of Human Communication.* New York: W. W. Norton and Co., 1967, pp. 240–248.
43. Watzlawick, Paul, op. cit., pp. 236–240.
44. Schaef, Anne Wilson. Presentation at Unity Church. St. Paul, Minn., 1976.
45. Williams, E. F. *Notes of a Feminist Therapist.* New York: Praeger Publishers, 1976, pp. 6–10.
46. Reynolds, Phyllis. Counseling from a feminist perspective. *Student Counseling Bureau Review* (University of Minnesota) vol. 26, September 1975, pp. 56–60.
47. Kronsky, Betty. Feminism and psychotherapy. *Journal of Contemporary Psychotherapy,* vol. 3, Spring 1971, p. 98.
48. Williams, E. F., op. cit., pp. 109–110.
49. Kronsky, Betty, op. cit., p. 97.
50. Schaef, Anne Wilson, op. cit.

12

HEALTH APPRAISAL OF LOW-INCOME WOMEN

BEVERLY L. McELMURRY

The chapter on health appraisal of low-income women by Beverly McElmurry begins with a review of the literature, followed by a study of rural, nonfarm women who were receiving public aid. The unique function of the nurse in the assessment of women's health and its potential value to society concludes the chapter.

The family lives in abject poverty I never dreamed could exist in this community. No indoor plumbing. Children attend middle class school; cannot adjust; cannot help but smell. One son retarded. Daughter, 11, promiscuous. One child, the result 'of union between father and daughter, placed in foster home. Cats and dogs in abundance. Mother stated dog had brought in a mangled coon. She roasted it for dinner.*

How would the mother in that home define "health"? The interaction of poverty and states of health is cause for concern in the community health field. Health professionals may be limited in dealing with the problem by the gap between their own largely middle-class health values and the health values of the low-income people they serve.

The intent of the research described in this chapter was to provide a nursing perspective of the way in which low-income women view health. This perspective accepted that "a person acts in accordance with his own experience in a particular situation; an examination of this experience is the necessary starting place for helping him to grow."[1]

Certain humanistic assumptions guided the approach to this chapter, among which are the following:

1. The full health potential of the relationship between a nurse and the recipient of nursing services depends on their interaction as whole human beings.

2. Every person, including the nurse and patient, is a unique interdependent combination of body, mind, emotions, and spirit. It is this unique combination that the nurse looks for when assessing the health status of low-income women.

3. The patient and nurse are colleagues. Such a relationship activates growth and mutual problem solving.

4. Health, for nurse and patient, is defined within the context of the life experience of each.

Poverty and the special health promotion and maintenance needs of women have an enduring quality that cautions the humanistic bents of nurse-investigators and dampens the desire to move rapidly into the specifications of nursing practice interventions for this patient population or to delineate swiftly the outcomes expected from such interventions. The data collection tool used in this study should be further refined. More opportunities to appreciate and respect low-income women are likely to result in more accurate specifications for group-anchored interventions.

---

*From notes of a student. Acknowledgment is given the nursing students who assisted with this study, especially Sue Clark, Pam Miller, and Lois Wilson. I assume full responsibility for the work reported in this paper.

The heart of developing clinical nursing in this area is, eventually, to propose nursing interventions that are testable. Such interventions may take the form of models for educational activities with low-income women, but it is premature to propose hypotheses before a descriptive base is established, either for an individual or for a group. This line of reasoning led Lefcowitz, in interlinking education, poverty, and health issues, to ask, "What change in health policy—financial and/or structural—will increase utilization among the less educated, given their relatively lower preference for health care?"[2]

To obtain a focus for developing nursing interventions and a set of related or expected patient outcomes, nurses must first comprehend the health status of low-income women and how these women express it.

Time spent with nursing students who cared for rural-area public-aid recipients helped me to develop preliminary hunches about the indirect ways in which low-income women express their sense of health and well-being. For example, a general or masked depressive state was frequently revealed by the passive-aggressive, manipulative manner in which the women related to those around them. A vicious cycle was evident: Unsatisfied affectionate love and human-intimacy tendencies left the women less trusting and spontaneous in relating to other people, who then responded negatively to their stiffness and distrust. The press of economic and social situations coupled with low educational achievement left the women with an underdeveloped sense of their physical and psychologic selves. Community health and support systems personnel sometimes worsened the cycle by rejecting or stigmatizing the women as undesirable.

These observations suggested the appropriateness of a more systematic study of low-income women through the development of a health appraisal form. In addition, students might use such a form as a tool for examining nursing practice.

The purpose of this study was to begin the development of tools and methodology with which to describe the reported and perceived health status of low-income, rural, nonfarm women.

REVIEW OF LITERATURE

The literature speaks more directly to the dimensions of poverty than to the health appraisal of low-income women. Chilman cautions that we know only part of what needs to be known about low-income cultures and that "not all the possibly relevant questions have been asked. Moreover, it seems as if research has focused chiefly on the weaknesses of the poor rather than their strengths."[3]

Chilman identifies the following problems of research with low-income or poverty groups: (1) the use of questionnaires when educational levels are so low that literacy is a problem, (2) the difference between statistic and pragmatic significance, (3) moving from group findings to individual diagnosis or predictions, and (4) failure to realize that behavior is complex and multidimensional.

National data on relationships between low income and health states are labeled as health characteristics but are in reality descriptions of illness. The national data from health interview and health examination surveys are essentially reports of illness, such as restricted-activity days, acute conditions, physical visits, and hospital episodes.[4] Researchers in nursing must work to develop outcome measures more appropriate to the health-related concerns involved in the proposal of nursing interventions for the promotion and maintenance of health.

Bergner and Yerby substantiated the need for descriptive data in their discussion of low-income barriers to the use of health services:

The poor behaved differently from the middle class and the affluent across a wide spectrum related to health care. Illness is defined differently. There is less accurate health information. The poor are less inclined to take preventive measures, and delay longer in seeking medical care. When they do approach health practitioners, they are more likely to select subprofessionals or the marginal practitioners often found in their neighborhoods.[5]

Many writers suggest that the life of low-income people is improved by raising their educational levels or instituting homemaker and child-care services. Such proposals often come from middle- and upper-class reformers who have never consulted the people whose lifestyle they propose to change. Likewise, many proposals to improve life for low-income people are piecemeal remedies rather than comprehensive plans. Milio, however, demonstrated the supportive role of health personnel in facilitating a group's identification of needed services and in becoming self-directive in designing and implementing its own health services.[6]

Bauer reported many health characteristics that differentiate low-income from higher-income groups.[7] Low-income people have more untreated conditions, a greater number of dental caries, poorer health, more prevalent chronic conditions, higher disability rates, less access to medical and dental care, greater reliance on clinics and emergency units for health care, and more hospital episodes. Bauer also reports that "aid recipients have poorer health than nonrecipients."[8] Pomeroy[9] found that welfare recipients report poorer health for themselves and their children than do nonwelfare people. Criteria for determining "good health" were not, however, developed in Pomeroy's sample.

Komisar[10] noted that the majority of adults on welfare were women. Women suffer most from a life of poverty.[11] Lesse also believes that American culture creates major stresses for women in the middle years of life.[12]

My experience, with or without a review of the literature, is that low-income women present a special concern to those involved in the delivery of health care services. Some evidence indicates a geographic dimension to the problem, since mothers in rural farm and nonfarm areas spend longer continuous periods on public assistance.[13]

Triplett reported the characteristics and perceptions of low-income women as they affected use of preventive health services.[14] Triplett did not focus on the perceived health status of the patients, but she did conclude that low-income women can be expected to talk freely about their health care experiences. In light of Polansky's[15] identification of verbal accessibility as a problem for low-income people, Triplett's study suggests that trained nurse-interviewers can be successful in obtaining interview data from research subjects.

Brinton looked at the value differences between nurses and low-income families but did not attempt to describe health. Rather, she included among her tools an instrument that compares the importance that nurses and mothers attach to various questions related to health.[16] The questions, however, do not provide a categorization or description of what constitutes a healthy state.

It can be concluded that research literature about low-income women is limited and sketchy. When related to health, it emphasizes not the presence of a healthy state but rather its absence.

LaBelle reviewed definitions of the term "health" and concluded that the definition used by a given group (such as nurses) gives direction to the research, service, and educational activities performed by that group.[17] The present inadequate conceptualization of the term "health" demonstrates the need to develop a complex construct. An individual state of health or well-being is characterized by subjective and objective aspects of behavior, which are influenced by physical, emotional, social, and environmental conditions. "A continuing problem," states LaBelle, "is the development of criteria and indices to measure health. The research problem reflects the constantly changing or adaptive components that are a part of health."[18]

METHOD

Low-income, nonhospitalized women receiving public aid were interviewed to determine their status in four dimensions of health: physical, psychologic, social, and environmental. Furthermore, the women were asked to identify, in their words, their state of health. Interviews were conducted by student nurses trained in basic techniques by the researcher. The data reported here reflect preliminary work in developing a health assessment interview guide.

TOOL

In the view of Yura and Walsh, the nursing process provides a general framework for examining clinical practice concerns and should be related to research endeavors.[19] Consistent with this outlook and with my earlier definition of health, the tool developed was used to obtain information about physical, psychologic, social, and environmental variables.

Examples from the interviewer's assessment guide are included here. Figure 12–1 shows major categories within each variable, as well as the type of question asked in each category. Figure 12–2 illustrates the nurse's conclusion and intervention record following assessment of health data. In essence, a patient health problem becomes a nursing concern if it is expected to respond to the type of action or intervention carried out by the nurse.

STUDY SAMPLE

Subjects selected for this program were derived from women receiving public aid in a selected rural, nonfarm, midwestern area. Their ages ranged from late adolescence to late adulthood. All were judged to be of normal intelligence.

Initially, 20 women were identified for the

PHYSICAL VARIABLE
Categories:
  Hygiene
  Examples of questions in this category:
    Routines
      e.g., Bath, complete   Y N   Regular   Y N   Frequency _____
    Difficulties or limitations
      e.g., Physical incapacity   Y N   Explain _____
    Independence
  Nutrition
  Rest
  Mobility
  Female health
  Systematic evaluation
  Restrictions
  Indirect influences

PSYCHOLOGICAL VARIABLE
Categories:
  Behavioral
  Examples of questions in this category:
    Alcoholic intake: Amount _____ Frequency _____
    Circumstances _____ Regularity _____
    Smoking   Y N   Amount per day _____
    Uses of leisure time (respondents circle appropriate descriptors)
    Flexibility in daily schedule   Y N
    Long- and short-term goals (options provided)
  Emotional
  Adaptive behavior
  Intellectual/academic
  Information input
  Perceptions
  Values and priorities

SOCIAL VARIABLE
Categories:
  Vocational/economic
  Examples of questions in this category:
    Attitudes toward responsibility and authority
      Resentment   Y N   (client's view)   Y N   (nurse's view)
      Respect   Y N
    Major concerns about work:
      Health
      Social
      Money
      Job itself
      etc.
    Health hazards and benefits associated with work _____
    Employment history
  Communication/interpersonal
  Family
  Indirect influences

ENVIRONMENTAL VARIABLE
Categories:
  Physical
  Examples of questions in this category:
    Housing
      Type: single-family, apartment, single room, etc.
      Provision: owned, rented
      Cleanliness and general sanitation: adequate, inadequate
      Heat: adequate, inadequate
      Air pollution   Y N
      Water pollution   Y N
      Excessive noise   Y N
      Waste disposal   Y N
  Social environment
  Indirect influences

Figure 12.1. Variables included in the health appraisal of women.

State of Health
    How this woman defines health _____
    How she describes health _____
    Determination that she is _____, is not _____ healthy and the reasons for this _____
    _____
    What she does to maintain or improve health _____
    When she does comply with recommended health practices and when she does not comply _____

Agreed Areas for Nurse and Patient to work on
    Area(s) identified by client _____
    Area(s) and/or problem(s) the nurse identifies _____

Possible Approaches
    Approach   Criterion/criteria for evaluating approach
    _____   _____
    _____   _____
    _____   _____
    _____   _____
    _____   _____

Implementation of Nursing Approaches
    Dates   List in order of priority
    _____   _____
    _____   _____
    _____   _____
    _____   _____

    Unpredictable happenings:
    _____
    _____
    _____
    _____

Nurse's Evaluation and/or Reformulation of Nursing Approach
    _____
    _____
    _____
    _____

Figure 12.2. Nurse's conclusions and intervention record after considering assessment data.

study, but data are reported on the 13 who remained in the case load for the full four-month period. The subjects' agreement to participate in the project was obtained.

DATA COLLECTION

Student nurses assigned to provide care to the women for four months, as part of a community health field experience, were the data collectors. It was their responsibility to determine at which point in their relationship with the study subjects it seemed appropriate to collect assessment information. Usually this followed a judgment that a trust relationship had been established between them. Some data were gathered over the entire period of time.

DATA ANALYSIS

Analysis of data from this pilot study is qualitative, reflecting an early stage of inves-

tigation in a relatively unexplored area. In their explanation of field methodology, Schatzman and Strauss captured the essence of the approach herein employed:

> Field method is more like an umbrella of activity beneath which any technique may be used for gaining the desired information, and for processes of thinking about this information.[20]
> [The] researcher . . . enters and relates himself to a human field in its natural state; that is, in its own time and place, and in its own recurrent and developing process.[21]
> "Method" is seen as an abstraction of the ways the researcher handles, or might handle, the many real situations, problems, and options which present themselves to him as he conducts his inquiry.[22]

FINDINGS

Women in the study sample thought of health predominantly in terms of the presence or absence of physical states usually associated with a disease. "Health" generally meant the absence of disease symptoms or of uncomfortable states, such as flu or colds. On the whole, women in the study evidenced little inclination to incorporate psychologic, social, or environmental components into the determination of her own health status.

Physical

General hygiene measures were adequate except for dental care, which rarely met recommended practices. Some women used only mouthwash in their dental regimen, and others reported brushing their teeth two or three times per week. Nearly all said that limited finances affected their hygienic states.

Concern for physical safety in the home varies among the subjects. Some of the women carefully removed dangerous materials from the reach of children, whereas others, for example, let their children live in the midst of furniture bulging with dangerous springs.

The study women were able to assume responsibility for self-care but most needed encouragement or suggestions from the nurse to increase their awareness of hygiene or safety factors important to health.

Generally, the women ate two to three meals per day. For snacks, they preferred breads and cereals. None reported taking nutritional supplements such as vitamins unless the doctor had specifically urged their use. As a group, the women did not self-medicate. Some hoped to lose weight but felt their financial situation limited diet choice.

Rest-sleep data produced little significant information. The only reported dissatisfaction was sleep interruptions from others, usually small children. However, the subjects rarely reported fatigue and did not report that sleep interruptions interfered with their overall sense of sufficient rest.

Most women in the study group were involved in daily household work and child-care activities. Few were sufficiently active to qualify for an activity level above "moderate," and the nurses were inclined to place them, as a group, in the sedentary category.

In the area of female health, the women were questioned about menstrual cycles, use of contraceptives, fertility, and breast self-examination practices. Five of the subject women used no contraceptives, five used oral contraceptives, one had an intrauterine device, and one had been sterilized. All had heard of breast self-examination, but nine never performed it. Two did it irregularly, one did every month, and another did every morning (she had previously had a breast biopsy). None of the women reported irregular menstrual cycles.

Generally, the body-systems evaluation of each woman revealed conditions already known to her and under medical treatment. One woman did have untreated dental problems. The lack of significant findings in this area is in itself interesting. It may be that the findings are consistent with the women's health concepts, since most of them viewed health as the absence of disease and sought treatment only for infections or dysfunctions. Also, the women in the study were primarily young adults, not yet subject to chronic health problems.

One of the subject women could not recall the last time she had seen a doctor, but 12 reported a medical examination within the last two years. Although most sought dental examinations every two years, one had not seen a dentist in eight years, and another had not seen one in four years. None participated in any health screening programs, either because the programs were not offered, the subjects were not aware of the programs, or they were not inclined to participate.

Psychologic

Data collected in this health component suggest possible further fruitful explorations.

About half of the study women smoked. Ten were satisfied with the way they spent leisure time, usually in the company of family or friends. As a group, the subjects reported few hobbies or other interests not directly related to homemaking.

One woman—an 18-year-old mother of a three-year-old child, with no husband in the home—reported boredom. Nine women had daily schedules related to homemaking and child-care activities. Most were financially dependent on another person or on public aid.

Short-term goals of most importance to the women were everyday needs (nine), money (seven), and maintenance (six). Most important long-term goals were money (seven), employment (seven), and everyday needs (six).

Attributes of the subject women that seem to deserve fuller exploration include determination, timidity, and self-concept. Data collectors portrayed the women as "hopeful" if they seemed determined to improve their situations (more positive in self-concept). A description of a woman as "timid" usually corresponded with poor self-concept.

The nurse-interviewers were asked to describe the women's positive and negative adaptive behavior. Six were described as present oriented, four as distrustful of others, seven as accepting of their situation and of the people in that situation, five as trusting, and four as manipulative.

Only one of the subject women reported finishing high school. None received vocational training, but two were completing their education via the general education degree (GED) program offered through the local school system.

More than half of the subject women made decisions on the basis of impulse, but the same number said they used reason to arrive at decisions. Five viewed their opportunities as limited, whereas two thought that their futures held plentiful opportunity. Nine saw their chances for creative self-expression as low.

A majority of the women (seven) reported that they would be influenced by input or counsel from professionals such as nurses. They would weigh this influence against that of family, friends, and social agencies.

Asked to identify values and priorities, the women placed highest values on family (eleven), health (eight), maintenance (eight), money (nine), and independence (six). Seven women placed no priority on education or learning, whereas eight stressed the importance of recreation. Half listed employment as a priority.

When asked to identify their roles, nine women listed "mother," five chose "individual," another five "homemaker," seven said "single parent," and another seven said "friend." "Student" was listed twice; "wife" once.

Occupation and Work History

Of the 13 women studied, only one was currently employed. A factory worker earning minimum wages, she had passed through many job changes. Most of the women had no paid vacation, no savings, and no retirement plans. Two were supported by their husband's income. The remaining 10 were receiving some form of public aid. Most of the subject women saw their financial situation as inadequate, although some felt it sufficient to sustain them.

Social/Emotional

Ten of the subject women were described as socially isolated in the realm of communication and interpersonal skills. The closest associations reported by this group were with immediate family members. The interviews revealed that three of the women thought their affectional needs were inadequately satisfied. Eight thought their need for achievement was unsatisfied, and four lacked satisfaction of security needs. Five needed greater approval from others, and the same number felt insufficiently recognized by others. Three sensed that they did not belong to a group with a significant identity in the community.

Only six of the women chose to discuss their sex lives. All six were sexually active. The impression gained from study of the data was that most were satisfied with their sexual partners. The women made all the decisions regarding method of contraception, with no discussion with or participation by the partners.

Five of the subject women were single, three were married, three were separated, and two were divorced. All shared what the interviewers regarded as a profoundly passive and dependent attitude toward the men in their lives, as demonstrated by decision making in their relationships.

Most of the women, whether married or single, expressed the desire to be successful as parents. Probed on details of child care or perception of children's needs, however, they were often vague. Most appeared unable to understand concepts of mobility, play and environmental needs, and distribution of age-appropriate responsibilities. Their backgrounds limited them in discussions of the physical, psychologic, and social needs of young and adolescent children.

Yet the mothers as a group exhibited a remarkable sense of pride in their children and a hopeful attitude toward the children's future development. This pride was evident, even though some of the children had created classroom problems sufficient to bring them to the worried attention of school personnel.

Most women in the study reported the family as a source of maintenance, reproduction, and socialization, but not as a source of status within the community. They had given little thought to parenthood beyond the fact that it gave them someone to love and care for.

The subject women had little interest in social issues and little contact with people of other races. They saw themselves as members of a low-income social stratification and acted accordingly. None reported voting, and none belonged to community organizations or took part in community activities. Only one woman was actively involved in a church. The impression of the group was that the churches of their communities were not involved with them.

Environmental

All of the women lived in rented housing facilities. Overall, housing was adequate except for furnishings, general cleanliness, and sufficient privacy for all family members.

SUMMARY

Asked to develop a model description of the women they had interviewed, the nurses agreed on the following:

Generally, the women had been raised in low-income families and were participating in a learned way of life. They considered it normal to have children at an early age. Their relationships with men reflected both a need to be loved and a desire for sexual activity as a form of entertainment. Sexually active women exhibited severe lack of adequate information regarding use of contraceptives.

As a rule, the women had not completed high school and were underdeveloped in job-related skills. Their dim sense of self was manifested in an apparent lack of ability to change their stations in life.

When means could be found to develop skills related to jobs or to home and child care, hopeful attitudes developed among the subject women. As a group, they were oriented to the present time.

The women lacked knowledge about nutrition and about the growth and developmental needs of children.

Television and social activities planned with immediate family members were primary sources of entertainment. The women said very little about close family members in their conversations with outsiders. It was the opinion of the interviewers that the women slept a great deal.

Continued refinement of the health assessment of low-income women may support the hunch that they exhibited masked depression arising from the situation in which they found themselves. It is unlikely that future exploration will uncover genuinely healthy situations among the poor, as long as "health" is tied to notions of productivity, self-sufficiency, and satisfaction with life.

IMPLICATIONS

The nurse's unique function in health state assessment is increasingly recognized as the base for subsequent health maintenance or health promotion actions. The assessment process is itself an interaction that alters the people involved in it. We may anticipate that the person whose health state is assessed will grow in his or her perceptions of what health means and will come to understand what health means to the nurses. The concept of "health" then becomes a heuristic device that can educate both the nurse and the patient.

This study sought to initiate an appreciation of the context in which low-income women viewed themselves and their health states. The description of the women's perceived and reported health status provides data for planning, implementing, and evaluating nursing practice. Nursing actions based on such data more accurately respond to the health needs of women in low-income situations. The ability of such women to obtain health care is partially due to economic restrictions, but it is also related to their ability to differentiate among health states, to find entry into the health care delivery system, and to determine where a particular quality or type of care can be obtained.

Nurses have ready access to the socially stigmatized, including low-income women. The extent to which a nurse can function as the advocate of such women in realizing access to good health care depends on how exact and sensitive that nurse is in assessing the woman's health status and practices.

References

1. Fischer, Constance T. Contextual approach to assessment. *Community Mental Health Journal*, vol. 9 1973, p. 38.
2. Lefcowitz, M.J. Poverty and health: A reexamination. *In* Kane, R.L., Kasteler, J.M., and Gray, R.M. (eds.) *The Health Gap: Medical Services and the Poor.* New York: Springer, 1976, p. 55.
3. Chilman, C.S., *Growing Up Poor.* Washington, DC: U.S. Government Printing Office, 1966, p. 9.
4. National Center for Health Statistics. *Current Listing and Topical Index to the Vital and Health Statistics Series, 1962–1975.* DHEW publication no. (HRA) 78–1301, April 1976.
5. Bergner, L. and Yerby, A.S. Low income and barriers to use of health services. *In* Kane, R.L., Kasteler, J.M., and Gray, R.M. (eds.) *The Health Gap: Medical Services and the Poor.* New York: Springer, 1976, p. 31.
6. Milio, Nancy. *9226 Kercheval: The Storefront That Did Not Burn.* Ann Arbor: University of Michigan Press, 1970.
7. Bauer, M. Health Characteristics of Low-income Persons. *Vital Health Statistics* vol. 10, 1972, pp. 1–51.
8. Ibid., p. 2.
9. Pomeroy, R. Comparison of Negro Mothers from Welfare and Low-Income Families. *Poverty and Human Resources* vol. 5, 1970, p. 46.
10. Komisar, L. Issues: Subsidies and women. *Poverty and Human Resources Abstracts* vol. 9, 1974, p. 46.
11. Washington, B.B. Women in poverty. *Poverty and Human Resources Abstracts* vol. 1, 1966.
12. Lesse, Stanley. *Masked Depression.* New York: Jason Aronson, 1974.
13. U.S. Department of Labor. Manpower report of the president, including a report on manpower require-

ments, resources, utilization, and training. *Poverty and Human Resources Abstracts* vol. 3, 1968, p. 124.

14. Triplett, J.L. Characteristics and perceptions of low-income women and use of preventive health services: An exploratory study. *Nursing Research* vol. 19, 1970, pp. 140–146.
15. Polansky, N.A., Borgman, R.D., and DeSaix, C. *Roots of Futility*. San Francisco: Jossey-Bass, 1972.
16. Brinton, D.M. Value Differences Between Nurses and Low-Income Families, *Nursing Research* vol. 21, 1972, pp. 46–52.
17. LaBelle McElmurry, B. *The Development of a Nursing Curriculum Design for Health Promotion and Maintenance*. Ann Arbor, MI: University Microfilms, No. 73–25, 598, 1973.
18. Ibid., p. 82.
19. Yura, Helen and Walsh, M.B. *The Nursing Process: Assessing, Planning, Implementing, Evaluating*. New York: Appleton-Century-Crofts, 1973.
20. Schatzman, Leonard and Strauss, A. *Field Research: Strategies for a Natural Sociology* Englewood Cliffs, NJ: Prentice-Hall, 1973, p. 14.
21. Ibid., p. vi.
22. Ibid.

ADDENDUM

The preceding chapter reflects my early work in women's health. Subsequent professional life changes following the first edition of *Women in Stress* has precluded further work with low-income rural women on public aid. However, a few observations are warranted on women's health, poverty, and nursing.

Since 1978, nurse researchers have evidenced activity in areas of women's health. A computerized literature search using terms relevant to the concern of this chapter (low income, women, health economics, and so on) and focusing on the last five years uncovered a little over 200 references. However, relatively few of the citations reviewed were articles written by nurses or articles addressing the health issues faced by low-income women in America. Research on women's health has yet to realize the goal of examining the health of women within the context of their lived experience over the lifespan. There have been great strides in networking researchers working in women's health and some progress in establishing conceptual bases for studies of women's health. Much of the work in women's health by nurses has been published in journals or books that have a relatively small circulation. Even the government's attempt to arrive at consensus on a women's health agenda for the 1980s has been questioned as suspect in a political environment where the "gender gap" has become a familiar criticism.

The area of women's health needs a great deal more attention in order to move from a focus on women's reproductive health to a real understanding of the experiential lifespan perspectives so important to women's health. An in-depth description of women of various ages and circumstances is a prerequisite to developing positive measures of health status as well as deficiency and illness measures. There is much that is not fully understood about women's health, and there is little interest in funding research on women's health. The funding available to women's health researchers makes them paupers in terms of research funding levels. The researchers are not unlike the women described by the term "feminization of poverty." Paula Kassell[1] explains the literal meaning of the term as making poverty appropriate for women.

The term that would express what has been happening to women and our rage about the shredding of the "safety net" is *the pauperization* of women, the term we should be using.[1]

The "nouveau poor," as predicted by Ehrenreich and Stallard[2] and Stallard, Ehrenreich, and Sklar,[3] will consist of women and their children by the year 2000, unless something is done to alter the trend of the 1970s. Nurses can find guidance about the data and research needs in women's health from the writings of Muller[4] and Moore.[5] The more comprehensive synthesis of what is needed is reflected in economist Muller's points about women and health statistics:

Future research could have as one focus the concept of women's health capital, evaluating it at different age levels and for different lifestyles, and studying its relation to utilization, the yield on alternative investments, and interactions with other forms of human capital. Another productive area of research would be the study of the distribution of health-related functions within the household, and opportunities for programmatic investment to improve household efficiency in production of health by diet, hygiene, and other measures. Women's encounters with the health care system should be examined to show what relationships exist between psychosocial aspects of these encounters and the treatment options, quality of care, and outcomes that are experienced by women. Dynamic aspects of women's health and health care could be approached by both longitudinal and cross-sectional studies, development of lifetime aggregates and sequences, and other life cycle-oriented statistics. Monitoring of women's participation in HMO's, health planning agencies and all innovative systems or institutions in the field of health is essential in evaluating system performance with respect to providing equality of opportunity. It also could be correlated with measures of system effectiveness in dealing with women's health problems and meeting humanistic norms in patient care.[4]

In summary, the health care of low-income women is a social issue. As such it has been difficult in the 1970s to discern progress in arriving at some resolution of the problems associated with ensuring health care for these women and their families. It is a monumental task just to appreciate the scope of the problem as evidenced by the U.S. Bureau of the Census[6] project to compile and analyze statistics pertaining to the status of women worldwide. What to do about the problems in any one discipline is even more problematic. Whatever, it seems preferable to work toward the development of a nursing response that recognizes problems such as accessibility and acceptability of the health services and that provides advocacy for the assumption of self-care competency.

References

1. Kassell, P. Names will never hurt us? *New Directions for Women,* vol. 12, November/December 1983, p. 2.
2. Ehrenreich, B., and Stallard, K. The Noveau Poor. *Ms* vol. 11, August 1982, pp. 217–224.
3. Stallard, K., Ehrenreich, B., and Sklar, H. *Poverty in the American Dream: Women and Children First.* Boston: South End Press, 1983.
4. Muller, C. Women and health statistics: Areas of deficient data collection and integration. *Women and Health,* vol. 4, Spring 1979, pp. 37–59.
5. Moore, E.C. *Public Health Reports Supplement: Women and Health, United States, 1980.* (DHHS Publication No. HRA-80-605. Washington, DC: U.S. Government Printing Office. September-October 1980, pp. 84.
6. Center for International Research, U.S. Bureau of the Census. Women in development project. Washington, DC, December 1983.

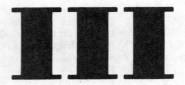

WOMEN'S LIFE
EXPERIENCES AND
THEIR RESOLUTIONS

This section discusses the life experiences women face and their resolutions, starting with physically abused women; continuing with the impact of rape, child abuse, infertility, and eating disorders; and ending with circumstances of women in pain.

13

WORKING WITH THE PHYSICALLY ABUSED WOMAN

CAROL VALENTI

Carol Valenti's chapter on physically abused women starts with the problem of definition—the label of "battered women." She continues with the identification of the factors involved in unhealthy relationships and proceeds to write of the interventions possible in both the health care system and society.

Anyone who approaches the area of family violence needs to have an appreciation of the complex nature of the problem. Any form of family violence is obviously a family problem, but it is also a personal, relationship, cultural, social, and legal problem. There are no easy solutions. Professionals working with many aspects of family violence find themselves at times feeling bewildered, frustrated, irritated, and perhaps even hopeless. Professionals must identify and deal with negative reactions to intense situations. Progress is being made in many parts of the country to assist those who find themselves caught in violent situations. The purpose of this chapter is to present material that shoud be helpful for professionals intervening when family violence, specifically violence against women, occurs.

LABELING THE PROBLEM

One should be aware of the possible damage in using the label "battered woman syndrome." The label "battered woman" has proved to be important in drawing attention to an area that has been ignored and under-assessed. It has also been important in gathering statistics and in doing research in this problem area. However, when professionals in a variety of settings attempt intervention, the label has the potential of misleading the professionals and possibly to harming the patient. It can mislead professionals into thinking that

they are dealing with a very different human problem. Seeing only the label can influence the helping person to ignore the specific dynamics involved in each situation. Physical abuse in one respect demonstrates the existence of a relationship problem. It is a complex problem that shares many variables with other types of relationship problems. If individuals have the expertise to work with relationship problems, they can work with women in physically abusive situations. Professionals far too often believe that they do not have the expertise to work with "battered women" and tend to refer them elsewhere for services. In many situations, making a referral can be a mistake. Individuals involved in helping professions should attempt to work with situations involving family violence in their own setting. Outside assistance should be requested by individuals who have had the courage to try to work with this problem. Information on community resources such as emergency housing, criminal prosecution, and financial assistance can be crucial to a woman caught in a violent relationship. Information should also be sought on factors that help perpetuate violent situations and on the concerns one should have for women who find themselves in violent relationships. Information such as this will serve as an important adjunct to professionals' existing abilities to work with individuals experiencing relationship problems.

Labeling also has the potential of harming the patient. An individual with the label "battered woman" may begin to view herself as different from or "sicker" than another woman who might be experiencing relationship problems without physical violence. This faulty perception can add to the amount of shame and embarrassment a woman in a physically abusive situation is already experiencing. There has been much damage done in the mental health field by the labeling of mentally ill patients. For many individuals it has been difficult to overcome the stigma involved in the frequent usage of such labels. We certainly have not reached this point with physically abused women, but we must be aware of the possible negative effects of labeling on those involved in violent situations.

FACTORS OR DYNAMICS INVOLVED IN UNHEALTHY RELATIONSHIPS

If professionals expect to be effective in working with relationship problems, they must be aware of factors or dynamics involved in the perpetuation of unhealthy relationships. One factor is one's personal or family background. It is generally believed that a large number of adults who find themselves in physically abusive situations have been exposed to models of family violence as children, the idea being that violence passes from one generation to another. Such individuals either were abused as children or witnessed violence between their parents. In a study done on three generations of abused children, the theme that violence passes through generations was supported.[1] The study concluded that the abused child might cope with abuse by identifying either with the aggressor or with the victim. As an adult, the formerly abused child might become either another violent member of society who abuses others or an adult victim of physical violence. The abused child may have learned that love equals being hurt, and abuse received as an adult reinforces this theme. A study done by Gayford in England on 100 abused women showed that 23 of the women and 51 of the abusing men had been exposed to models of family violence as children.[2] Added to the learned belief that love equals being hurt is the fact that violent situations can become familiar. It should be stressed that physically abusive situations are never acceptable to the victim. However, it is understandably difficult for individuals who have been exposed to violence all their lives to leave a violent situation if they think there is a high likelihood that they will be in a similar situation again.

Another variable at work in helping to perpetuate unhealthy relationships, although it takes a particular turn in physically abusive situations, is the low self-concept of the people involved. There are many situations in which the woman develops an intimate relationship with her self-concept intact. The devastating effects, however, of even one beating, along with the psychologic abuse that is usually involved, can be devastating to her self-worth. There are other instances in and out of physically abusive situations in which the individuals come to the relationship with a diminished self-concept. A woman in this instance may have a tendency to choose an inadequate man with the hope of being able to improve him. An inadequate man is defined here as one who is chronically unemployed, chemically dependent, or in trouble with the law. By improving this man, the woman can validate her own worth. The woman's self-concept is then reflected in the accomplishments or failures of her partner. Eventually, the woman realizes the impossibility of the task that she has set for herself but stays with the man because she experiences such a personal sense of failure. In many instances in which physical abuse is occurring, the abusing man admits to the fact that he perceives the woman as being more adequate than himself—occupationally, socially, and educationally. If the man lacks good verbal skills, feels threatened by the woman, and is also violent, he may strike out at the woman. Striking out by the man in these situations can be done in an effort to maintain the superior role that he has been socialized to believe he must maintain in order to qualify as a man. The more inferior and frightened a violent man becomes, the more likely he may be to strike out at his partner. In one of his studies, sociologist Richard Gelles discovered that family violence was more prevalent when the husband's occupational and educational status was lower than his wife's.[3]

Another factor that helps perpetuate unhealthy relationships for women is the socialization of women. There is strong emphasis in our culture on the importance of being a good wife and mother. One of the functions of a good wife and mother is taking almost total responsibility for keeping the family together. Women many times feel a tremendous sense of failure if they are unable to keep the family unit together, no matter what the cost. The situation becomes even more intense if pressure is put on the woman by her family and friends to stay and "grin and bear it." Particularly when physical violence is present within a family system, having detrimental effects on the children as well as the adults involved, encouraging the woman to stay seems, indeed, unhealthy and foolish.

The financial bind that women often find themselves in can be a strong force that helps keep them in unhealthy relationships. In our society it has been common for a woman to choose marriage or involvement with a man at an early age. This can mean not only that she is now without a profession but also that she has never worked outside of the home. If dependent children are involved, a woman at times is at a loss as to how she can independently support herself, let alone the children. Leaving a physically abusive situation often engenders tremendous fear of physical reprisal by the abusing party. It may mean that the woman has to leave everything she knows and owns and accomplish much with dependent children and no money. Where, then, does the physically abused woman go with her children for safety? The homes of friends and relatives are usually not acceptable, for the abusing party will often look first for the woman at such locations. Women who live in communities that have shelters for them and their children are indeed fortunate, for often shelters are the only safe place to which a woman can escape.

In physically abusive relationships, fear can be an overwhelming factor that makes it difficult for the woman to make the choice of leaving her situation. Often the woman has been threatened with a knife or a gun and has been told she will be killed, possibly along with her children, if she attempts to leave. If there is no safe place for the woman to go, she may feel trapped in an impossible situation.

For many individuals, the thought of a relationship ending mainly means that the person will be alone. Fear of the loneliness that might result from such a separation can keep both men and women in relationships that they have defined as unhealthy. Both men and women sometimes feel that being in a bad relationship is better than being alone. When the fear of loneliness is so great that it will force someone to stay in an unhealthy relationship, individuals can and perhaps should become more aware of the dynamics involved in their personal fears. Such an awareness can help individuals

to see their situation more clearly and to make better choices for themselves in relationships.

Many times people stay in unhealthy relationships because they hope that the unpleasantness will disappear. A relationship is rarely all bad. There are often good times as well as traumatic times, and ambivalence about terminating the relationship can certainly stem from such mixed experiences. In physically abusive situations, a woman is often treated well after a beating. Her partner often does special favors for her or her children or buys them presents. Frequently this is the only time the physically abused woman is treated in such a positive manner. There is the hope that after such a pleasant experience the physical abuse will not happen again.

Another justification given by individuals for remaining in a bad situation is, "But I love him/her." Such a statement made after individuals have defined a relationship as unhealthy for them can be indicative of what they think they deserve in life. The motivation for leaving a bad situation is low if individuals believe they do not deserve or will never find anything better.

Chemical dependency is often involved in unhealthy relationships. Reliable data are not available on how often chemical dependency is involved in physically abusive situations, but it is generally thought to be high. Chemical usage by the abusing party has generally been regarded as the cause of violence. There is a growing belief, however, that many men may drink as an excuse or justification for becoming violent.[4] After the violent incident, both the assailant and victim can blame the behavior on alcohol. It is often assumed that, if an individual has been drinking, he is not responsible for his behavior. The use of chemicals by the victim in violent situations needs to be examined and can be a factor in making it difficult for a woman to leave an unhealthy relationship.

One must have an appreciation of the tremendous amount of energy it takes a woman to plan and execute a move away from a family situation, particularly if there is violence. Living in a psychologically and/or physically abusive situation erodes a woman's self-concept. Eventually, she begins to believe the cruel, disparaging remarks and may begin to believe that somehow she deserves the physical abuse as well. The more worthless and depressed a woman feels, the less energy she has and the more difficult it becomes to harness that energy to plan and carry out a move. Support and help from outside resources is sometimes the only way a woman is able to make a move away from a violent situation.

INTERVENTION

Effects of Attitude on Behavior

Professionals can and should attempt to intervene in family situations when violence is present. One's attitudes toward violence, and specifically violence toward women, is an important consideration in any discussion of intervention, for attitudes have a direct effect on one's behavior.

Dealing with physical abuse evokes certain attitudes and feelings in professionals that might not be apparent when working with other types of problems. Often there is an implicit and at times unrecognized attitude by professionals that, if a woman does not define physical abuse as a problem or does not display a readiness to act, or both, she is somehow "sicker" than another woman who might not be ready to get out of an unhealthy, nonviolent relationship. Holding such attitudes can affect professionals' behavior. At times, individuals in the helping profession urge a woman to leave a physically abusive situation before she is ready to do so. By taking such a stance, professionals can lose the woman to their services or influence her to leave a situation before she is psychologically ready. In the latter situation, there is a high likelihood that she will either return to the same situation or find herself in a similar situation.

There appears to be a personal and perhaps even societal attitude that, at some level, violence against women, particularly if the perpetrator is her husband, is acceptable, understandable, or at least justifiably provoked by the woman. Attitudes such as this have been reflected in a study conducted at Michigan State University.[5] In this study, fights were staged and observed on a city street. In the first three situations, a woman was being attacked by a woman, a man was being attacked by a woman, and a man was being attacked by a man, respectively. In all of these situations, a male bystander came to the rescue of the victim. In the last staged situation, a woman was being attacked by a man. No male bystander came to the rescue of the victim in this situation. The experiment was repeated several times with the same results. Many people can recall the tragic Kitty Genovese murder in New York City, in which not one of the 38 witnesses attempted to intervene.[6] When the witnesses were questioned, many of them said that they did not intervene because they thought the attacker was the victim's husband. Implicit in such a tragic, frightening lack of response may be the attitude in our society that the use of violence against women within the family system is acceptable or understandable.

Another shocking development in our society and that of Europe is the growing commercial trend in which the motif of violence against women is used to advertise and successfully sell clothing and records. A revealing article in *Time* magazine entitled "Really Socking It to Women" describes how prominent fashion photographers and advertising people, as well as record companies, are using violence to sell their products.[7] It also describes how *Vogue* magazine abroad and in America has used situations depicting violence against women to stimulate sales of their products. There have been pictures showing women as killers and victims and one in which a woman's head is being forced into a toilet bowl. American *Vogue*, in a 12-page spread, shows a man intermittently caressing and menacing a female model. The grand finale occurs when the man smashes the woman across the face. On the next page, the female model is pictured affectionately nudging the abusing man. The Jon Anthony jumpsuit that the model wears in this picture spread has sold beautifully. Needless to say, the manufacturer of the jumpsuit thinks the ad was successful. The most distressing question to be asked is, Why can violence and maltreatment of women stimulate sales in a predominantly female market?

This *Time* article also describes a store window in a Boston boutique. Displayed in the window was an apparently dead woman with blood running out of her mouth tumbling out of a garbage can with a pair of men's shoes on her head. The sign in the window read "We'd kill for these." One could certainly offer innumerable cultural, sociologic, or sexist reasons for the use of this form of advertising. One thing that cannot be denied is that trends such as this are promoting and perpetuating the attitude that violence against women is acceptable and, in some cases, even enjoyed by the victim. Promoting such attitudes in any manner will drastically affect society's and one's individual motivation to assess and intervene when violence against women ocucrs.

Professionals working with family violence must become aware of their personal attitudes toward violence, specifically violence against women, and reflect on how these attitudes affect their behavior. This awareness can be accomplished by providing opportunities for indivduals in the helping professions to come together and talk openly about their thoughts and feelings on the subject and to acquire information on and insight into some of the factors involved in the perpetuation of family violence. Only after helping people have reflected on their personal attitudes are they ready to consider some of the specifics involved in intervention.

Helping Process

The helping process is a framework that can be used effectively by professionals to assess and intervene. I define the helping process as professional activity with the purpose of assisting individuals, couples, or families with emotional states or practical situations that they have defined as a problem and have a desire to act on. It is the professional's responsibility to help the individual, couple, or family define the problem and to either help them assess their readiness for action or attempt to motivate them toward action for change. It is not the professional's responsibility to decide unilaterally what a problem is to the individual, couple, or family or when and how they should act on the problem. These are rules or concepts that many of us hold to be true in working with people. It is particularly important to emphasize them in any discussion on violence against women.

When using the helping process, the professional must first discover whether physical abuse is occurring in a situation and then ascertain whether the individual, couple, or family is defining such abuse as a problem. When the professional is working specifically with a woman, she may regard other problems in her life, such as chemical dependency of her spouse or of herself or other family problems, to be of more concern to her than physical abuse. It is clearly the professional's role to identify whether violence is occurring and never to lose sight of it when working with a woman or her family but at the same time to respect the woman's position in defining such violence as a problem.

There are many situations in which women do define physical abuse as a problem. The next step in using the helping process is to assess her readiness to act on the situation. Often, even though the woman sees her situation as a problem, she does not demonstrate a readiness to act on it. As previously discussed, there are many factors and dynamics that help perpetuate unhealthy, physically abusive relationships and that directly affect a woman's readiness to act. The professional should help the woman to discover what dynamics and factors are involved in her resistance to change. It is also appropriate for the helping person to give the woman feedback on the negative effect that the situation may be having on her. The professional must never go beyond this point and force or pressure the woman to leave the situation before she is ready to leave.

Intervention in the Health Care Setting

The health care setting provides many opportunities for assessment and intervention when violence against women is occurring. Health care settings include emergency rooms, physicians' offices, outpatient clinics, and inpatient hospital units. As discussed in an earlier chapter, women are frequent users of health care services. They often go to physicians or other health personnel for birth control, pregnancy, and gynecologic problems; they also take their children to health care facilities for treatment. Whenever a social or family assessment is done in a health care setting, consideration should be given to relationships within the family. If there is any indication of problems in these relationships, it is necessary to ask in a sensitive way whether there is any physical abuse. When the woman's symptoms are anxiety, depression, or various somatic complaints, one should thoroughly assess her social and family situations. There have been many situations in my experience in which, even though the presenting problem has been anxiety or depression, the real but concealed problem has involved physical abuse. Women also come to a health care setting for treatment of injuries. It is always appropriate for the physician or allied health professional to ask the cause of injury. If there is reason to think that the woman might have been assaulted, it is appropriate to ask her in a sensitive manner whether she has been assaulted, and if so, by whom.

There is usually a great deal of shame and embarrassment associated with being caught in a violent situation. One should not expect a woman coming to a health care facility for help to offer information about physical abuse without some assistance by a professional. Even after sensitive questioning, the woman seeking help might give an untrue or defensive answer. In addition to shame and embarrassment, there are other factors that might inhibit a woman's response to questioning about physical abuse. Often the woman is fearful of the consequences if she tells someone what has been happening. She also might believe that it is useless to tell anyone because nothing could possibly be done to make the situation any better. The woman might also be reluctant to talk about physical abuse for fear that she will be regarded as "sick" for remaining in the relationship. No matter what the response of the woman, the most important thing is that the question has been asked. Even if the woman is not ready to define abuse as a problem or to act on the situation, by asking the question, the professional has opened the door for her. If and when the woman is ready to talk about her situation, she knows there is a place for her to go.

In my practice, I have identified certain considerations in approaching a woman about the possible existence of family violence. In view of the previous discussion on the feelings of abused women, it is important to make any questions as nonthreatening as possible. It helps put a woman at ease, when the professional is questioning about violence, to tell the woman that this is a common problem in the health care setting and that she is not alone in her experiences. If the woman does admit to physical abuse, consideration must be given to her physical safety. The woman should be told about the professional's concern for her safety. She should also be asked if she is afraid of being severely hurt. It takes only a few seconds in a violent situation for the victim to sustain serious bodily harm. If the woman does admit to fear of severe bodily injury, she should always be believed, no matter how extreme or unbelievable her story may seem. A woman who comes to a health care setting for treatment of injuries should be asked if she wants to return home. The woman might be too frightened to return to a situation in which the abusing partner can attack her again. At a time such as this, it is essential to be aware of community resources that could be of assistance to the abused woman.

There are situations in which both women and their children are being physically abused. A professional must remember this important consideration. It is appropriate and necessary to ask a woman whether the children are being abused. If information is received about child abuse, the professional must fulfill possible legal responsibilities in reporting this to the proper agency. Mandatory reporting of child abuse might force the woman to do something about her situation before she is psychologically ready to do so.

Another important consideration in interviewing a woman who has been physically assaulted is to inform her that she has the right to file criminal charges. The author has interviewed women who did not know that it is a crime for a husband or boyfriend to beat his partner. Knowledge of procedures for criminal prosecution is essential to help the woman if she wishes to press criminal charges. Often the woman is reluctant to initiate criminal proceedings because of the overwhelming fear of reprisal by the abusing party. Informing the woman of her rights and of the procedures for prosecution is an appropriate activity of the professional. The woman should never be forced or pressured to follow this course, however.

Group Approach to Intervention

In my experience, women's therapy groups have been an effective means of attempting to intervene when relationship problems exist. It is not advisable to put together in a group only women who have been physically abused and then label the group a "battered women's group." As previously discussed, there can be detrimental outcomes to such labeling. Rather, women experiencing a wide range of relationship problems, physical abuse being only one of them, should be considered for this group experience. There are many advantages to having a group with a mixture of problems. It is therapeutic for all group members to see the similarities and differences among themselves regardless of their situations. It helps to reduce the isolation barrier of women in physically abusive situations if they can see themselves as being similar to other women in different situations. Individuals who are experiencing relationship problems or who have a diminished self-concept generally believe, for a variety of reasons, that they have little self-power and few rights; they do not think that they deserve to have emotional feelings or express their needs. These factors are often present whether or not physical abuse is occurring. These are issues that can be addressed through a group approach. Group process can be used to help individuals who practice and learn new ways of relating to other significant persons in their lives.

In emphasizing the group experience for women, it is particularly important to state that the women do not have to leave unhealthy relationships in order for personal growth or change to take place. In my practice, I have observed that women can change as a result of a group experience regardless of their personal situations. Through a group experience, women begin to develop their ability to share feelings with others and thus begin to trust and accept the help of other people in and outside of the group in stressful as well as pleasant times. It is generally believed that there are certain pros and cons relating to the ways in which outside relationships affect group process. Considering the extreme isolation of some of these women, it is exciting to see them develop meaningful relationships for perhaps the first time in their lives. The possible negative effects on group process seem minimal in comparison to these growing friendships.

Another area of personal growth for women I have observed in a group experience, again regardless of the participant's personal situation, is the development of a stronger self-concept and thus the beginnings of healthier behavior. This development is very much connected with the first area discussed, for from the building of trusting relationships also comes a better opinion of oneself. There are declarations that women can make to promote a more positive self-concept. Setting limits within a relationship on the type of behavior that will be tolerated is such a declaration. Women do reach the point when they state that further physical violence will not be allowed. Sometimes this limit-setting is accomplished by the real threat of separation or even by the threat of physical reprisal by the woman. Women who make decisions to seek employment or job training or who enroll in school also find that they eventually begin to feel better about themselves. Another behavior that helps promote a healthy self-concept is asking for what one wants and needs in a relationship. This behavior can be initiated, practiced, and learned within a group context.

As mentioned at the beginning of this chapter, working in this problem area can become quite frustrating to the professional. It is undoubtedly more frustrating to work in settings where the professional, rather than the woman, is identifying the problem. Although it is likely in these situations that the woman might not be ready to do anything about her situation, questions regarding family violence still need to be asked. Individuals in a helping profession, therefore, must identify and deal with their own frustrations and irritations. It might be helpful if professionals in a variety of settings dealing with family violence formed support groups for themselves. These groups could provide not only a good oportunity for the expression of thoughts and feelings but also the impetus for discovering new and better approaches for dealing with this complex problem area.

References

1. Silver, Larry, Dublin, Christina, and Lourie, Reginold. Does violence breed violence? Contributions from a study of child abuse syndrome. *American Journal of Psychiatry*, vol. 126, September 1969, pp. 152–155.
2. Gayford, J.J. Wife battering: A preliminary survey of 100 cases. *British Medical Journal*, vol. 1, January 1975, pp. 194–197.
3. Edmiston, Susan. The Wife Beaters. *Woman's Day*, March 1976, p. 61–63.
4. Ibid.
5. Borofsky, G.I., Stollack, G.E., and Messe, L.A. Sex differences in bystander reactions to physical assault. *Journal of Experimental Social Psychology*, vol. 7, 1971, pp. 313–318.
6. Edmiston, Susan, op. cit.
7. Really Socking It to Women. *Time*, February 7, 1977, pp. 58–59.

General References

Straus, Murray, Geller, R., and Steinmetz, Suzanne. *Behind Closed Doors: Violence in the American Family.* New York: Anchor Books, 1980.
Walker, Lenore. *The Battered Woman.* New York: Harper and Row, 1979.

14

IMPACT OF RAPE ON VICTIMS AND FAMILIES: TREATMENT AND RESEARCH CONSIDERATIONS

LINDA LEDRAY
SANDER LUND
THOMAS KIRESUK

Linda Ledray, Sander Lund, and Thomas Kiresuk discuss rape's impact on the victims and their families in this chapter. They begin with the incidence of rape and community attitudes toward rape. The research study serves as the basis for revealing the impact of physical trauma on the victim and the social and psychologic impact on the victim and her family. The treatment intervention is described, and the chapter closes calling for more research in this area.

Rape is a problem of great national, local, and personal concern. A rape has far-reaching effects on a woman's social, psychologic, and physical being, often leading to involvement with the police, the court system, medical personnel, and counselors. This chapter deals with some of these issues. It includes the incidence and reporting of rape, the impact of rape on the woman and her family or significant other, the postrape experience, and some of the recent changes in the medical and legal system that make the system more responsive to the needs of the victim.

This chapter also outlines some of the difficulties related to clinical research in the area of sexual assault, suggests some strategies for surmounting these obstacles and developing useful research designs, examines some of the themes that might be important in such research, and describes a research project conducted at Hennepin County Medical Center in Minneapolis that addresses some of the issues raised in the foregoing discussion.

INCIDENCE AND REPORTING OF RAPE

According to FBI statistics, there were over 82,000 forcible rapes in the United States in 1980.[1] This represents an 8 per cent increase since 1979, a 45 per cent increase since 1976, and a 94 per cent increase since 1971. There was a slight decrease in the numbers of reported rapes until 1984 when an increase of 6.7 per cent occurred over the previous year. In 1984, 84,230 rapes were reported.[2] The number of rapes reported is consistently lower during the winter months of each year and peaks during the summer months. Forcible rapes have increased at a higher rate than any other *Crime Index* offense in the past 10 years. There also appears to be a shift in the incidence of reported rapes from the major urban areas to the suburbs. Whereas 39 per cent of the reported rapes for 1980 occurred in cities with populations over 250,000, in 1976 this figure was 42 per cent. The suburbs reported an increase of 11 per cent from 1979 to 1980, and rural areas reported an increase of 10 per cent during this period.

Although rape is the most frequently committed violent crime in the United States, the *Uniform Crime Report* states that rape is reported to the police less often than any other *Crime Index* offense.[2] Officials cannot be certain if this increase is due to better reporting, an actual increase in the incidence of rape, or a combination of the two. Even if better reporting is responsible for the higher statistics, officials estimate today that only one out of every four to 10 rapes is reported.[3] These figures also then indicate that an additional 246,000 to 738,000 women are actually raped every year. This means someone is being raped every second of every day, including this very moment, somewhere in the United States. Reporting is lowest in major urban areas with high population densities and low income levels.[4, 5] It appears that many rapes go unreported because of the pervasive myths regarding rape and rape victims generally held in our society. These myths tend to disparage the victim and to demonstrate sympathy for the assailant.[6-8] It is probable that rapes also go unreported because of the humiliation and depersonalization of the victim by police, medical personnel, and the legal system.[9-11]

COMMUNITY ATTITUDES

Pervasive but unfounded myths about rape have been long accepted as fact and have a profound effect on the way that society views the rapist and rape victim, on the way that the victim sees herself, and on the number of rapes that are reported. The acceptance of these myths appears to be the result of a lack of understanding of the nature of forcible rapes.

One such myth is that rape is usually an impulsive act that occurs because the woman acts or dresses seductively and that rapists are driven mad with sexual desire and cannot help themselves. This view has been discredited by the research of Amir and others, who have shown that rapists plan their rapes and that their intent is often aggressive rather than sexual.[12] Amir's research also questions the

commonly held belief that rape is a sex crime and supports the belief that rape is an assault, an act of aggression by one person against another. The findings of Price concur and show that the rape victim is reacting to an aggressive act of violence rather than a sexual act.[13]

A paradoxical twist of this myth has been reported by Jones and Aronson, who find that, the more socially respectable the victim, the more she is seen to be at fault by society. Rape victims are faulted more if they are either a virgin or married than if they are divorced. The authors interpreted these data as evidencing the belief in a "just world," where people get what they deserve. According to this theory, if a victim is perceived as respectable, there is a greater cognitive need to attribute fault to her actions, because fault cannot be attributed to her character.[14] This theory is based on Lerner's just-world hypothesis[15, 16] and the cognitive dissonance theory.[17]

Rape myths include beliefs that women enjoy or secretly desire to be raped, that nice girls do not get raped, that rapes occur only in dark alleys, and that a woman cannot be raped unless she is willing ("a woman can run faster with her skirt up than a man with his pants down"). These and many others are discussed and refuted by Amir,[18] Brownmiller,[19] Medea and Thompson,[20] and many other reputable scientific investigators. However, these myths continue to be believed by otherwise intelligent, knowledgeable individuals, and, no matter how unfounded, they have a profound effect on both the victim's view of herself and the family's or significant other's view of the victim.

IMPACT ON THE VICTIM

Rape is a violent crime with physical, social, and psychologic consequences that are often of great magnitude. However, until recently there has been little concern about the impact on the victim. Rape has been considered a crime by one man against the property (wife or daughter) of another man.[21]

The way a woman responds to rape depends to a great extent on her prior adaptive capacity, coping style, and social support.[22] Certainly the 1495 rape victims seen by the Sexual Assault Resource Service (SARS) between 1978 and 1981 reacted in a variety of ways and to various degrees. Preliminary research, although limited, provides some insights into the nature of the physical, social, and psychologic suffering of the victim regardless of age, race, occupation, or personal history.

Physical Trauma

The physical trauma is perhaps best documented because of records kept by hospitals. The rape victim may have sustained injuries from being beaten and other forms of physical violence, as well as from forceful intercourse leading to vaginal and rectal trauma. From the limited statistics available it appears that the need for hospitalization after a rape is low. Hayman and Lanza reported that only 1 per cent of the rape victims seen in a Washington, DC, hospital needed to be hospitalized, and only 3 per cent needed emergency room treatment for severe injuries.[23] Hennepin County Medical Center in Minneapolis found that 18 per cent of the rape victims treated from 1977 to 1980 had been beaten severely enough to require medical treatment. Statistics are not readily available on the number of deaths related to or subsequent to rape, since these are usually reported by the police as homicide. However, fear of death or serious injury is often the greatest concern of the woman at the time of the incident.[24, 25]

Statistics show that the risk of pregnancy following a rape is low, about 1 per cent; as is the risk of contracting venereal disease, less than 4 per cent but increasing. However, these are both of great concern to a woman following a rape. It is difficult to ascertain the actual risk of becoming pregnant or contracting venereal disease after a rape, because the statistics available are based on the small percentage of women who report the incident and receive care after the rape. This care usually includes prophylactic penicillin to prevent venereal disease and prophylactic diethylstilbestrol to prevent pregnancy.[26] The above statistics would undoubtedly be much higher were they to include the many victims, possibly 13 out of 14, who fail to report the rape, receive no prophylaxis, and are therefore much more vulnerable to both venereal disease and pregnancy.

Other, often long-term physical problems may occur. These include changes in eating habits and in sleeping patterns, often owing to recurrent nightmares.[27]

Social Impact

The social impact of rape on the victim is not documented in systematized research; however, implications can be drawn from case studies. Rape has been recognized as a time of crisis for the victim. However, it differs from other crises, because the victim's usual support system is more likely to be disrupted.[28, 29] The victim may be isolated after rejection by the husband, family, friends, lover, or all four, because of their preconceptions regarding her role in the rape.[30] Peters and Medea and Thompson found that many victims voluntarily withdraw socially and emotionally from all contact with friends and family, while they are at the same time afraid to be alone.[31, 32] Brownmiller has shown that rape may often be used by the man as a means of conquering, suppressing, and subjugating the female to his authority or of punishing her.[33]

Case studies document incidents of victims being evicted from their apartments following rape, because the landlord was upset when the police arrived and the landlord believed it to be a drug bust. Other victims may move to another city, either voluntarily or after being ordered to leave home. For many this move represents a way to escape the social disgrace still associated with rape.[34] If the rape occurred in their home they may fear that the rapist will return and therefore they move to ensure their safety.[35] The literature alludes to some long-term effects of the socially disruptive consequences of rape; however, the extent and prevalence have not yet been determined.

Psychologic Impact

Although the physical and social impact of rape is great, the psychologic trauma is the most devastating.[36] Research studies of the psychologic impact of rape are just beginning to appear in the literature and evidence a pattern of response, which Burgess calls the "Rape Trauma Syndrome."[37] This pattern is usually divided into three phases. Phase 1, the *acute reaction,* is characterized by shock and disbelief, physical symptoms, gross anxiety, emotional breakdown, and disorganization and disruption in the normal pattern of behavior and function. Phase 2, the *outward adjustment,* includes resolution of the acute anxiety, denial and suppression, and return to normal function at work, school, or home. This usually occurs a few days to a week after the incident. Phase 3, that of *integration and resolution,* often goes unnoticed. It is characterized by the onset of depression, the need to talk about the experience, anger at the assailant and at oneself and eventually a realistic appraisal of one's view of oneself. Depression is indeed one of the most pervasive and significant psychologic symptoms encountered in rape victims.[37a, b, c, d]

Case studies have revealed the existence of

long-term psychologic effects of rape. Some of the long-term traumas noted are recurrent nightmares, depression, phobia to men, fear of being alone, fear of being outside if the rape occurred outside, fear of being inside if the rape occurred inside, sexual fears, fear of crowds, fear of people behind them,[38] and fear of looking provocative.[39] In Operation De Nova, a Hennepin County Juvenile Division program in Minneapolis, it has been found that the first sexual experience of 70 per cent of the juvenile prostitutes was either rape or an incestuous relationship.[40] This finding raises additional questions about the long-term effects of rape.

Burgess also identified what she calls a compound reaction. This was noted in individuals with current or past physical, social, or psychiatric difficulties and consisted of additional symptoms such as depression, psychosis, and suicidal behavior.[41] Two rape victims seen in the Hennepin County Medical Center emergency room in a six-month period have attempted suicide subsequent to their rapes.

IMPACT ON THE FAMILY OR SIGNIFICANT OTHER

Borges,[42] Peters,[43] Medea and Thompson,[44] and Brownmiller[45] all recognize that the attitude about rape and the reaction of the family or significant other to the rape incident are of great significance to the rape victim, but they give no clear indication as to how or the extent to which this is significant. Emergency room nurses at Hennepin County Medical Center have found that often the first question asked by the rape victim is, "Should I tell my husband/parents/boyfriend?" and, if so, "How should I tell them?"

Mental health professionals have accepted for some time that the family is an interacting social system. Whatever affects one member has an effect on another member. The rape victim, as a member of a social system, interacts with family and friends. However, very few research data are currently available regarding the family's/significant other's reaction to a rape or how their reaction affects the victim.

Many families decide to keep the rape a secret. This practice may "protect" both victim and family immediately, but case studies show that problems may arise in therapy at a later date.[46] From these case studies we have learned that families are often inconsiderate and rejecting, blame the victim, and misplace their anger at the rapist onto the victim instead of providing the support she so desperately needs.[47] Although no statistics are currently available, Brownmiller states that husbands often divorce their wives after a rape, further escalating the trauma and isolating the victim.[48] Burgess concurs that the adverse reaction of the significant other is often part of the further traumatization of the victim after the rape.[49]

One would expect that the traumatization of the victim would end when the rape incident ends. This is not always the case. All too often, the trauma is compounded during what should be treatment.

TREATMENT OF THE VICTIM

The treatment needs of rape victims include medical intervention, psychologic intervention, and legal intervention by the police and perhaps the courts.

Medical Intervention

Fortunately, only 30 per cent of rape victims receive minor injuries, small lacerations, or bruises, and only 3 per cent sustain injuries requiring treatment or hospital admission.[50] Still, a primary concern of many victims is medical care. The medical needs of rape victims extend beyond the care of injuries. The components of good medical care following a rape include (1) care of injuries; (2) testing for and prevention of sexually transmitted disease; (3) pregnancy risk evaluation, testing, and preventive care; (4) evidentiary examination with proper documentation and maintenance of the proper chain of evidence; and (5) psychosocial crisis intervention.

Although progress has indeed been made in the past 15 years, unfortunately many hospitals across the country have still not developed protocols for the care of sexual assault victims and will not see them. Other hospitals may see rape victims, but their protocols do not include all five components just mentioned. Sexually transmitted disease testing, pregnancy testing, and crisis intervention are the most often neglected areas. As a result, rape victims are either turned away or do not get complete care. Some of those who are turned away do go elsewhere for care; others get no help at all. A 1985 survey completed in a large midwestern city concluded that only 20 per cent of rape victims who were asked to go to another hospital actually did so.[51]

Hospital administrative and clinical personnel indicated three primary concerns in deciding to refer rape victims to other institutions rather than providing care at their own emergency rooms. Many hospitals saw only a few (one or two) rape victims a month. As a result, with the rotating shifts typical of E.R. staffing patterns, they felt unable to provide their personnel with adequate experience to become proficient at collecting evidence and maintaining the proper chain of evidence. In addition, since it is not possible to predict when these few victims would come to the E.R., it was not possible to have extra nurses available. One sexual assault examination may take over 5 hours; 2 hours is an average length of time. Small emergency rooms felt unable to provide the necessary nursing care to complete the examination. The third concern was the likelihood that both the E.R. nurse and physician would be required to appear in court to testify about their role in the evidence collection. This would require a significant additional time commitment. These are indeed issues of concern in hospital management.

In response to these problems, the Sexual Assault Resource Service in Minneapolis developed a new nursing position, a sexual assault nurse clinician (SANC). This nurse is now available on call to go to local private hospitals whenever a rape victim comes in. The E.R. staff are responsible for initial triage and care of any physical injuries. This is done prior to the SANC's arrival. Once on the scene, the SANC completes the evidentiary examination; the sexually transmitted disease testing and prevention; and pregnancy risk evaluation, testing, and preventive care and provides initial crisis intervention and referral to local community rape centers for supportive follow-up care. In addition, the SANC is available to see the rape victim on two additional occasions for follow-up sexually transmitted disease and pregnancy evaluation and care. She is also available to testify as an expert witness should the case go to court.

A major advantage of the SANC program is that once initial training is complete this program can operate with funded paid staff, not volunteers, on money available through the county attorney's office in over one half of the states across the country. In most areas this money is unutilized, and rape victims are not getting the services they so desperately need. Equal access to medical care for the rape victim remains an important problem to resolve. It is hoped that this new nursing position will be a major step in that direction.

Psychologic Intervention

Interventions specific to the needs of the rape victim have also just recently been identified. The Sexual Assault Resource Service in Minneapolis has identified seven components essential to meeting the counseling needs of rape victims and a treatment model based on these needs.[37a]

These counseling needs include the following. First, the counselor must be nonjudgmental and must recognize that it is the subjective experience of rape that is important. It is not the counselor's job to determine if the woman was "really" raped. Beyond all else, the victim needs to be believed, not questioned or blamed. Whatever she did or did not do, it was the best decision she could make at the time, in her particular situation. It is not the counselor's role to judge her but rather to reassure her that she is not to blame.

Second, it is important to be an empathetic, accepting, and respectful listener to whom the woman can express her feelings when she is ready to do so—the key point being "when she is ready." The response of victims can vary from being happy to be alive to withdrawal and extreme anger. These feelings may be expressed at various points in time. The counselor should not expect any particular response from the victim but rather should be available to listen and respond to the woman on her terms, as she is ready to deal with issues.

Third, it is important to respond to the woman as a normal, healthy individual who is presently in a state of emotional disequilibrium subsequent to a serious life crisis. She will need reassurance that what she is experiencing is a normal response to rape. She must be made to understand that it does not mean she is "crazy" and that the feelings will eventually pass. She must know that the issues will be resolved.

Fourth, the counselor must assist the woman to regain or maintain control of herself and of her situation. The counselor can best do this by ensuring that the victim knows she has the ability to make choices, by helping her identify the alternatives, and by providing her with the information necessary for her to make educated choices.

Fifth, the counselor must treat the woman as separate from the rape. She is not a "raped woman," who will always be a "raped woman." She is a woman who has been raped and who now has significant issues to resolve. The rape has not changed who she is; it was a very traumatic life experience that happened to her and that she must now deal with.

The sixth component is that the counselor must help the woman identify and deal with the responses of those people in her social support system. It is important to review the possible responses of these people, both positive and negative, so that she is better prepared for their reactions. Unfortunately, the responses are not always positive and supportive, but it is more difficult for the victim when negative responses come as a surprise and she does not understand the underlying dynamics involved.

Seventh, the counselor must address issues of personal safety. While we can never be completely safe and invulnerable to a rape, there are things we can do to make ourselves less vulnerable. There are choices we make every day, and it is important to be aware of the impact of these choices on our vulnerability.

Legal Intervention

The other agency with which the victim will most likely have immediate contact is the police department and later perhaps the courts. She must decide whether she wishes to press charges and to fill out a police report. Her credibility may be questioned. The police, not believing the rape charge, may change the charge to a lesser offense. The police report goes into specific detail regarding the rape incident and includes questions about intimate sexual contact that are difficult to answer, especially when addressing a disbelieving, insensitive man.[52] A strong effort is presently underway to change both the attitudes of the police and police treatment of the victim. Many cities have established special sexual assault squads with well-trained, sensitive policemen and policewomen.[3]

Should the victim decide to prosecute and should the assailant be apprehended, the victim must then undergo the ordeal of the courtroom. In many states her character is literally put on trial. Her credibility, morality, and past sexual conduct are questioned.[52] Not only must she relive the experience in detail but she must do so in a public courtroom where members of the press may be present to report the incident in the media.

Even after she undergoes this ordeal, the chances of obtaining a conviction are very low. Nationally about 40 per cent of those taken to court are convicted.[53] The situation is not as bleak in Hennepin County, where for the past two years the Sexual Assault Services have made a concerted effort to change the legal system and protect the rape victim rather than only the rapist. The present conviction rate in Hennepin County is 75 per cent, one of the highest in the nation. This has been possible because of a coordinated effort among the police, courts, and medical/counseling personnel.

COORDINATION OF SERVICES

Rape is a law enforcement, legal, and medical problem. The groups of professionals involved cannot work in isolation and expect to solve a problem they do not have all the resources to deal with. To function effectively, an interlocking system must be established with mutual support and cooperation among these professionals and the agencies they represent.

In the past, each of these groups worked independently. The police brought the victim to the hospital and later completed their report on the incident. The hospital treated any injuries and did routine venereal disease and pregnancy tests. When the woman chose to prosecute, the courts later became involved.

The result of this situation in 1970 was that in the entire state of Minnesota, only 23 charges of rape were made and only 12 of these resulted in convictions. The police did not understand rape and in many instances did not believe a rape had actually occurred, as evidenced by their changing the charge to breaking and entering or burglary. When the police did make an arrest for rape, often after expending considerable time and effort to apprehend the suspect, the courts could not prosecute because of the lack of evidence. In many instances there was nothing to base the case on; it was the woman's word against the suspect's. The physicians and nurses in emergency rooms had no idea what evidence would be useful, how to collect it, or what to do with it if it was found. So the evidence was lost or considered inadmissible in court because it was improperly handled. Victims did not want to prosecute because of revictimization in the courtroom; nor did they choose to call the police or see medical personnel, because of the lack of understanding and empathy others had experienced and reported.

When this situation was finally identified and the problem recognized, a concerted effort was made by legal, medical, and law enforcement groups to discuss the issues in interagency meetings. Their goals were not only to improve their own understanding and handling of the rape situation but, even more importantly, to learn from each other and integrate and coordinate their efforts so that they could provide support and assistance to each other and deal more effectively with victims of sexual assault.

The police received training to increase their understanding of the rape situation and the needs of rape victims. The police and the courts worked with hospital personnel to develop an evidentiary examination that would allow physicians and nurses to collect evidence that could later be used in court. The hospitals trained interested physicians and nurses to collect this evidence and provide support to victims of rape. When necessary, they would go to court and testify as expert witnesses. Because these professionals were now providing a very useful service, their frustration was greatly diminished and replaced by a satisfaction with the service they were providing.

Since 1970 the county attorney's office has made dramatic changes that have greatly enhanced the total impact of services to victims of sexual assault. This began with the establishment of the Sexual Assault Program, a division of the county attorney's office. Its efforts have led to changes in the laws relating to criminal sexual conduct, making them much more comprehensive, humanistic, and nondiscriminatory and, most importantly, making it easier to more appropriately charge and prosecute offenders. In addition, the laws now protect the victim and do not allow her character to be put on trial. The county attorney also issued a directive that offenders would be charged with the sexual crime; they would not be allowed to plead guilty to a lesser crime and have the sex charge dropped.

Under the present coordinated services, the following is a typical case:

A 24-year-old white woman, Mrs. Mary K., was brought to the Hennepin County Medical Center emergency room at 11:30 P.M. by two policemen. She had called the police after an unknown man had broken into her ground-floor apartment and raped her. Her husband was out of town.

Upon arriving at the emergency room she was tearful and frightened. The policemen were both understanding and sympathetic. While one comforted her, another identified her as a rape victim to the nurse in charge of the emergency room. She was taken immediately to a quiet section at the back of the emergency room specifically set aside to deal with rape victims. The nurse who had been trained to deal with rape victims remained with her throughout the medical-legal examination. While the evidentiary examination was being completed, the rape crisis counselor on-call arrived.

The emergency room nurse introduced Mary to the rape counselor, who Mary would later learn would be available to meet with her for up to one year. Mary was afraid to go home, so the counselor found her a safe place to spend the night.

The next day the rape counselor called Mary and arranged to pick her up and take her to the police station to complete the police report. Based on Mary's statement and the evidence collected by the emergency room staff, the police were able to apprehend the offender, who later pleaded guilty. The counselor would have accompanied Mary to court had this been necessary. The counselor met with Mary and her husband weekly for the next two months to discuss their feelings about and reactions to the rape. She also met Mary at the hospital on her return visits to see if she had contracted venereal disease or was pregnant. After the first two months they decided the visits could be less frequent, although they continued to meet for the next 10 months and terminated the meetings one year after the incident.

Mary and her husband moved to a new location shortly after the incident. Mary was still a little uncomfortable when her husband was out of town; otherwise, their lives had returned to normal.

Once these groups integrated their services, other groups working with victims and offenders became involved in the Sexual Assault Task Force. Representatives from various community agencies met regularly to share information and concerns. The agencies represented included hospitals, rape crisis centers, police, the county attorney, homes for battered women, counseling services for victims and offenders, Department of Corrections, Court Services, and witness assistance programs. By meeting on a regular basis to share interests and concerns, to solve problems, and to continually coordinate their programs, these groups can offer more effective services to offenders, victims, and families or significant others.

Since this coordination has occurred, the number of cases of sexual assault charges has increased from 23 in the entire state of Minnesota in 1970 to 136 in Hennepin County alone in 1976. This compares with a 1 per cent increase in a neighboring county, where no changes in the system occurred. While only 50 per cent of the cases were convicted in 1970, 75 per cent of the cases were convicted in 1980. Only 10 per cent of these ever had to go to court. The evidence was so well established that the defendant pleaded guilty, greatly decreasing the trauma to the victim. The Minneapolis police state that at least 70 per cent of the case is made by the evidence presently collected by hospital personnel. The coordination of efforts and the integration of programs are recognized by all involved as essential in providing the services that must be available to victims and their families or significant others.

The more closely the sexual assault situation is examined the more we are faced with a dearth of systematic research about the impact of rape and needs of rape victims and their families or significant others, who are also affected by this experience and must deal with their feelings as well as those of the victim.

OBSTACLES TO CLINICAL RESEARCH IN THE AREA OF SEXUAL ASSAULT

Like most human problems, sexual assault is a topic that has little potential for study in the controlled conditions of laboratory research. Neither the event, nor the conditions of the event, nor the characteristics of any of the main actors are subject to the control of the investigator, and as a consequence most research in this area is descriptive, involving ex post facto analysis of rapes. Threats to validity owing to poor control of spurious sources of variation are legion, and the inappropriateness of research designs that incorporate experimental safeguards means that many of the conclusions generated from such research must be interpreted with caution.

The efficacy of various approaches to the treatment of victims of sexual assault, however, is a subject that can be addressed with greater methodologic confidence. Once a victim of sexual assault has been identified and has sought services, it is possible to institute appropriate research controls (that is, random assignment of victims to treatment conditions that embody various kinds of therapy modes of untested effectiveness) to mitigate the effects of contaminating variables.

A major obstacle to effective research in this area accrues from the absence of a body of useful empirical generations from previous research. Not only are there no generally accepted theories and principles to guide research, but also the field is often still obfuscated by popular myths, half-truths, and untested convictions, which must be dealt with before formative research can begin. Inquiry must literally start at the most rudimentary level.

Related to this is what might be called the problem of definition. Meaningful research requires a clear specification of the variables under study. In research regarding sexual assault, this is impeded by the absence of previous research to (1) point out the important variables to study and (2) provide a commonly accepted definition for further inquiry.

A severe threat to the validity of research regarding sexual assault comes from the difficulty in drawing unbiased samples for study from the true universe of sexual assault victims. In the first place, not all instances of sexual assault come to public attention. For a variety of reasons, many of those who are victims of such attacks do not report it, which means that it may never be possible to make an unbiased estimation of the essential characteristics of victims of sexual assault. This problem may be mitigated in the future as rape is destigmatized and positive efforts are made to construct means to facilitate the entrance of rape victims into the human services delivery system.

With regard to clinical research in this area, the problem of the nonrepresentativeness of those who seek services as opposed to the whole universe of those who are victims of sexual assault is not so acute. The function of clinical research is to determine the efficacy of a given treatment for those who receive services. However, a related problem is that, because of the nature of sexual assault, many victims refuse or are unavailable to participate in research. Often this means that clinical research generalizations are founded on work focused on a small and probably nonrepresentative segment of the universe of rape victims. The various "quasi-experimental" designs catalogued by Campbell and Stanley do not solve the problem but are helpful in highlighting which assumptions are required in various designs for statistical inference to be valid.[54]

Rape research is also greatly hindered by the special circumstances attendant on sexual assault. One special issue, alluded to earlier, is that rape involves violence, humiliation, and potential stigmatization of the victim. Because of the special vulnerability of the victim and because research may exacerbate the aftereffects of rape (and may also bring attention to the victim that she wishes to avoid), special safeguards are necessary to insure that the research procedures are innocuous regarding the victim's recovery and do not contribute to potential stigmatization.

In addition, because sexual assault is a crime, any research in this area must be managed so that it does not compromise the legal processes. Confidentiality is always a crucial issue, but particularly in this instance it is vital that client records be guarded with absolute security. Also, records, if they are liable to be used in a legal case, must be kept so that they do not inadvertently compromise the prosecution of the perpetrator of the sexual assault.

Measures

One critical consequence of the absence of a cohesive body of past research data in the area of treatment of victims of sexual assault is that there are few measurement devices specific to this area. Investigators may borrow or adapt measures from fields with related emphases (e.g., crisis intervention), but, since there is no guarantee that such measures actually assess variation in appropriate variables reliably, the results may, to one extent or another, be compromised.

Related to the above issue is the fact that the absence of measures means that there are no baseline data on the recovery of rape victims from assault. There has been little empirical validation of the kinds of problems experienced by rape victims, and overall there are no commonly accepted empirical standards for evaluating treatment accorded to victims of sexual assault. Without such information, it is problematic for clinicians, community, and policymakers to assess the impact of rape treatment programs.

A technical difficulty regarding most measurement in the area of treatment of sexual assault is that most of the measures employed thus far have been reactive; that is, the method and content of the measure are apparent to the subject and in consequence may alter her attitudes and behavior regarding the assault and her recovery from it. Even in routine social research, reactive measures have been shown to bias outcomes.[54] In the turbulent setting of rape therapy research, where the victim may be confused and disoriented in the immediate after-effects of the assault, all reasonable effort must be made to control the effects on results of intrusive research methodology.

RESEARCH STRATEGIES

The existence of the above problems and others related means that the conduct of rape treatment research in the coming years will be guided and controlled by a series of issues and needs.

Exploratory—Multivariate Designs

Since systematic empirical inquiry regarding the causes, constituents, and consequences of sexual assault is only now beginning, a major emphasis in the field will be on establishing the parameters of the field, identifying the most important variables for study, developing common definitions of concepts, devising special research methodology, and constructing empirical models that can be employed in wide subsequent research. In this process there is a need for both wide-ranging exploratory studies and tightly focused field experiments. The exploratory studies help the field develop a clinical focus, common vocabulary, and formative theoretical framework. The field experiments provide small amounts of empirical information that can be woven into the general theoretical formulations. At both the macro and micro levels, it is important that the designs include provision for the study of the effects of multiple variables.

As research gets underway, it is vitally important that an information network be formed among rape researchers and that central offices be established to coordinate activities, evaluate research, identify needs, and facilitate development of theoretical and empirical generalizations. The impetus for research in this area comes from various sources, and those who will conduct the research represent almost all of the major academic and human service disciplines. Redundant actions and wasted effort (not to mention potential hostility among disciplines) will probably occur unless those involved in studying and preventing sexual assault can link themselves to an entirely new and unencumbered communication system. A helpful sign is that the National Institute of Mental Health has established and funded the National Center for the Study and Control of Rape.

Measurement

The lack of meaningful measures in the area of sexual assault will be alleviated, at least in part, as a natural consequence of the implementation of theoretically meaningful and technically sound research designs, the development of technically sound measurement being an inevitable aspect of the implementation of effective research. At least two strategies are possible with regard to development of meaningful measures to assess the effectiveness of treatment of rape victims.

Standard Measures

The usual procedure in clinical rape treatment research has been either to borrow measures from related fields like crisis intervention or to develop questionnaires and measurement forms specifically for the immediate situation. The difficulty with the former is that instruments developed for other purposes may not be sensitive to the essential processes involved in the treatment of victims of sexual assault. The difficulty with the latter is that program-specific measures tend to be of variable psychometric quality, are not norm-referenced, are difficult to interpret, and are difficult to generalize with other research findings. Examples of standardized measures that may be appropriate to research in sexual assault are the Hopkins Systems Checklist, the Holmes Stress Inventory, the Menninger Health Sickness Rating Scale, and the Self-Rating Symptom Scale.

An essential prerequisite for the development of fixed-content measures of the efficacy of the treatment accorded victims of sexual assault will be the identification and specification of the constructs that are important in the therapy process. Some such constructs will, of course, generalize from other field measures, but some will be specific to recovery from sexual assault. Most needs will be identified through the successive formulation, testing, and reformulation of research hypotheses. Once such constructs are identified, "indicators" (usually scales intended to reflect variation in behavior or attitudes) may be selected (or constructed) to signify changes in the quality or quantity of variables being measured. These scales can then be evaluated to determine their reliability (the degree to which they measure whatever it is they measure consistently) and validity (the degree to which they measure whatever they are supposed to measure), and statistical norms may be developed to show how the scopes of the measure vary when generated from populations with various characteristics.

Individualized Goal Attainment Measures

The development and validation of meaningful standard measures will inevitably be a lengthy process. One form of assessment appropriate to determine the effectiveness of the services provided victims of sexual assault is already in existence. This is individualized goal attainment (IGA) measurement. A characteristic of this form of measurement is the determination of treatment outcome according to the attainment of specific, predetermined clinical goals that have been tailored to fit what is known both about the client and about the probable effects of the proposed treatment. With roots in idiographic psychology, psychotherapy research, and management science, IGA measurement currently is constituted by a loosely comparable set of goal-setting methodologies. Perhaps the best known of these is goal attainment scaling,[55] which at last count had been formally implemented by over 300 human service organizations throughout the world. Goal attainment scaling is a flexible, patient-specific technique for quantitatively assessing attainment of specific, predetermined goals. Goal attainment is measured on a grid-shaped form called a goal attainment follow-up guide (Fig. 14.1). Such a form consists of a succession of discrete five-point scales, each of which represents an individual patient concern arrayed along a qualitatively ordered series of possible outcomes. The nature of these outcomes ranges from "most unfavorable outcome thought likely," to "best anticipated success," with the expected level of success at the middle level. The content of each scale is determined prior to treatment and is tailored to the needs, capacities, and expectations of the person receiving the services. There is a variety of strategies possible for determining the content of a goal attainment follow-up guide. One strategy is for a clinician, or group of clinicians, to fill in the content without patient participation. Another strategy is for a clinician and patient to determine the content through negotiation. A third strategy is for the patient alone to determine the content.

At a predetermined time following the construction of the goal attainment follow-up guide, the patient is contacted and, on the basis of each scale of the follow-up guide, the degree to which the specified goals have been achieved is determined. From this information it is possible to calculate a goal attainment score. A goal attainment score is generated through a formula that transforms the weighted ratings on the individual scales on a follow-up guide into a single overall numerical value. A goal attainment score of 50.00 indicates that, on the average, a patient has exactly attained the "expected outcome" level on the goals scaled. A score of more than 50.00 indicates that expectations have been exceeded, and a score of less than 50.00 indicates

Level at Intake: ✔
Level at Follow-up: *

Score at Intake: 29.4
Score at Follow-up: 62.2
Goal Attainment Change Score +32.8

GOAL ATTAINMENT-FOLLOW-UP GUIDE

Scale Heading and Weights

Scale Attainment Levels	SCALE 1: Fear of going out by myself ($w_1 = 3$)	SCALE 2: Fear of pregnancy as a result of assault ($w_2 = 3$)	SCALE 3: Relationships with others ($w_3 = 2$)	SCALE 4: Sexual relationships ($w_4 = 3$)	SCALE 5: Sleep ($w_5 = 3$)
much less than the expected level of results	So fearful of going out that I stay in the house all the time. ✔	Afraid of pregnancy, but have done nothing to find out if I am pregnant.	Avoid all contact with other people I feel so ashamed.	Avoid sex altogether.	Unable to sleep at night.
somewhat less than the expected level of results	Fearful of going out, but will go out for necessary errands, i.e., grocery store, work, etc., if someone is with me.	Have made an appointment to find out if I am pregnant. ✔	Avoid all contact with other people except family because I feel so ashamed. ✔	Have had sex, but enjoy sex less than 25% of the time. ✔	Able to sleep 2–3 nights a week. ✔
expected level of results in — months	Fearful of going out, but will go on errands alone (i.e., to grocery store, work, etc.).	Have gotten results of pregnancy test. If pregnant, have not made a decision regarding this.	Feel ashamed at times. Have contact with my family and 1 other person in spite of my feelings.	Have had sex, and enjoy sex 26–50% of the time. *	Able to sleep 4 or 5 nights a week.
somewhat more than the expected level of results	Fearful of going out, but will go to additional activities 2–4 times per week. *	Am pregnant, and have decided what to do about pregnancy. *	Feel ashamed at times. Have contacts with my family and 2–3 other persons in spite of my feelings. *	Have had sex, and enjoy sex 51–75% of the time.	Able to sleep 6 nights a week.
much more than the expected level of results	Fearful of going out, but will go to additional activities 5 or more times per week.	Have taken action on decision regarding pregnancy.	Feel ashamed at times. Have contacts with my family and 4 or more persons in spite of my feelings.	Have had sex, and enjoy sex more than 76% of the time.	Able to sleep 7 nights a week. *

Technical Aid to Goal Attainment Scale as originally developed by Dr. Thomas Kiresuk and Dr. Robert Sherman. Copyright © 1979 Linda E. Ledray, R.N., M.A., Director, Sexual Assault Resource Service and Minneapolis Medical Research Foundation, Inc. All rights reserved.

Figure 14.1. Sample clinical guide: Sexual Assault Resource Service (SARS).

they have not been met. A distribution of goal attainment scores typically approximates a normal curve, with a mean of about 50.00 and a standard deviation of about 10.00. This makes it possible to use parametric statistical procedures to analyze results.

Systematic investigations regarding the reliability[56, 57] and validity[58, 59] of goal attainment scaling have found them to be within accepted psychometric parameters.[60] The special relevance of goal attainment scaling to clinical research regarding sexual assault relates to the current absence of accepted measures of the impact of rape and the corresponding need to determine appropriate problem areas and recovery rates. The goal attainment follow-up guides constructed for clients of rape treatment centers will serve as a depository of information regarding what must be done to alleviate the consequences of rape for a victim and how long it takes to do it.

Attrition

As in most field studies, the utility of data collected in clinical rape research will depend largely upon success in recruiting appropriate subjects and following them up in an appropriate and timely fashion. If a significant portion of the sample leaves treatment or declines follow-up, the research will have to contend not only with asymmetric cells and a computationally difficult method of analysis, but also with logical limitations on the inferences that can be drawn regarding treatment effects. The topic under investigation is very sensitive; most research methods are somewhat intrusive; and the length and intensity of commitment required of victims in a study are sometimes demanding. These factors, together with the manifest need to avoid even the subtlest pressure on subjects to participate in a research project, mean that attrition of the sample may become a serious threat to the integrity of a study. Fortunately, there is some evidence that victims of sexual assault who seek, or are brought to, medical services are typically willing, even enthusiastic, to help find more effective means to assist other rape victims. For example, during a survey of rape victims who were receiving services at Hennepin County Medical Center, 25 out of 25 approached said they would participate in a study that involved multiple follow-ups, randomized assignment to different kinds of treatment, and potential family involvement in therapy. Although this finding is a hopeful sign for the future of

research in this area, it seems self-evident that our success will vary according to our ability to devise and implement special means to mitigate the effects of sample attrition. A straightforward means to reduce attrition is to ensure both that the research has a realistic potential to add to what is known about treatment of rape victims and that the purpose and methods of the study are clearly communicated to the potential participant. People seem more likely to participate in a project when they are convinced that it is worthwhile and they understand how it works. Victims will also be more likely to participate if their prior commitment is elicited through the use of a consent form and if the research procedures are either intrinsically rewarding to the subject or are linked to events that are rewarding. Particularly in longitudinal studies, follow-up success can often be increased if the application of the research measures are linked to some form of treatment intervention. Minimizing paperwork, ensuring that staff members are sensitive and efficient, and assuring patients of absolute confidentiality will also help increase participation.

Of course, no field study will ever prevent all attrition of research subjects. One means to mitigate the bias occasioned by the differential loss to the study of subjects is to implement a very aggressive follow-up policy for a small, randomly selected subset of the sample. Although often too costly to adhere to on a large scale, making every effort to follow-up a limited number of subjects provides a means to estimate the characteristics of those who reject or are unavailable for follow-up. Such findings can be used during data analysis to correct for the effect on results of differences between subjects who do and do not receive follow-up.

Sensitivity

Few crimes are as physically and psychologically deleterious to a victim as is sexual assault. The pain, horror, and confusion occasioned by rape greatly increase the vulnerability of a subject to further injury and require that special safeguards be implemented to see to it that her recovery is in no way hindered by the research. To ensure, for example, that victims are able to make a truly "informed consent" regarding participation in a given piece of research, presentation of the consent form and subsequent initiation of research procedures should be delayed until the immediate turmoil surrounding the attack has subsided and the victim has a chance to examine the research critically. As an additional safeguard, the content of the consent form can be reviewed at every follow-up so that the victim will have ample opportunity to withdraw from the study.

It is vitally important that follow-up contacts be absolutely confidential and as unobtrusive as possible. No one should be contacted regarding the victim's participation in the study without her explicit approval. Follow-up workers should be matched with victims on racial and ethnic variables and should dress in a style that blends with the victim's neighborhood and lifestyle. If the victim does not wish the follow-up to take place in her home, arrangements should be made for an interview at another site and free transportation provided. Concern that follow-ups will interfere with the victim's full recovery is mitigated by the findings of a study by Halley and Baxter.[61] In this research, patients of Hennepin County Mental Health Service who had previously been followed-up to determine treatment outcome were surveyed again to assess reaction to the previous follow-up. Over three-quarters reported being pleased with the previous follow-up and many had shown a marked clinical improvement subsequent to follow-up (suggesting that research follow-ups are not contraindicated clinically and may even have salutary side effects).

A source of great concern for those who participate as subjects in research regarding rape treatment is that their records remain strictly confidential. To protect each subject's right to privacy, all records must be treated as privileged communications. Storing research data in locked files in locked rooms (or, if the data are stored in an automated information system, seeing to it that appropriate security measures are adhered to) is a good beginning, but in addition steps should be taken to ensure that the research workers who have access to the data are unable to determine the identity of the subject. One means to do this is to store records according to a randomly selected identification number, with all identifying information (e.g., name, address, telephone number) deleted. A master list identifying each subject can be maintained by the coordinator of the research, but after a subject's active involvement in the research is over (and it is no longer important to be able to identify a subject as an individual) the link between the identification number and the subject's name is destroyed. This makes it impossible to identify the subject at any future time, either inadvertently or by design.

THEMES IMPORTANT IN CLINICAL RESEARCH REGARDING SEXUAL ASSAULT

Overall, relatively little seems to be known about how people recover from the trauma of sexual assault.

Treatment

The most obvious and pressing research topic in this area relates to determining the relative effectiveness of various methods of helping rape victims recover from their attack. Often rape victims receive little more than perfunctory medical care following the assault, but sometimes they also receive intense, long-term, crisis-oriented counseling. The relative (comparative) effects of these two forms of treatment are not known and clearly require investigation.

Once base rates have been established regarding effectiveness, it will be important to inquire as to how the treatment process is influenced by the characteristics of those who render treatment. As Strupp[62] observed regarding psychotherapy, it is no longer legitimate to treat therapy as a "blackbox" that will have the same effect on all patients. Complex problems require complex solutions, and, just as each patient is individual in terms of needs and capacities, each service provider is individual in terms of therapeutic philosophy and skill level. The central task in clinical research regarding sexual assault will be to find the optimal means to match different kinds of treatment and different kinds of treatment providers with specific patient problems. Questions must be answered in a variety of areas:

1. *The assault.* How is the victim's recovery affected by the characteristics of the assault and the assailant (e.g., the degree of violence of the attack, the number of attacks, the relationship of the attacker to the victim, the physical location of the attack)?

2. *The victim.* How is the victim's recovery affected by the characteristics of the victim herself (e.g., her age and background, her attitude toward rape, her previous sexual experiences, her previous level of "mental health")?

3. *The treatment.* How is the victim's recovery affected by the characteristics of the treatment she receives (e.g., long-term or short-term, medical alone or medical plus counseling, immediate or delayed)?

4. *The therapist.* How is the victim's recovery affected by the characteristics of the person

who provides treatment (e.g., professional or paraprofessional, level of skill and training style, therapeutic opinions and attitudes, degree to which therapist is similar to victim in terms of personal characteristics)?

5. *Other circumstances.* How is the victim's recovery affected by the immediate circumstances of the assault and its aftermath (e.g., the victim's financial/vocational situation, the sort of treatment received from police and medical personnel, the existence of a support group or family or friends)?

The overall course of clinical research regarding rape will be guided by past research, by experiential observations of those already in the field, and by evolving theoretical formulations. Initially, most research will be summative in nature, dedicated to determining whether particular forms of clinical intervention are worth continuing. As effective treatment modalities are identified, research will become increasingly formative, aimed at refining and improving clinical practices and determining situations in which they are most likely to have maximum impact.

Family Involvement

Although the act of rape is usually a solitary event for the victim, recovery often takes place in the midst of a complex social network composed of family, friends, and casual acquaintances. Little is currently known about how this support system can influence a victim's recovery from sexual assault. Common sense would suggest that an open, loving, and supportive family that allows expression of anger and rage would provide the backup needed by a rape victim at a time when she would feel most vulnerable and unloved. Yet some families would clearly have a potential for being destructive in the aftermath of an assault (e.g., might blame the victim for the attack), and others might need therapeutic guidance to know how best to assist the victim.

Many questions must be answered. Should families be involved in planning and providing treatment for a rape victim? If so, how soon after the attack should they be brought in? What kind of families should not be involved? What should be done with victims who have no immediate support system? (Can artificial support systems be created?) If the victim has an enduring outside relationship with a male (husband/lover/boyfriend), how, if at all, should this person be involved in treatment? Clearly, different victims in different situations have different needs and different potential for benefiting from services. Research into the complex interaction of the various factors described above is needed to develop guidelines for rape treatment definitions.

Goal Setting

One specific, practical, and easily implemented means to maximize the impact of treatment of victims of sexual assault may simply be to involve them in clinical goal setting. There is substantial evidence that client goal setting has a facilitative effect on mental health therapy.[37a, 63-65] It will be important to determine if such an effect is also operative with regard to therapy for victims of sexual assault. The clinical functions of patient goal setting are varied, depending on the needs of the patient and the therapeutic style of the counselor. Often patient goals stimulate treatment motivation; sometimes they are a means to keep treatment focused on particular issues; other times they are a catalyst for communication; and yet other times they facilitate mutual examination of expectations. Severe and intransient discrepancies between counselor and patient goals have been a rarity in the experience of the authors; to the extent that disagreements occur, they typically serve as a basis for further discussion and negotiation. Davis[66] describes the basic process at work as "target tropism:" the inherent tendency for a person to try to move toward any goal held up for her or him. Whatever the underlying mechanism, the success of goal setting as a treatment facilitator in mental health opens a clear line of research in the rape treatment field.

Conclusion

Although an ageless social problem, rape has recently become a topic of grave public concern with the recent resurgence of the feminist movement and the subsequent legislation enacted by Congress (P.L. 94–93, Title III, Part D) establishing the National Center for the Prevention and Control of Rape. However, although rape crisis centers have been established in various cities, sexual assault remains a topic about which there is little formal research. Knowledge that exists comes largely from descriptive studies, agitation by women's advocates, and political debate.

The substance of the available information deals with such topics as the effects of immediate intervention and crisis support, prevention of sexual assault, and changes needed within the legal system. Little attention has been paid to determining the hopes and aspirations of rape victims, to trying to anticipate their patterns of recovery, or to developing counseling guidelines. Nor has sufficient attention been paid to the way a family reacts to sexual assault, to the nature of a family's aspirations and intentions, or to changes in the family structure over time. Recently, there have been serious efforts to study and alter attitudes toward rape, but no link has been established between attitude formation and its effects on the behavior of the rape victim and her family.

References

1. U.S. Department of Justice. *Uniform Crime Report for the United States.* Washington, DC: U.S. Government Printing Office, 1976.
2. The Victim in a Forcible Rape Case: A Feminist View. *The American Criminal Law Review, A Symposium: Women and the Criminal Law,* American Bar Association, Section of Criminal Law, no. 2 (Winter 1973):347.
3. Flakne, Gary (ed.) *Sexual Assault: The Target is You.* Minneapolis: Hennepin County Attorney's Office, 1976, p. 13.
4. Amir, Menachem. *Patterns in Forcible Rape.* Chicago: University of Chicago Press, 1971, pp. 27–39.
5. MacDonald, John M. *Rape: Offenders and Their Victims.* Springfield IL, Charles C Thomas, 1971.
6. Brownmiller, Susan. *Against Our Will: Men, Women and Rape.* New York: Simon and Schuster, 1975, pp. 28–308.
7. Amir, Menachem, op. cit., pp. 17–29.
8. Medea, Andra, and Thompson, Kathleen. *Against Rape: A Survival Manual for Women.* New York: Farrar, Straus, and Giroux, 1974, pp. 1–28.
9. Hayman, Charles. What to do for victims of rape. *Medical Times,* Vol. 101, June 1973, p. 49.
10. Peters, Joseph J. Social, legal, and psychological effects of rape on the victim. *Pennsylvania Medicine,* February 1975, pp. 34–36.
11. Carbary, Lorraine Judson. Treating terrified victims. *Journal of Practical Nursing,* February 1974, pp. 20–22.
12. Amir, Menachem, op. cit., pp. 129–194.
13. Price, Vern. Rape victims: The invisible patients. *Canadian Nurse,* April 1975, p. 30.
14. Jones, C. and Aronson, E. Attribution of fault to a rape victim as a function of respectability of the victim. *Journal of Personality and Social Psychology,* vol. 26, June 1973, pp. 415–419.
15. Lerner, M. J. The desire for justice and reactions to victims. *In* Macaulay, J., and Berkowitz, L. (eds.) *Altruism and Helping Behavior.* New York: Academic Press, 1970, pp. 205–229.
16. Lerner, M. J. and Simmons, C. H. Observers' reactions to the innocent victim. *Journal of Personality and Social Psychology,* vol. 4, 1977, pp. 203–210.
17. Bern, D. J. and McConnell, H. C. Testing the self-perception explanation of dissonance phenomena: On the salience of pre-manipulation attitudes. *Journal of Personality and Social Psychology,* vol. 14, 1977, pp. 203–210.
18. Amir, Menachem, op. cit.
19. Brownmiller, op. cit.
20. Medea and Thompson, op. cit.
21. Brownmiller, op. cit., p. 18.
22. Hilberman, Elaine. *The Rape Victim.* Washington, DC: American Psychiatric Association Committee on Women, 1976, pp. 33–39.
23. Hayman, C. R. and Lanza, D. Sexual assault on women and girls. *American Journal of Obstetrics and Gynecology,* vol. 109, Feb. 1971, p. 50.
24. Hanss, Joseph W. Another look at the care of the rape victim. *Arizona Medicine,* vol. 32, August 1975, p. 634.
25. Price, op. cit.
26. Hayman and Lanza, op. cit.
27. Peters, op. cit., p. 36.
28. Hilberman, op. cit., p. ix.
29. Burgess, Ann Wolbert. Crisis and counseling requests of rape victims. *Nursing Research,* vol. 23, May-June 1974, 196–202.
30. Hilberman, op. cit.
31. Peters, op. cit.
32. Medea and Thompson, op. cit., pp. 101–110.
33. Brownmiller, op. cit., pp. 49, 283–308.
34. Hanss, op. cit.
35. Burgess, Ann Wolbert, and Holmstrom, Lynda L. Rape trauma syndrome. *American Journal of Psychiatry,* September 1974, p. 983.
36. Hayman and Lanza, op. cit., p. 48
37. Burgess, op. cit., pp. 981–985.
37a. Ledray, Linda E., and Chaignot, Mary Jane. Services to sexual assault victims in Hennepin County. *Evaluation and Change,* Special Issue, 1980.
37b. Ledray, Linda E.: Counseling victims of rape: A nursing challenge. *Perspectives in Psychiatric Care,* in press.
37c. Frank, Ellen, Turner, Samuel, and Duffy, Barbara: Depressive symptoms in rape victims. *Journal of Affective Disorders,* vol. 1, 1979, pp. 269–277.
37d. Resick, Patricia A., Calhoun, Karen S., Atkeson, Beverly M., and Ellis, Elizabeth M. Social adjustment in victims of sexual assault. *Journal of Consulting and Clinical Psychology,* vol. 49, 1981, pp. 705–712.
38. Ibid.
39. Price, op. cit., p. 30.
40. Interview with Debbie Anderson, Director, Sexual Assault Services, Hennepin County, Attorney's Office, Minneapolis, June 1976.
41. Burgess, op. cit., p. 985.
42. Borges, Sandra S., and Weiss, Kurt. Victimology and Rape. *Issues In Criminology,* vol. 8, 1973, pp. 71–115.
43. Peters, op. cit.
44. Medea and Thompson, op. cit.
45. Brownmiller, op. cit.
46. Peters, op. cit.
47. Price, op. cit.
48. Brownmiller, op. cit., p. 124.
49. Borges and Weiss, op. cit., p. 99.
50. Ledray, Linda E. Indian Community Sexual Assault Treatment Program. Unpublished paper, 1985.
51. Ledray, Linda E. Sexual assault and rape: Confronting the problem. *In* Wold Susan J. (ed.). *Community Health Nursing: Issues and Topics.* New York: Prentice-Hall, in press.
52. Peters, op. cit., pp. 34–36.
53. Price, op. cit., p. 29.
54. Campbell, Donald T., and Stanley, Julian C. *Experimental and Quasi-Experimental Designs for Research.* Chicago: Rand McNally, 1966.

55. Kiresuk, Thomas J., and Sherman, Robert E. Goal attainment scaling: A general method for evaluating comprehensive community mental health programs. *Community Mental Health Journal*, vol. 4, 1968, pp. 443–453.

56. Sherman, Robert E., Baxter, James W. and Audette, Donna M. An examination of the reliability of the Kiresuk-Sherman goal attainment score by means of components of variance. Unpublished report, Program Evaluation Resource Center, Minneapolis, Minnesota, 1974.

57. Garwick, Geoffrey. An introduction to reliability and the goal attainment score. Unpublished report, Program Evaluation Resource Center, 1972.

58. Sherman, Robert E. Content validity argument for goal attainment scaling. Unpublished report, Program Evaluation Resource Center, 1972.

59. Garwick, Geoffrey. A construct validity overview of goal attainment scaling. Unpublished report, Program Evaluation Resource Center, 1972.

60. Davis, Howard R. Four ways to goal attainment: An overview. *Evaluation*, vol 1, 1973.

61. Halley, Coleen, and Baxter, James. Client perception of evaluation at Hennepin County Mental Health Service. Unpublished report, Program Evaluation Resource Center, 1971.

62. Strupp, Hans H. The outcome problem in psychotherapy revisited. *Psychotherapy: Theory, Research and Practice*, vol 1, 1964, pp. 1–13.

63. Jones, Susan and Garwick, Geoffrey. Guide to goals study: Goal attainment scaling as therapy adjunct? *Program Evaluation Report Newsletter*, vol. 4, July-August 1973, pp. 1–3.

64. LaFerriere, Lorraine, and Calsyn, Robert. Goal Attainment Scaling: An effective treatment technique in short term therapy. Ph.D. diss., Michigan State University, 1975.

65. Smith, David L. Goal attainment scaling as an adjunct to counseling. *Journal of Counseling Psychology*, vol. 23, 1976, pp. 22–27.

66. Davis, Howard R. Change and innovation. *In* Feldman, Saul (ed.) *Administration in Mental Health Services*. Springfield, IL: Charles C Thomas, 1973.

15

CHILD ABUSE

GEORGIA MILLOR
LA VOHN JOSTEN

This chapter on child abuse written by Georgia Millor and La Vohn Josten begins with the statistics regarding this area of concern and a review of the literature by researchers in the field. The role of the nurse in a special project designed as a treatment intervention for mothers at risk, including a case study, is detailed.

Child abuse and neglect are two consequences of family dysfunction. Neglectful parenting and abusive parenting are considered by some professionals to be at opposite ends of the spectrum of acceptable parental response to the demands of childrearing.[1] However, for the purposes of this chapter, neglectful and abusive childrearing patterns will be considered as a single maltreatment syndrome and henceforth will be called child abuse.

Although multiple theoretical formulations and models exist to explain the causal roots of family violence and child abuse,[2-11] stress is one of the factors repeatedly included as a structural or process component of these models. Child abuse is thought to occur when the family's cognitive, affective, and economic resources are inadequate to cope with either intrafamily or external family demands. In a comparative study of 70 abusive and 70 control families, abusive families displayed "chronic and intense conflict between children and parents . . . and showed repeated efforts to maintain dysfunctional family and marital ties."[12] The control families, in contrast to abusive families, were able to mobilize their own emotional resources and use external sources of support in coping with parent-child or marital conflicts.

Nurses frequently have contact with families during periods of stress and are often the first persons to have contact with an abused child in the home, school, or health care setting.[13]

Thus, nurses are key professionals in the processes of early identification of high-risk families and identification of suspected abused children, and in the treatment of the victims, their siblings, and parents. The success of nursing interventions in these processes is contingent upon knowledge of the factors associated with abuse and the dynamic inter-relationships of these factors in producing or exacerbating stressful family environments. Nurses must also understand usual patterns persons exhibit when coping with stress as well as understand the factors that enhance coping. With this knowledge, they can use the nursing process to develop and implement care aimed at both facilitating the family's coping efforts and reducing the risk that child abuse will occur or reoccur.

Helfer[6] proposed that three components are necessary in order for child abuse to occur: (1) the potential for abuse, (2) a special child, and (3) a crisis or series of crises. The potential for abuse includes poor parenting received by the parents, poor marital relationships between parents, poor social support systems, and lack of knowledge regarding normal child growth and development. The abused child may be thought of as "special" (whether this is imagined or real) owing to prematurity, to chronic illness, or to being temperamentally difficult or bothersome. The triad of factors that contribute to family dysfunction and subsequent child abuse will be described following a discussion of the definition and incidence of abuse.

Common to all cases of abuse is a child who has suffered or is at risk for suffering some type of injury. The injury can result from a purposeful action or from the absence of any action when purposeful action is necessary for the child's well-being. The injury can be physical, emotional, intellectual, sexual, or social. The degree of damage may be so minute that it is impossible to detect or so severe that the child dies. Examples of various forms of child abuse include those that lead to readily definable injury: a four-year-old who is hit repeatedly in the abdomen until the spleen ruptures; a toddler whose legs are twisted until the bones break; an infant who is shaken so severely that the brain begins to bleed; an infant who is inadequately fed, stimulated, or loved, so that his body or mind does not grow. Other forms of abuse result in injuries that are more difficult to detect: an adolescent girl whose father fondles her genitals; a toddler who is left alone in the parents' apartment for a period of time; a seven-year-old who is not allowed to go to school because the child's mother does not like to be alone. Common to all of these examples is an act or the absence of an act that results in a child's receiving either physical, emotional, sexual, or intellectual injury.

The true number of children who are abused each year in the United States is not known. The reasons for this include failures to identify childhood trauma or neglect as child abuse, reluctance of persons to report suspected cases, inadequate evidence to validate all reported cases, and inadequate treatment resources.[14, 15] Based on data collected from May 1979 to April 1980 from 600 participating agencies in 26 counties in 10 states, the National Incidence Study[16] projected that 652,000 unduplicated cases of child abuse occur annually. Of these, only 43 per cent are substantiated by children's protective service agencies. The estimated and actual numbers of child abuse reports have risen appreciably from 289,837 in 1975[17] to 711,142 reports in 1979.[18]

It has been thought that the average age of the abused child is under four years.[19–22] However, Fisher and Berdie[23] found that 36 per cent of the 1976 American Humane Association reported cases were between 10 and 18 years of age. The National Incidence Study[16] stated that the incidence of reported abuse increased with age: 17 per cent of cases were under 5 years old; 36 per cent were between 6 and 11 years; and 47 per cent were between 12 and 17 years. The interaction between age, severity of child abuse, and fatalities continued to be associated with children under five years old.

Child abuse is a potentially lethal syndrome; an estimated 1300 abused children die yearly.[16] Although preschool children account for 17 per cent of reported cases, they sustain 74 per cent of fatalities.[16] The child between one and six months old seems particularly vulnerable, for abuse is the second-ranking cause of death for this age group.[24] Death of a sibling owing to injuries or neglect without a plausible history of accidental trauma or illness may be the first indication that abuse is occurring in a family.[25] The duration of ongoing abuse prior to a substantiated diagnosis ranges from one to three years,[22] and recidivism is common among reported families.[26]

Who are these parents who have injured so many children? Characteristics of abusive parents reflect commonalities among all parents. Abusive parents represent all educational levels, social strata, and ethnic groups.[27–29] Education ranges from partial grade school to advanced postgraduate degrees, and IQs range from the 70s to the 130s.[30] Although abuse crosses all socioeconomic levels, the highest incidence of reported cases tends to occur in the lowest levels, that is, below $7000 annual income[16] or among families receiving public assistance.[31] Low income and high unemployment are particular sources of economic stress that are considered to contribute to abuse.[32, 33] Very often the father is absent from the home or unemployed;[34, 35] when he is employed, his occupational status is typically lower than his level of skill.[36] The majority of abusing parents are married and living together at the time of abuse, and parental ages tend to fall within the early to mid-twenties.[20, 22, 27, 37] Galub[38] states that in three fourths of abuse cases natural parents are involved in the child's mistreatment and that mothers are more often responsible for abuse than fathers, probably because they spend more time with the children. Empiric data to support Galub's presumption are not conclusive. In each of three studies of abusive families, equal numbers or percentages of mothers and fathers were identified as the perpetrators.[37, 39, 40] Other perpetrators in these studies included stepfathers, mothers' boyfriends, and adolescent siblings.

Identification of the perpetrators is viewed by some as contrary to the therapeutic goal of improving family functioning and unity.[1, 14, 37] The identification of the perpetrator seems essential, primarily in those cases brought before family court, to determine who will receive child custody. Generally, although one parent is the active abuser, the other parent tends to passively sanction the mistreatment.[41]

The concept of role reversal, that is, the parent expecting the child to take care of the parent, has also been set forth as a factor in abuse by parents. It appears that some parents perceive their children from birth as having adult powers for deliberately displeasing or judging them.[28, 42] Aggression is often used by parents for dealing with these seemingly disapproving infants.[43] Other studies add that abusing parents are unable to empathize with their children.[1, 44]

It has also been reported that abusive parents frequently possess feelings that reflect a poor self-concept.[45-47] Clinical observation of abusive parents reveals that parental inadequate self-esteem is a common problem. Numerous studies of abusing parents indicate that they were themselves victims of some form of abuse as children.[6, 38, 48] The presence of low self-esteem in abusive parents is readily understandable if, throughout their younger years, their own parents raised them in a manner that conveyed to them that they were worthless, bad, mean, and deserving of physical or emotional mistreatment. As young adults, the inability of these individuals to use their parents as supportive persons may further contribute to the development of unfavorable self-images, or to the inability to sustain positive relationships with others, or both. The cumulative effect of low self-esteem is thought to contribute to the development of inadequate coping resources in adulthood, which leaves these parents vulnerable to feelings of poor self-esteem when they experience events such as unemployment. The nurse needs to recognize that a history of childhood mistreatment is an indicator that parents may mistreat their own children, particularly when the family is experiencing stress in other aspects of life. Social support may mediate the impact of stressors on these families.

However, social isolation is a common feature of life for abusive families.[12, 49-51] Elmer[19] noted that abusive families had few contacts with persons outside the family; abusive mothers rarely belonged to church, PTA, or other social groups and had almost no close friends. Abusive mothers also stated they had no other adults in the family on whom they could count for help, as they were isolated from their extended families. Green and colleagues[49] noted that abusive mothers described their spouses as being emotionally unsupportive concerning childrearing; the mothers also reported alienation from their parents related to their childhood experiences of rejection, criticism, and physical punishment. Thus, kin were viewed as unavailable for childrearing assistance. In a case study report,[52] intergenerational relationships between parents and grandparents were hostile and sporadic; neither parent saw their biologic parents as sources of support despite clinical observations of warmth and nurturance between the maternal grandparents and the two toddlers. In a seven-year study of 674 abused children and 500 control subjects, Lenoski[51] reported two significant findings associated with social isolation: abusive families had fewer pets and fewer listed phone numbers (10.5 per cent) than did control families (88 per cent). Frequent household moves were also reported for abusive families.[53] Residential mobility is a family pattern that removes parents from the influence of kin or neighbors who may provide social support or positive role models for learning acceptable ways to raise children. Residential mobility may also contribute to isolation from social workers and nurses who can detect dysfunctional family relationships and suggest strategies for coping with situational crises.

Some researchers have proposed that abusing parents share misconceptions about childrearing. When a child is not able to satisfy the needs of his or her parents, punishment and even abuse often occur.[54] These parents often expect more of their children than the children are able to give, physically, intellectually, or emotionally. On a questionnaire given to a group of parents receiving public health nursing services, 7 per cent of whom were known to have abused or neglected their children, 25 per cent of the parents indicated that they expected their child to be toilet trained by one year old, and 50 per cent expected their child to know right from wrong at one year old or sooner.[55] This assumption about unrealistically high parental expectations for child behaviors has been widely accepted in abuse causality models. However, an investigation of developmental expectations among three groups of parents (14 abusers, 15 neglecters, and 12 control parents matched on sociodemographic variables) revealed that the abusing and neglecting parents were less knowledgeable than control parents were about when a child should achieve specific developmental milestones.[56] Abusive parents expected their children to achieve developmental milestones later rather than earlier than age norms for the average child. The findings of this study and of its previous research[56] suggest that abusing and neglecting parents may have both unrealistically high and unrealistically low expectations of their children's behavior. The role of the nurse in providing information about normal growth and development and about how parents can respond to irritating child behavior in a nonabusive manner is essential in the promotion of child safety and improved parent-child relationships in abusive families.

Independent of demographic and parental characteristics, knowledge about the abused child must be considered in order to determine why one child is abused and another is not, within the same family. Although previously cited age differences are associated with the incidence of abuse, sex differences are generally unreported. Various studies suggest that the child is a stressful presence and may indeed elicit harmful childrearing behaviors.[30, 49, 57-60]

Zalba[42] reported a high incidence of child abuse among children born premaritally, extramaritally, or from unplanned pregnancies. Prematurity, low birth weight and psychosocial failure to thrive have been associated with the incidence of child abuse.[61-63] However, a critical analysis of these and similar studies suggested that the newborn's health status alone is an inconclusive predictor of who is at risk for abuse.[64] "Bonding failure" has been offered as an alternative explanation for infant maltreatment.[65, 66] Prospective studies have not substantiated the simple "bonding failure" hypothesis.

For many of the biologically at-risk infants, the mother's pregnancy or delivery may have been difficult, and when combined with neonatal separation and concomitant lack of opportunity to get to know their babies, these events may contribute to sustained mother-child stressful interactions. In a longitudinal prospective study of 275 mothers, 32 mothers did not provide adequate care to their infants within the first three months.[58, 68] Perinatal complications alone did not distinguish between the 32 mistreating mothers and a group of 33 mothers who provided high-quality child care.[49, 67] The group designation was based on observer ratings of mother-child interactions and on results of the Child Care Rating Scale administered during home visits when the infants were three, six, and nine months old. However, the Brazelton Neonatal Inventory scores[69] for orientation, irritability, and consolability discriminated between the two groups of infants. The mistreated infants scored low on prosocial behaviors. The mistreating mothers were found to be psychologically unable to "recognize their own and their children's needs for autonomy and their own ambivalence" concerning pregnancy and mothering.[58] The investigators concluded that the mistreating mothers were unable to manage the complexities of attachment to and separation from their babies that made these dyads vulnerable to abuse.

Rather than looking at the individual characteristics of the parents, children, or environmental sources of stress in a linear relationship to child abuse, investigators are focusing attention on the interactive dynamics between parents and abused children, in an attempt to understand the parental childrearing responses to potential or actual aversive child behaviors.[46, 48, 70] An investigation of the influence of the abused child's temperament characteristics on parent-child interactions appears to be a useful clinical and research approach to identifying the special child.

Temperament is defined as the manner in which a child interacts with the sociocultural environment, or how a child behaves. This behavioral reactivity is considered constitutional and has a particularly stable pattern from infancy through early childhood.[71-73] The measurement of temperament provides an assessment of nine formal reactivity categories: activity, rhythmicity, approach versus withdrawal, adaptability, intensity, threshold of responsivity, distractibility, persistence, and mood. The ratings for these categories are used to determine the child's temperament style; the three distinct temperament styles are slow-to-warm-up, difficult, and easy. The difficult child's behavioral reactivity profile includes high activity; irregularity in sleep, feeding, or elimination; withdrawal from new situations; slow adaptability to change; negative mood; and high intensity in social interactions. The child with a difficult temperament style is at risk for developing behavioral or psychiatric disturbances during childhood,[74, 75] at risk for developing disturbances in parent-child relationships,[76-80] and at risk for abuse.[30, 58]

Children's temperaments or reactivity patterns were among the health, personality, and intellectual characteristics evaluated in a longitudinal study of 100 injured infants, conducted by Elmer at an urban medical center.[19, 82] Infants 13 months of age or younger who were radiologically examined for bone injuries were classified as abused or accidentally injured, based on clinical evidence and a family history of the traumatic event. From within these two groups, 17 pairs were available and matched with respect to age, race, sex, and socioeconomic status eight to nine years later. A third group, of 25 uninjured children, hospitalized at about the same ages as the other children, was recruited into the study as another comparison group for the eight- to nine-year follow-up evaluation. Gregg reported that the injured infants with the temperament characteristics of high activity, negative mood, and low distractibility "maneuvered themselves into accident situations" with objects, stairs, and heights.[81] Additionally, nonabusive mothers tended to describe their babies more favorably than did abusive mothers, even when the research observer rated the temperaments of several of the nonabused infants as predominantly negative.

At the time of injury and at the one-year follow-up, the Thomas and Chess[73] interview method of assessing temperament was used. At the one-year and eight-and-a-half year follow-up evaluations, the temperaments of the abused children were significantly different from those of the matched comparison children in the accidentally injured and uninjured groups.[19, 82] At age eight to nine years, the differences between pairs in the three groups for most of the reactivity characteristics were less obvious, which suggests that maturation may modify those characteristics that are likely to produce an accidental injury or to elicit abusive maternal behaviors. Also, the specific categories of behavioral data were not identical to the earlier-age measures. Abused children were perceived by their school teachers as having more nervous mannerisms than had the other two groups rated by teachers. There were also significant differences by group in maternal ratings of the children's behaviors, using a brief questionnaire called "Your Child–Most Children." Abused children were rated as angrier than most children their age; the maternal ratings for perseverance and explorative behavior were higher for accidentally injured children than for abused or uninjured children.

In an exploratory descriptive study of 60 abused children, Green, Gaines, and Sandgrund[49] reported that the abuse-provoking child within the families was perceived by mothers as the most aggressive and demanding of their children. De Lissovoy reported that mothers of abused children aged two to seven years perceived their children as "alert, not

calm, excitable, active, demanding, and restless."[57] On the basis of the negative adjectives chosen by abusive mothers, de Lissovoy concluded that these children were capable of actively eliciting harmful parental responses.

Herrenkohl and Herrenkohl[83] examined behavioral differences between abused children and their nonabused siblings (n = 379). They found that in approximately half of the families one child, and in one fifth of the families two children, were targets of abuse. The target children, compared with their nonabused siblings, were described negatively by their mothers (thick-headed, clumsy, crabby) and as having childrearing difficulties (eating problems, temper tantrums, head banging, moodiness). The mothers reported having less control over the target children than over their nonabused siblings. These differences between target children and nontarget siblings were significant at $p \leq 0.01$.

Terr[36] conducted a six-year longitudinal study of family dynamics in 10 families observed during treatment for child abuse. On the basis of home observations, she noted that children can contribute to their own mistreatment by responding to parents with retaliatory behaviors. Terr observed, "In each case the abusing parent had a specific fantasy about the abused child that brought on the violent action." She stated that only when "displacement was fluid" were the other children in the family also harmed. In a group of 41 severely abusive families, Young[25] observed seven families, in each of which only one child was the target for abuse; the siblings of the seven target children were neglected. This finding was corroborated by Nurse[41] in her examination of 45 abusive families in which the target child had a special or preferential meaning to the abusive parent and was viewed indifferently by the passive spousal partner.

In keeping with Helfer's[6] three conditions essential for child abuse, Millor developed and tested a theoretical framework (Fig. 15.1) for studying the relationships between mothers' ratings of their children's temperaments, the levels of bother elicited by temperament behaviors, and self-reports of their childrearing behaviors.[9, 35] The central assumptions of this self-role definition of the stressful situation framework are (1) the child is an active organism who, through interactions with parents or siblings, influences the family's sociopsychologic environment; (2) reciprocal expectations for role performance exist among family members; (3) temperament characteristics influence

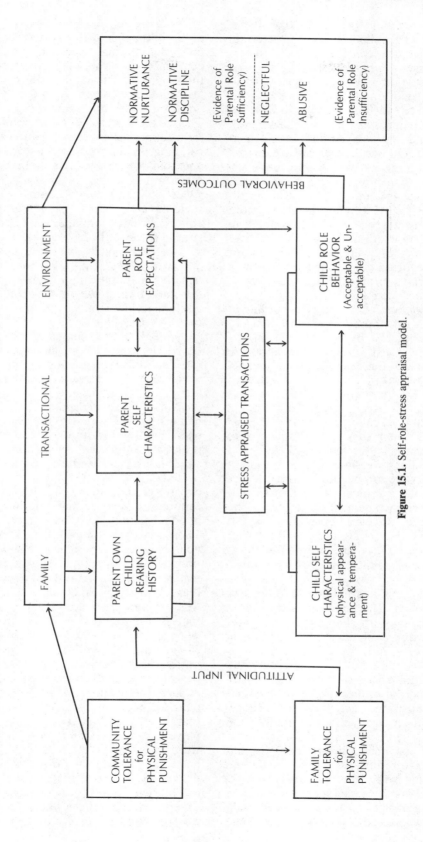

Figure 15.1. Self-role-stress appraisal model.

role performance; and (4) the lack of fit between the child's temperament and parental expectations is a source of tension and fosters stressful transactions in the family. Abuse and neglect provide prima facie evidence of parental role insufficiency and family crises.

Millor's study[35] focused on identification of temperament characteristics that distinguish the target child in abuse families from a nonabused sibling. It was hypothesized that the temperament of the target child indicates characteristics that contribute to his or her being viewed as "special," and that this child experiences more frequent punishment or more harsh punishment than a sibling. Mothers in abusive families were interviewed within two to sixteen weeks following the first incident of child abuse reported to and substantiated by a county children's protective service agency. The sample included 10 abusive and 10 nonabusive control families, matched according to age of the target abused child and years of education completed by the mother in the abusive family. Each family had at least two children between the ages of three and 74 months, for a total of 20 pairs of children (n = 40). There were similar numbers of boys and girls in each of the groups of abused and matched nonabused children and their siblings. Mothers rated their children's characteristics using the infant (ITQ),[84] toddler (TTS),[85] and preschool (BSQ)[86] versions of temperament scales, which were modified to include ratings for level of bother or pleasure reactions mothers felt toward each temperament item. The temperament styles, easy versus difficult, did not distinguish the target children from other children. However, there were significant paired differences (Wilcoxon equality of ranks test, 1-tailed p < 0.05) on three of the nine temperament categories and on five of the nine bother categories. The target abused children were less adaptable to changes in their caregivers or environment than were children in the other three groups, were less persistent in play behaviors than their siblings, and had higher thresholds to stimuli than both control groups of children. Bother ratings for the temperament categories activity, adaptability, mood, persistence, distractibility, and the total level of bother score were higher for the target children than for their siblings. These discriminating negative ratings of the target children were consistent with other reports in the literature of children's behaviors that contribute to excessive demands on their mothers' abilities to cope with usual childrearing situations.

The scores of Disbrow's Ways Parents Handle Irritating Child Behaviors[46] and Chamberlin's Childrearing Checklist[87] revealed significant differences between target children and their siblings. The target children were yelled at, spanked or slapped, scolded, told not to do something, or shamed more frequently. They were distracted from or physically restricted for misbehavior less often and received cuddling, kissing, praise, or were played with and told stories by their mothers less often. High bother scores and difficult temperament styles correlated significantly with maternal scolding and punitive responses to irritating child behaviors for target children only. The study provided theoretical and empirical support for Millor's hypothesis that one child in abusive families is appraised in a discriminately negative or bothersome manner, and that for this target child the mother-child social and disciplinary interactions are less favorable than those for a sibling.

Family structural characteristics, such as maternal or paternal age and years of school, race, marital status, socioeconomic status, maternal employment, and numbers of children did not differ significantly between abusive and control families in Millor's study.[35] The dynamic relationship between the abusive parents' childrearing histories and their current problems coping with the routine demands of childrearing appeared to contribute to the reported differences in mothers' behaviors. More abusive mothers than controls experienced disruptions in their families during early childhood (1-tailed McNemar's test, p = 0.03). There was only one abusive family in which neither parent experienced childhood disruptions owing to parental divorce, adoption, or foster care placement. Few abusive mothers recalled pleasant childhood activities that they were trying to recreate for their own children; four mothers and two fathers in six families were abused or neglected as children. In the 10 nonabusive families, only two fathers reported childhood disruptions and none of these parents experienced abuse or neglect. When maternal education and family income were matched, more mothers in nonabusive families than mothers in abusive families were employed or volunteered in positions where they were involved in children's activities and were learning, formally or informally, about child development or were acquiring job skills to match their desires for upward social mobility. The parents' resources seemed more effective for coping with a father's unemployment and other sources of environmental stress in these nonabusive control families. Given the small sample size and specificity of family eligibility criteria, these findings are not generalizable to the larger population of abused children or their mothers.

Millor's study suggests that the presence of an adversely perceived child is a continuous source of transactional stress. For parents with the potential for abuse, physically harmful or punitive childrearing interactions may escalate toward this special child and result in an incident of suspected abuse that is reported by health professionals to children's protective service agencies.

Another approach to understanding the relationship between stress and child abuse uses the life change events model.[48, 88, 89] The theoretical assumption of this model is that life change events represent nonspecific psychosocial stressors. When the number of events that occur within a critical period of time is high, the person's coping resources may become diminished and the person then becomes at risk for adverse social or health outcomes (or both), including child abuse. The significance of stress as a factor contributing to child abuse within this model has been substantiated.

Justice and Duncan[7, 89] administered the Social Readjustment Rating Scale to 35 abusing parents and to 35 control subjects. In assessing the degree of stress experienced by the study group, Justice and Duncan[87] gave the questionnaire to the abuser and to his or her spouse because of their belief that if both parents are involved in the family both are involved in the abuse. They found that the abusive families in the year preceding the abuse incident had suffered more stressful events than nonabusive families and that those events were more severe. The overwhelming frequency and intensity of stressful events adversely affected the parents' ability to deal constructively with even minor stress and made them vulnerable to responding in a destructive manner. The abusive parents were also more likely to feel a sense of rivalry with the other members of the family, including the child, as to which member was going to get his or her needs for nurturance met within the family system. If the child is not meeting the parents' needs, he or she is a readily available object toward whom the parents may vent their frustrations when overwhelmed by stress.

Conger, Burgess, and Barrett[88] administered the Social Readjustment Rating Scale to parents in 20 abusive and 20 control families.

Seventy per cent of the abusive parents attained moderate to high life change events scores. The mean life change scores for all abusive parents were significantly higher than for control parents (Wilcoxon signed ranks test, $p < 0.025$). Although personal injury or illness was the only event that significantly more abusers (40 per cent) than control parents (15 per cent) experienced prior to the abuse incident, control parents were "more likely to experience positive life changes, e.g., outstanding personal achievement."[88] Reporting a history of being abused as a child and moderate to severe life change characterized 41 per cent of the abusive parents, but none of the control parents reported this combination of stressors. The average number of children per family was three, and the median age for all children was 6.5 years.[90] For those families who retained custody of their children over a number of years since the initial or most recently reported abuse event, parents continued to display nonreciprocal interactional patterns with their children, some of whom were young adolescents.

In their prospective study of factors that contribute to maternal mistreatment of young children, Egeland and his colleagues administered a battery of psychologic tests, including a modified Social Readjustment Rating Scale, to 267 primiparous mothers from low socioeconomic backgrounds.[48, 58] The weighted life change scores for the 32 mistreating mothers were higher than those for the 33 high-quality care providing mothers; their group mean scores were 10.59 and 6.03, respectively.[48] In further analyses of the relationship between high stress and abuse, 51 (19 per cent) of the total mothers' scores were above the cut-off score selected to represent high stress. In this subsample, 12 mothers were also in the mistreating group. The characteristics of the highly stressed mistreating mothers that distinguished them from the highly stressed adequate care mothers and from the entire sample included high scores for anxiety concerning maternal role, aggression and defensiveness, low scores for social responsiveness to their infants, and less openness to sources of social support. It was the interaction of maternal and child variables in these highly stressed dyads that predicted the mistreating mothers.

Authors of theories of response to stress give further insight into the relationship between stress and child abuse. Gelles[4] suggests that people learn how to deal with stress within their families of origin and tend to use the modes of adaption to stress used by their parental models, including physically restrictive or harmful childrearing behaviors. Understanding the family characteristics that facilitate positive crisis adjustment is essential if the nurse is to help abuse-prone families. Hill[91] states that these characteristics include "family adaptability, family integration, affectional relations among family members, good marital adjustment of husband and wife, companionable parent-child relationships, family council type of control in decision making, social participation of wife and previous successful experience with crisis." It is apparent that many of these characteristics are in opposition to the characteristics ascribed to abusive families. LeMasters[92] adds that certain features of the crisis affect the family's success in mastery of the event, including "(1) the nature of the crisis event; (2) the state of organization or disorganization of the family at the point of impact; (3) the resources of the family; and (4) its previous experience with crises."

Although the pathways of causal relationships that produce abuse are not clear, most professionals in the field of child abuse agree that abusive parents lack the coping repertoire to perform their roles adequately, as expected by health professionals or by society in general. Change is an inherent process in child and family development; the frequency and nature of social and environmental demands on parents change over time also. Nursing care for abusive families must be based on knowledge of adaptive processes. Specific nursing interventions that are process oriented include reducing parental knowledge deficits about children's temperaments, normative development milestones, and childrearing behaviors; supporting caregiving and social interactions that are sensitive in pacing and reciprocal to children's behavioral cues; encouraging release of parental anger and clarification of confusion about potential or actual abusive events; and encouraging parental use of available social supports from within their extended families or by the community. By helping parents cope more constructively with potential sources of stress, nurses play a key role in reducing the family's vulnerability for child abuse.

Public health nurses involved in the Special Families Care project designed a process-oriented treatment plan for use with families whose mothers' historic backgrounds put them at risk for child abuse.[93] Not only did the special nursing interventions reduce the incidence of child abuse in the treatment group (n = 23) compared with

similar families (n = 32) that did not receive intensive nursing, but also the infants in the treatment group physically grew at expected normal rates and passed all items on the Denver Developmental Screening Test at the age of two years. Only two children in the treatment group compared with seven in the comparison group were placed in foster homes.[94] The evaluation of outcome data also suggested that parenting skills improved and more mothers developed positive social support networks in the treatment group than in the comparison group. The Special Families Care Project was able to demonstrate that intensive nursing services, sensitive to changing needs and resources of high-risk families, made a clinically significant contribution to improved family functioning over a two-year period.

Therapeutic programs that combine counseling of the parents and counseling or play therapies for children are more effective in restoring family integrity and reducing recidivism than are those programs that provide only parent counseling.[26] The peer play behaviors of abused children and their social interactions with adults are distinctly different in manner and themes from those of normal children.[95, 96] Play therapy helps abused children to express their fears and fantasies about physical assault, rejection, and separation from their parents.[97]

In addition to facilitating normal play and social behaviors among children, caregivers in play programs can also model mothering skills. Role modeling is one method of teaching abusive parents to break intergenerational patterns of poor parenting. This method is not limited to play programs and can easily be incorporated into the role of clinic and public health nurses.[98, 99] The nurse may also use process recordings of children's play behaviors or mothers' ratings on temperament scales, or both, to identify temperament patterns that may contribute to interactional difficulties. The nurse can use this information to help mothers adapt their childrearing behaviors to fit their children's temperaments. As the goodness of fit between mother and child improves, their vulnerability for subsequent abusive interaction may be reduced.

Nurses at the Minneapolis Health Department assisted families with many of the problems abusive families experience. Data on 845 families receiving public health nursing services from the Minneapolis Health Department were analyzed for the presence and improvement of the following parental problems: history of abuse of a child; inadequate parenting received by parents; inadequate emotional support; inadequate cognitive functioning ability; abuse of one parent by the other; mental health including inadequate self-concept, personal immaturity, poor emotional control, and chemical dependence; lack of knowledge of normal growth and development; major stress or stresses in the past year; rejection of a child; and inappropriate use of services.[100] Within six months of the initiation of public health nursing services, 71 per cent of the families showed improvement in the area of at least one problem. The areas that showed the largest percentage of improvement included lack of knowledge of normal growth and development, inadequate support, inadequate self-concept, and coping with stress. These data suggested that public health nurses were most effective when their interventions included teaching and supportive counseling.

To clarify the role of the nurse in helping the family who is vulnerable to or actually experiencing child abuse, an outline for the nursing process is presented subsequently, followed by a case situation using the process outline. During or after many of the life change events or stressors listed on the Social Readjustment Rating Scale,[101] the family would also have contact with a nurse. The most obvious life events include death of a spouse, death of a close family member, personal injury or illness, change in health of a family member, pregnancy, sex difficulties, and death of a close friend. One mode of coping with stress may be to develop illness symptoms. The nurse having contact with a parent who is seeking medical care and is diagnosed with psychosomatic illness should also be concerned. Mogielnicki and colleagues[102] reported on three cases in which functional symptoms were used by the parents as a mode of coping with impending child abuse.

Although more than one nurse had contact with the family presented in the case situation, the activities of only one of the nurses involved in the case are described. In actual work settings, which nurse performs which activity may vary, depending on the unique features of the work setting and the community.

NURSING PROCESS OUTLINE: STRESSFUL EVENT[55]

1. Data to be collected.
   a. Meaning of current stressful event to this family.
   b. Other stressful events that this family has experienced in the past year.
   c. Level of family functioning at the time of the most recent stressful event.
   d. Family style in coping with stressful events.
   e. Strengths family has that will aid them in coping constructively with the stressful event.
   f. Resources available and acceptable in the family's environment that will support their efforts to cope.
   g. Level of family functioning in the weeks and months following the stressful event.
2. Sample data collection questions.
   a. Have you ever lost anyone close to you?
   b. Have you yourself or anyone close to you been ill or hospitalized in the past few years?
   c. At the time (specific stressful event) occurred, what was going on with your family?
   d. What kinds of things did you enjoy doing together?
   e. When something upsetting happens to your family what do you usually do?
   f. Who is the person most helpful to you when you are upset?
   g. How has your life changed since (specific stressful event) occurred?
3. Sample nursing diagnosis.
   a. Family denies impact of stressful event.
   b. Family is unable to meet basic needs for food, rest, or shelter since occurrence of stressful event.
   c. Family members blame each other for causing stressful event.
   d. Family refuses to accept assistance in coping with stressful event.
   e. Family has made a constructive plan to cope with stressful event.
4. Sample objectives for nursing care plan.
   a. Family will resolve their feelings about the stressful event.
   b. Family will cope with the stressful event.
   c. Family will be able to re-establish homeostasis within the family unit.
5. Sample nursing care plan.
   a. The nurse will give the family members an opportunity to express their feelings about the stressful event including its effect on them as a group as well as individuals.
   b. The nurse will help the family members identify strengths and resources among themselves that will aid them in coping with this stressful event.

c. The nurse will help the family members identify methods of coping that they have used effectively in previous stressful events and that would be appropriate in this situation.

d. The nurse will help the family identify and use constructive methods of coping to replace previously used nonconstructive methods.

e. The nurse will refer the family to resources that can facilitate constructive coping with the stressful event.

6. Sample expected outcome criteria.

a. Family is able to meet their basic needs for food, rest, and shelter.

b. Each adult family member makes supportive statements to other family members.

c. Family is able to manage activities necessitated by the stressful event.

CASE SITUATION

Frank Smith, a 46-year-old fireman, was severely burned in a factory fire. He was hospitalized but died 36 hours after admission. His wife, Martha, is 38, a full-time homemaker, and mother of four children: Bill, 21, married with two children; Harvey, 17, a senior in high school; Jim, 14, a sophomore in high school; and Frank, Jr., 9, in the third grade. A month after the father's death, the school nurse brought Frank, Jr., to the hospital emergency room with a broken arm, which he had when he arrived at school that morning. Upon examination, Frank, Jr., was found to have numerous welts on his back and chest. A diagnosis of suspected child abuse was made.

What could either the hospital or the school nurse do to help this family better cope with the father's death and decrease the likelihood of abuse occurring? The first step was to determine the meaning of this stressful event to the family. A sympathetic interviewer used open-ended questions to ascertain the role played by the father in the family and subsequently the roles of the other family members. Most persons seek reasons or explanations for the cause of an event that go beyond the facts of the event itself. Many persons believe that it is God's will; others think that they have always had bad luck and that this is simply another example of it. Some families are very vocal about their beliefs. Some beliefs are comforting; some are upsetting. If a family's beliefs are the former, it may add to their ability to cope with the event.

One of the things the nurse assessed was who made the decisions in the family, which

helped to clarify the dependency needs of the family. If Mr. Smith made all the decisions and none were made by each or mutually, Mrs. Smith will feel more stressed by the decisions she will now be facing. Also, if Mr. Smith made all the decisions, Mrs. Smith may have played a dependent role in the family system and perhaps is less confident in her decision-making ability. In addition to the father's role in family decision making, the affectional ties of all family members, including the father's relationship with the children, are significant. Obviously, the children needed help in dealing with their father's death. If they were perceived by the mother to have been closer to their father, she may resent them if they now turn to her for comfort.

Persons who have resources available to help in a crisis will more likely use positive methods of coping. By asking about persons perceived to be helpful to the family, one hopes to determine the availability of persons who are willing and able to support the family through the crisis as well as the family's willingness to accept that help. As previously noted, abusive families tend to be isolated families.

The nurse also assessed whether the family's coping abilities had been decreased by previous stressful events. As stated earlier, many families who have experienced numerous stressful events may experience more child abuse. If stressful events have occurred, it is helpful to determine the family's method of coping with those crises as a clue to how they may cope with this crisis. One wants to determine if the family is able to reach out for help if their methods of coping are ineffective. Knowledge of the acceptability and the mode of expressing negative feeling within the family system is also helpful. Is crying accepted? When upset, does anyone go out and get drunk? The nurse had data about how the family responded during Mr. Smith's hospitalization, and the especially significant data included initial family response to the accident, including their ability to manage the necessities of life for themselves, that is, food, rest, transportation, and arrangements necessitated by the accident such as insurance papers and notification of other family members.

The nurse also had data on their ability to support each other emotionally. If extended family members or friends or both were present, did they increase or decrease the family's ability to function? Was Mrs. Smith able to be at all supportive to her children, or did she expect them to take care of her during this stressful event? The nurse also had data on the family's concept of their ability to cope. Healthy families recognize that they can cope with some crises, but if the crises are too severe, they seek help. Families who are over-confident may be denying the significance of the stress, which may lead to later difficulties, or may be afraid to accept help because of problems they have with trusting helping persons. Other families may convey the belief that they are incapable of managing the crisis and expect others to take care of them completely. Either situation puts the child at risk for neglect or abuse.

The school nurse had additional data on the Smith family, which aided in her assessment of the impact of Mr. Smith's death on the family. She had information on previous stressful events that this family had experienced. The school records contained such data on the family as residential moves, absences by Frank, Jr., because of illness, and other problems Frank, Jr., had had. Abused children often have problems getting along with their classmates or teachers, because they are either overly aggressive or withdrawn. The school nurse knew whether the family had shown appropriate interest in Frank's performance in school. The unrealistic expectations that many abusive parents have of their children may be reflected in excessive concern about the child's grades.

Nursing Diagnosis

Whether a hospital nurse, school nurse, or public health nurse has assessed the previously described data, she will be able to make a nursing diagnosis about the impact of Mr. Smith's death on the family's ability to function. Several possible diagnoses include the following: (1) Mrs. Smith is unable to express her feelings about Mr. Smith's death; (2) Mrs. Smith has unrealistic expectations of Frank, Jr.—she looks to him for comfort; (3) the family is unable to make decisions, e.g., those necessitated by Mr. Smith's death.

Nursing Care Plan

Specific activities the nurse might wish to include in her nursing care plan aimed at the overall objective of helping this family cope constructively with Mr. Smith's death include helping the family with the necessary decisions by referring them to someone such as the hospital chaplin, family minister, social worker, or other person acceptable to the family or, if the time is available, helping them herself. The person helping the family with decision making should help them clarify which decisions need to be made immediately and which can be delayed. She should help them to identify the various alternative decisions. She should help each family member feel comfortable in expressing his or her opinions on the possible alternatives and establish for the family that all opinions are to be respected. She should help them reach a consensus regarding a decision. Throughout the process, she should identify the positive behaviors exhibited by each family member, including their willingness to participate in the decision-making process. The latter is especially important, since it shows the persons involved that another person recognizes the difficult situation they are experiencing and it may decrease their feelings of isolation.

Specific activities by the nurse aimed at helping Mrs. Smith express her feelings about her husband's death call for a great deal of sensitivity. She must recognize Mrs. Smith's right to not express them or to select someone else with whom to share them. Mrs. Smith may have acquired cultural problems that might dictate how to behave in this situation; that is, perhaps her cultural group is stoic rather than expressive at the time of a death. However, the nurse has the responsibility of making Mrs. Smith aware that she can express her feelings to the nurse. In order to give Mrs. Smith this message, the nurse must do more than ask Mrs. Smith how she feels about her husband's death. She must be ready to accept those feelings, which might range from "I'm glad; he was a terrible person," to overwhelming grief. She must also provide a private place where both she and Mrs. Smith can sit without interruption. At times, the nurse is the best person to do this, especially if the nurse has had previous supportive contact with the family. At other times, it may be better for the family minister or a friend or relative to serve this role, but the nurse has the responsibility of seeing that someone is available to help Mrs. Smith.

Having someone available immediately and over the next year to help Mrs. Smith express her feelings may help with the problem caused by the unrealistic expectation that her young son will be able to comfort her. This problem as well as the fact that Mrs. Smith was very dependent on Mr. Smith place Frank, Jr., in a precarious position. He is too young to replace his father, and his mother could respond to his inability to take his father's place by abusing him. The activities of all the nurses and other professional personnel involved in helping the Smith family must be coordinated. In many cases, the public health nurse coordinates the family's care. Other activities of the public health nurse include the following: on-going assessment of the family's ability to cope with Mr. Smith's death, sympathetic listening to help the family through the grief process, and intervention as needed if other stressful events occur. All the activities mentioned, because they are aimed at helping the Smith family to use constructive coping mechanisms, may help in preventing the stressful event of the abuse of Frank, Jr.

When a child is seen in the emergency room because he or she has been abused, there are things the nurse can do to decrease the negative impact of this event on the family. Since Mrs. Smith was not present when Frank, Jr., was brought to the hospital, the first step would be to notify her. Abusive parents need the same caring concern that the relatives of any person admitted to the emergency room need. They are concerned about how serious the injuries are and feel very guilty because their anger resulted in their child's injury. The nurse should recognize and positively reward Mrs. Smith for being concerned about Frank, Jr. Most abusive parents have feelings of low self-worth. The feeling common to many abusive parents is "I must be a terrible parent to do this to my child," which adds to their low self-esteem. Treating the parents with respect, involving them in the child's care, as well as recognizing and rewarding them for the positive behaviors observed by the nurse, are important activities the nurse in the emergency room can perform in the treatment of a family in which abuse is suspected.

Cases of suspected physical abuse are required to be reported to the legally mandated reporting agency in all states, which is usually the child protection unit of the local welfare department. The nurse or the physician must tell the parents that a report is being made. Most abusive parents, because of their experience of being abused themselves, find it difficult to trust people. Basic to the establishment of a trusting relationship is honesty; thus, it is essential that the parents be told that a report is being made.

Being reported for child abuse is frightening. The nurse should recognize that the parents will be very concerned about what will happen to them and their child as a result of the report; thus, the consequence of the report should be made clear. For example, the nurse might say, "Tomorrow a social worker will be calling you to arrange a time to come and talk with you. She knows you do not want Frank, Jr., to be hurt again. She and we are going to try to help you so it doesn't happen again."

If Frank, Jr., were hospitalized because of his injury, the hospital nurse would also have an important role in helping this injured family. Neill and Kauffman have identified eight goals for the hospital nursing care of abused children and their families.[103]

1. Setting a tone of treatment rather than one of punishment
2. Promoting a sense of parental adequacy
3. Supporting strengths of the parent-child relationship
4. Decreasing the trauma of hospitalization for child and parent
5. Identifying needs of parents and child and sharing these with the team
6. Promoting the child's return to wellness
7. Implementing principles of crisis intervention
8. Modeling for parents and the child alternative ways of handling behavior, feelings, and interactions with others

Because parents who have abused their children have experienced frequent rejection and criticism (for example, have been abused themselves as children or have had negative life experiences), they are extremely sensitive to behaviors that indicate the professional staff's approval. Nursing care plans that are aimed at the goals identified by Neill and Kauffman should decrease the likelihood of the parents' having experiences with the professional staff that will lower their feelings of adequacy as parents. At times, professional staff members, because of their competence and efficiency, believe that they are, and actually are, giving better physical or emotional care or both to the child than the parents are able to give. The professional responsibility of teaching child care to the parent can also add to the parental sense of inadequacy. When one is being taught, one frequently gets the message that the person teaching is better or more adequate than oneself. Persons with low self-esteem sometimes cannot tolerate that additional blow to their self-esteem. Some persons respond verbally with a statement such as,

"What do you know? He's not your kid." Others withdraw from further contact with persons they think are being critical of them. This is one of the reasons some abusive families do not visit their abused child in the hospital. It is too painful for them emotionally.

The hospital nurse needs to acknowledge to the abusive parents their parental expertise—for example, the parents' knowledge of their child's likes and dislikes. The nurse should first explain to the parents what she must do for the child. Then, by asking the parents to help her plan the approach to this nursing activity, she is recognizing their importance and value in this situation. By involving the parents in many of the care activities, the nurse can set up a situation in which the nurse and parents are equals, each of whom brings something special to the situation. The nurse should also be comfortable sharing with the parents some of her mistakes or frustrations if they occur while she is interacting with the child. By sharing her mistake and how she would handle it next time, she is role-modeling an area with which many abusive parents have difficulty, that is, learning from one's mistakes.

Most, if not all, parents who have abused or neglected their children can benefit from the services of a public health nurse. The hospital nurse should refer the family to the public health nurse shortly after the child is admitted to the hospital. This will give the public health nurse time to initiate a long-term supportive relationship with the family before the child goes home. The public health nurse can also assess the impact of the current stressful situation, that is, the hospitalization of the child as well as the stress of the investigation on the total family. Of special importance is the effect of this stressful event on the parents' ability to care for their other children. The public health nurse plays an important role in coordinating the services the family is receiving as well as in assessing the impact of those services on the stress the family is feeling. In addition, the nurse can advocate within the service system for the family, provide supportive counseling, and teach parents how to care for the child and themselves.[104] The nurse, although recognizing many needs in the abusive family, realizes that improvement can occur only over time.

CONCLUSION

Stressful interpersonal transactions or a series of life change events that deplete a family's adaptive resources can cause any family to have problems in adequately meeting its members' needs. Parents who, because of inadequate role models, have learned ineffective modes of coping with stress, or whose life experiences have made them feel inadequate, and whose environments do not include supportive persons to aid in successful coping are vulnerable to losing self-control in response even to routine daily hassles. Children, especially those who are perceived as noncompliant with parental expectations or difficult to nurture, are at heightened risk for abuse during periods of family stress. By using their knowledge of the relationship between stress and the potential for child abuse, nurses can deliver care aimed at promoting the families' adaptive responses to sources of stress and thus can decrease the likelihood that children will be abused.

References

1. Rosenberg, J., and Cook, J. A. Differences in parenting and subsequent character structure development in child abuse and child neglect. *Journal of Pediatric Psychology*, vol. 1, Spring 1976, pp. 72–75.
2. Belsky, J. Three theoretical models of child abuse: A critical review. *Child Abuse and Neglect*, vol. 2, 1978, pp. 37–49.
3. Bittner, S., and Newberger, E. Pediatric understanding of child abuse and neglect. *Pediatrics in Review*, vol. 2, 1981, pp. 197–207.
4. Gelles, R. Child abuse and psychopathology: A sociological critique and formulation. *American Journal of Orthopsychiatry*, vol. 43, July 1973, pp. 611–621.
5. Gelles, R. Violence in the family: A review of research in the seventies. *Journal of Marriage and the Family*, vol. 42, November 1980, pp. 873–885.
6. Helfer, R. E. The etiology of child abuse. *Pediatrics*, vol. 51, Pt. II, April 1973, pp. 777–779.
7. Justice, B., and Justice, R. *The abusing family*. New York: Human Sciences Press, 1976.
8. Parke, R. Child abuse: An overview of alternative models. *Journal of Pediatric Psychology*, vol. 3, 1978, pp. 9–13.
9. Millor, G. K. A theoretical framework for nursing research in child abuse and neglect. *Nursing Research*, vol. 30, March/April 1981, pp. 78–83.
10. Straus, M. Stress and physical child abuse. *Child Abuse and Neglect*, vol. 4, 1980, pp. 75–88.
11. Young, M. Multiple correlates of abuse: A systems approach to the etiology of child abuse. *Journal of Pediatric Psychology*, vol. 1, Spring 1976, pp. 57–61.
12. Serrano, A., Zuelzer, M., Howe, D., and Reposa, R. Ecology of abusive and nonabusive families. *Journal of Child Psychiatry*, vol. 18, 1979, pp. 67–75.
13. Michalek, J. B. Nursing and child protection. *In* Newberger, E. (ed.) *Child Abuse*. Boston: Little, Brown and Company, 1982, pp. 217–233.
14. Davoren, E. *The Battered Child in California*. San Francisco: Rosenberg Foundation and San Francisco Consortium, March 1973.

15. Newberger, E., and Bourne, R. The medicalization and legalization of child abuse. *American Journal of Orthopsychiatry*, vol. 48, October 1978, pp. 593–607.

16. *National Study of the Incidence of Child Abuse and Neglect (Executive Summary)*. DHHS Publication No. (OHDS) 81-30329. Washington, DC, 1981.

17. DeFrancis, V. American Humane Association published highlights of national study of child abuse and neglect reporting for 1975. Child abuse and neglect reports. DHEW Publication No. (OHDS) 77-30086. Washington, DC: National Center on Child Abuse and Neglect, February 1977.

18. American Humane Association. *National analysis of official child neglect and abuse reporting for 1979*. DHHS Publication No. (OHDS) 81-30232. Washington, DC: National Center on Child Abuse and Neglect, 1981.

19. Elmer, E. *Children in Jeopardy: A Case of Abused Minors and Their Families*. Pittsburgh: University of Pittsburgh Press, 1967.

20. Holter, J., and Friedman, S. Principles of management in child abuse cases. *American Journal of Orthopsychiatry*, vol. 38, January 1968, pp. 127–136.

21. Martin, H., and Beezley, P. Behavioral observations of abused children. *Developmental Medicine and Child Neurology*, vol. 19, June 1977, pp. 373–387.

22. Solomon, T. History and demography of child abuse. *Pediatrics*, vol. 51, April 1973, pp. 773–776.

23. Fisher, B., and Berdie, J. Adolescent abuse and neglect: Issues of incidence, intervention and service delivery. *Child Abuse and Neglect*, vol. 2, 1978, pp. 173–192.

24. Schmidt, B., and Kempe, C. H. The pediatrician's role in child abuse and neglect. *Current Problems in Pediatrics*, vol. 5, March 1975, pp. 3–47.

25. Young, L. *Wednesday's Children*. New York, McGraw-Hill, 1964.

26. Cohn, A. Essential elements of successful child abuse and neglect treatment. *Child Abuse and Neglect*, vol. 3, 1979, pp. 491–496.

27. Lieber, L., and Baker, J. Parents anonymous—self-help treatments for child abusing parents: A review and evaluation. *Child Abuse and Neglect*, vol. 1, 1977, pp. 133–148.

28. Steele, B. Parental abuse of infants and small children. *In* Anthony, E. J., and Benedek, T. (eds.) *Parenthood*. Boston: Little, Brown and Co., 1970, pp. 449–477.

29. Steinmetz, S. Violence between family members. *Marriage and Family Review*, vol. 1, May 1978, pp. 2–17.

30. Elmer, E., and Gregg, G. Developmental characteristics of abused children. *Pediatrics*, vol. 40, Pt. I, October 1967, pp. 596–601.

31. Pelton, L. Child abuse and neglect: The myth of classlessness. *American Journal of Orthopsychiatry*, vol. 48, October 1978, pp. 608–617.

32. Kotulak, R. Studies link joblessness stress to abuse, illness. *Chicago Tribune*, Section 1, December 19, 1982, p. 10.

33. Satten, D. B., and Miler, J. K. The ecology of child abuse within a military community. *American Journal of Orthopsychiatry*, vol. 41, 1971, pp. 675–678.

34. Gil, D. Physical abuse of children: Findings and implications of a national survey. *Pediatrics*, vol. 44, 1969, pp. 857–864.

35. Millor, G. K. A comparative description of children's temperaments and maternal childrearing behaviors in abusive and neglectful families and normal fami-lies. Doctoral dissertation, University of California, San Francisco, December 1982 (University Microfilms International, No. 84-00, 022).

36. Terr, L. A family study of child abuse. *American Journal of Psychiatry*, vol. 127, November 1970, pp. 125–131.

37. Zuckerman, K., Ambuel, J. P., and Bandman, R. Child neglect and abuse. *Ohio State Medical Journal*, vol. 68, July 1972, pp. 629–632.

38. Galub, S. The battered child: What the nurse can do. *RN*, vol. 31, December 1968, pp. 42–45; 66–68.

39. Green, A. Child-abusing fathers. *Journal of American Academy of Child Psychiatry*, vol. 18, Spring 1979, pp. 270–282.

40. Weston, J. The pathology of child abuse: Summary of abuse cases. *In* Helfer, R. E., and Kempe, C. H. (eds.) *The Battered Child*, 2nd ed. Chicago: University of Chicago Press, 1974, pp. 61–86.

41. Nurse, S. Familial patterns of parents who abuse their children. *Smith College Studies in Social Work*, vol. 35, 1964, pp. 11–25.

42. Zalba, S. R. The abused child: A survey of the problem. *Social Work*, vol. 2, 1966, pp. 3–16.

43. Morris, M., and Gould, R. Role reversal: A necessary concept in dealing with the battered child syndrome. *In The Neglected/Battered Child Syndrome*. New York: Child Welfare League of America, 1963.

44. Melmick, B., and Hurley, J. Distinctive personality attributes of child abusing mothers. *Journal of Counseling and Clinical Psychology*, vol. 33, 1969, pp. 746–749.

45. Blumberg, M. Psychopathology of the abusing parent. *American Journal of Psychotherapy*, vol. 28, January 1974, pp. 21–29.

46. Disbrow, M., and Doerr, H. *Measures to Predict Child Abuse: A Validation Study (Final Report)*. Seattle: University of Washington, August 1982.

47. Rosen, B. Self-concept disturbance among mothers who abuse their children. *Psychological Reports*, vol. 43, August 1978, pp. 323–326.

48. Egeland, B., Breitenbucher, M., and Rosenberg, D. Prospective study of the significance of life stress in the etiology of child abuse. *Journal of Consulting and Clinical Psychology*, vol. 48, 1980, pp. 195–205.

49. Green, A., Gaines, R., and Sandgrund, A. Child abuse: Pathological syndrome of family interaction. *American Journal of Psychiatry*, vol. 131, August 1974, pp. 882–886.

50. Kempe, C. H. Approaches to preventing child abuse. *American Journal of Diseases of Children*, vol. 130, September 1976, pp. 941–947.

51. Lenoski, E. *How physically abusive parents differ from their controls*. Paper presented at The Battered Child Symposium, sponsored by the National Center for Child Abuse, Denver, CO, September 30, 1974.

52. Crain, L. S., and Millor, G. K. Forgotten children: Maltreated children of mentally retarded parents. *Pediatrics*, vol. 61, January 1978, pp. 73–79.

53. Lauer, B., Ten Broeck, E., and Grossman, M. Battered child syndrome: Review of 130 patients with controls. *Pediatrics*, vol. 54, July 1974, pp. 67–70.

54. Steele, B., and Pollock, C. A psychiatric study of parents who abuse infants and small children. *In* Helfer, R. E., and Kempe, C. H. (eds.) *The Battered Child*, 2nd ed. Chicago: University of Chicago Press, 1974, pp. 89–133.

55. Minneapolis Health Department. *Parenting assessment and intervention tool*. Minneapolis, 1977.

56. Twentyman, C., and Plotkin, R. Unrealistic expectations of parents who maltreat their children: An educational deficit that pertains to child development. *Journal of Clinical Psychology*, vol. 38, July 1982, pp. 497–503.

57. de Lissovoy, B. Toward the definition of 'abuse provoking child.' *Child Abuse and Neglect*, vol. 3, 1979, pp. 341–350.

58. Egeland, B., and Brunnquell, D. An at-risk approach to the study of child abuse. *Journal of American Academy of Child Psychiatry*, vol. 18, Spring 1979, pp. 219–235.

59. Friedrich, W., and Boriskin, J. The role of the child in abuse: A review of the literature. *American Journal of Orthopsychiatry*, vol. 46, October 1976, pp. 580–590.

60. Reidy, T. The aggressive characteristics of abused and neglected children. *Journal of Clinical Psychology*, vol. 33, October 1977, pp. 1140–1145.

61. Klein, M., and Stern, L. Low birth weight and the battered child syndrome. *American Journal of Diseases of Children*, vol. 122, July 1971, pp. 15–18.

62. Koel, B. Failure to thrive and fatal injury as a continuum. *American Journal of Diseases of Children*, vol. 118, October 1969, pp. 565–567.

63. Stern, L. Prematurity as a factor in child abuse. *Hospital Practice*, vol. 8, May 1973, pp. 117–123.

64. Leventhal, J. Risk factors for child abuse: Methodologic standards in case-control studies. *Pediatrics*, vol. 68, November 1981, pp. 684–690.

65. Lynch, M., and Roberts, J. Predicting child abuse: Signs of bonding failure in the maternity hospital. *British Medical Journal*, vol. 1, 1977, pp. 624–626.

66. Ounsted, C., Oppenheimer, R., and Lindsay, J. Aspects of bonding failure: The psychopathology and psychotherapeutic treatment of families of battered children. *Developmental Medicine and Child Neurology*, vol. 16, 1974, pp. 447–456.

67. Egeland, B., and Vaughn, B. Failure of "bond formation" as a cause of abuse, neglect and maltreatment. *American Journal of Orthopsychiatry*, vol. 51, January 1981, pp. 78–84.

68. Brunnquell, D., Crichton, L., and Egeland, B. Maternal personality and attitude in disturbances of childrearing. *American Journal of Orthopsychiatry*, vol. 51, October 1981, pp. 680–691.

69. Brazelton, T. B. *Neonatal Behavioral Assessment Scale*. Philadelphia: J. B. Lippincott, 1973.

70. Frodi, A., and Lamb, M. Infants at risk for child abuse. *Infant Mental Health Journal*, vol. 1, Winter 1980, pp. 240–247.

71. Carey, W. B., and McDevitt, S. Stability and change in individual temperament diagnoses from infancy to early childhood. *Journal of American Academy of Child Psychiatry*, vol. 17, Spring 1978a, pp. 331–337.

72. McDevitt, S., and Carey, W. B. Stability of ratings vs. perceptions of temperament from early infancy to 1–3 years. *American Journal of Orthopsychiatry*, vol. 51, April 1981, pp. 342–345.

73. Thomas, A., and Chess, S. *Temperament and Development*. New York: Brunner/Mazel, Inc., 1977.

74. Carey, W. B. Clinical applications of infant temperament measures. *Journal of Pediatrics*, vol. 81, October 1972, pp. 823–828.

75. Thomas, A., and Chess, S. *Dynamics of Psychological Development*. New York: Brunner/Mazel, Inc., 1980.

76. Campbell, S. G. Mother-infant interaction as a function of maternal ratings of temperament. *Child Psychiatry and Human Development*, vol. 10, Winter 1979, pp. 67–76.

77. Kronstadt, D., Oberklaid, F., Ferb, T., and Swartz, J. Behavior and maternal adaptations in the first six months of life. *American Journal of Orthopsychiatry*, vol. 49, July 1979, pp. 454–464.

78. Milliones, J. Relationship between perceived child temperament and maternal behaviors. *Child Development*, vol. 49, 1978, pp. 1255–1257.

79. Scholom, A., Zucker, R., and Stollak, G. Relating early child adjustment to infant and parent temperament. *Journal of Abnormal Child Psychology*, vol. 7, September 1979, pp. 297–308.

80. Ventura, J. N. Parent coping behaviors, parent functioning, and infant temperament characteristics. *Nursing Research*, vol. 31, September-October 1982, pp. 269–273.

81. Elmer, E. *Fragile Families, Troubled Children: The Aftermath of Infant Trauma*. Pittsburgh: University of Pittsburgh Press, 1977.

82. Gregg, G. Clinical experience with efforts to define individual differences in temperament. *In* Westman, J. C. (ed.) *Individual Differences in Children*. New York: John Wiley and Sons, 1973, pp. 307–321.

83. Herrenkohl, E., and Herrenkohl, R. A comparison of abused children and their nonabused siblings. *Journal of the American Academy of Child Psychiatry*, vol. 18, Spring 1979, pp. 260–269.

84. Carey, W. B., and McDevitt, S. Revision of the infant temperament questionnaire. *Pediatrics*, vol. 61, May 1978b, pp. 735–738.

85. Fullard, W., McDevitt, S., and Carey, W. B. *The toddler temperament scales*. Unpublished 1978 information sheet and test forms.

86. McDevitt, S., and Carey, W. B. The measurement of temperament in 3–7 year old children. *Journal of Child Psychology and Psychiatry*, vol. 19, July 1978, pp. 245–253.

87. Chamberlin, R., Szumouski, E., and Zastowny, T. An evaluation of efforts to educate mothers about child development in pediatric office practices. *American Journal of Public Health*, vol. 69, August 1979, pp. 875–886.

88. Conger, R., Burgess, R., and Barrett, C. Child abuse related to life change and perceptions of illness: Some preliminary findings. *The Family Coordinator*, vol. 28, January 1979, pp. 73–79.

89. Justice, B., and Duncan, D. Life crisis as a precursor to child abuse. *Public Health Reports*, vol. 91, April 1976, pp. 110–115.

90. Burgess, R., and Conger, R. Family interaction in abusive, neglectful and normal families. *Child Development*, vol. 49, December 1978, pp. 1163–1178.

91. Hill, R. Generic features of families under stress. *In* Parad, H. J. (ed.) *Crisis Intervention: Selected Readings*. New York: Family Service Association of America, 1972, pp. 32–52.

92. LeMasters, E. E. Parenthood as crisis. *In* Parad, H. J. (ed.). *Crisis Intervention: Selected Readings*. New York: Family Service Association of America, 1972, pp. 111–117.

93. Christensen, M. L., Schommer, B. L., and Velasquez, J. An interdisciplinary approach to preventing child abuse. *MCN*, vol. 9, March-April 1984, pp. 108–112.

94. Velasquez, J., Christensen, M. L., and Schommer, B. L. Intensive services help prevent child abuse. *MCN*, vol. 9, March-April 1984, pp. 113–119.

95. Gaensbauer, T., and Sands, K. Distorted affective communications in abused/neglected infants and their potential impact on caretakers. *Journal of American Academy of Child Psychiatry*, vol. 18, Spring 1979, pp. 236–250.

96. George, C., and Main, M. Social interactions of young abused children: Approach, avoidance and aggression. *Child Development*, vol. 50, June 1979, pp. 306–318.

97. Mann, E., and McDermott, J. Play therapy for victims of child abuse and neglect. *In* Schalfer, C., and O'Connor, K. (eds.) *Handbook of Play Therapy*. New York: John Wiley and Sons, 1983, pp. 283–307.

98. Morris, A. Conducting a parent education program in a pediatric clinic playroom. *Children Today*, vol. 3, November-December 1974, pp. 11–14; 36.

99. Stainton, C. Non-accidental trauma in children. *The Canadian Nurse*, vol. 71, October 1975, pp. 26–29.

100. Josten, L. Positive parenting: The nurse connection. *In Maternal and Child Nursing in the 80's: Nursing Perspective*. Baltimore: University of Maryland, 1981, pp. 106–111.

101. Holmes, T., and Rahe, R. The social readjustment rating scale. *Journal of Psychosomatic Research*, vol. 11, 1967, pp. 213–218.

102. Mogielnicki, R. P., Mogielnicki, N. P., Chandler, J. E., et al. Impending child abuse: Psychosomatic symptoms in adults as a clue. *Journal of the American Medical Association*, vol. 237, March 14, 1977, pp. 1109–1111.

103. Neill, K., and Kauffman, C. Care of the hospitalized abused child and his family: Nursing implications. *MCN*, vol. 1, March-April 1976, pp. 117–123.

104. Josten, L. Out of hospital care for a pervasive family problem . . . child abuse. *MCN*, vol. 3, March-April 1978, pp. 111–116.

16

THE STRESS OF INFERTILITY

SANDRA LINDELL

KATHLEEN DINEEN

Sandra Lindell and Kathleen Dineen begin their chapter on the stress of infertility with the religious, cultural, and social perspectives of infertility. This is followed by the statistics on infertility and the method of establishing the diagnosis. The chapter concludes by discussing the interventions available and the nurse's role.

"A childless woman is a monstrosity; we are born to be mothers. I too want to sacrifice myself, and I am often absorbed in gloomy thoughts these days: Will there never be a little one to call me mother?"

BALZAC, TWO WOMEN

RELIGIOUS, CULTURAL, AND SOCIAL PERSPECTIVES

One need not delve far into the historic consideration of woman to appreciate the significance of a verdict of infertility. Religious, cultural, and social value systems have established an obvious and strong relationship between fertility and worthiness. In the Old Testament, Genesis instructs humanity to "go forth and multiply." Other early religious forms revered the mother-goddess, her ability to give birth and to breastfeed, as well as her mysterious monthly cycles. In ancient Indian beliefs, woman was regarded as "the renewer of the race, the field in which man sows his seed."[1] In light of such definitions, infertility came to be interpreted as punishment from an angry deity and subsequent pregnancy as a gift. Furthermore, there are religions that teach that a woman's salvation is contingent on an ability to produce children, and there are societies that allow annulment if a woman is infertile.[2] Worldwide, cultures have always had symbols and rites to celebrate fertility,

some of which persist today. Although not as obvious as feasts and rituals worshiping a prolific harvest or the birth of a baby, the present-day custom of throwing rice at the bride and groom is, indeed, a vestige of an ancient custom, wishing the couple fertility. Other contemporary forms of celebrating include the new father's passing out cigars and the traditional baby shower for the mother-to-be.

The passage of generations has certainly not diminished the fact that childbearing and childrearing are regarded as woman's ultimate fulfillment of her biologic and social role. According to Menning,[3] the belief that everyone should have children is widely held in American society, which tends to be family-centered, with emphasis on the "normal" family constellation of mother-father-children. A fascination with children and anticipation of parenthood seem to be universal responses. In fact, customs, art, literature, the law, education, public opinion, and the communications media of radio and television all support the norm of motherhood and family.

The meaning of the diagnosis of infertility to a woman is multifaceted, as it includes aspects attached to her definitions of femininity, sexuality, and self-worth. Infertility may be seen as a development crisis, a failure to achieve a developmental milestone. Erickson[4] referred to the stage of generativity, believing

167

that parenthood is a biologic drive and its absence is experienced as some degree of personal impoverishment. While motherhood provides an opportunity for a woman to identify more closely with her own mother in pregnancy and childbearing, parenthood provides a unique opportunity to re-experience her own development as she facilitates her child's movement through the myriad developmental tasks of growth. For many, the separation of sexuality from motherhood is a difficult task. Motherliness is a normal component of femininity and a woman's psychosexual maturity. Deutsch[5] believes that coitus is, above all, an act of reproduction in the woman's mind. It is the beginning act that can end in the birth of child. As such, it is the first step of motherhood. Inability to follow through with reproduction and parenthood is, therefore, interpreted as a loss, a major life crisis for many women. Kraft[6] has noted that, for other women, pregnancy may fill a psychological need which is independent from the desire to parent an individuating child. Pregnancy may temporarily satisfy the internal feelings of emptiness experienced by some women or, idealized, it may subconsciously provide for unfulfilled childhood needs.

Rossi proposes that culture has given men no choice where work is concerned; they must work to attain the status of adult. Woman's equivalent assignment has been maternity. "There is considerable pressure upon the growing girl and young woman to consider maternity necessary for the woman's fulfillment as an individual and to secure her status as an adult."[7] Benedek,[8] who has studied the psychology of women, discusses the instinctual origins of motherliness. While the girl is growing up, she believes, the ego ideal incorporates the aspiration to feed and to be a good mother. Schechter[9] states that, through their childbearing abilities, women find their place in the continuum of the chain of generations. With such emphasis on the value of motherhood, it is little wonder that there exists a definite cultural and psychologic resistance to the nonfecund woman. Even less surprising is a woman's feelings of being different, of missing a major part of life, when she must come to grips with her inability to reproduce. Additional proof of the high value placed on fertility are the many euphemistic terms (most of negative connotation) applied to infertility: sterility, barrenness, fertility impairment, genital dysfunction, nonparenthood, childlessness, nonfecundity. Each of these phrases is taken from the infertility literature, and all seem to imply "less than whole."

THE MATTER OF CHOICE

In 1965, Rainwater published a fascinating research study of the factors underlying a person's goal of family size, of the social norms applied in evaluating family size, and of factors influencing effective use of birth control. This study, as well as research in many different societies, "suggests that . . . men and women have fairly clear ideas about the number of children that would be more gratifying and suitable for them. Most develop ideas about how many is too many, too few, just right."[10] This finding graphically points out the fact that adults take their fertility for granted. Society's programming is concerned with pregnancy prevention. With advances achieved in contraceptive technology, today's couples view fertility as a facet of life that is under their control, to be activated at will.[11] After all, family planning, in its broadest sense, includes the choice of whether or not to have children, how many, and when.[12] It is true that much of the current childlessness is voluntary. This turn of events can be related to major social changes, particularly those concerned with sexual mores and contraception. There has also been a growing acceptance of a woman's right not to want to parent, as career opportunities for women and women's success in careers have increased. In 1975, there was threefold more women stating an intention to remain childless than there were in 1964.[13] However, the salient point in this discussion is that these women were expressing a choice; and, for most people, the decisions revolving around childbearing and childrearing are just that: a matter of choosing whether and when, not if. What a rude awakening to have this choice denied.

CLASSIFICATIONS OF INFERTILE WOMEN

One must distinguish between two groups of infertile women, for their psychologic reaction to and possibilities of subsequent adaptation to their nonfecundity are different. The first of these groups includes those who are diagnosed as infertile prior to adolescence and, therefore, had that knowledge prior to consideration of family planning. The second group is that composed of women whose diagnosis was made in adulthood in relation to the attempt to conceive a child or to carry a pregnancy to term. The central focus for understanding the trauma and adaptation in both instances is the concept of body image "which reflects feelings about physical well-being, fantasies about what can be physically endured, as well as one's actual physical intactness or defectiveness."[14] In explanation of disturbances of body images, Kolb[15] states that a physical handicap present from the time of birth will become a part of the body image, as will the limitations it imposes. However, a handicap, or even an illness or physical injury, incurred later in life, is a threat to the stability of one's previously established body image. Thus, discovery of infertility is an intense narcissistic blow. The adult woman must make major revisions in her body image and self-concept. For many, this struggle brings their very identity into question. Schechter[16] likens the readjustment to that demanded of an amputee, as the adult experiencing this trauma has lost the ideal of herself as a biologic parent.

A woman's motivations for parenthood will be reflected in her reaction to infertility. In light of the cultural-societal-religious pressures presented, such motivations can be seen to include a desire to conform to outside pressure, to experience the rite of passage into adulthood, to relive a childhood of one's own, to compete with one's parents, to fulfill sex-role expectations, to experience pregnancy or to recapitulate a previous pregnancy, and to ensure genetic continuity.[17] The inability to fulfill any one of these needs may be internally defined as traumatic loss, a sense of missing a most important part of living.

DEFINITION AND STATISTICS

The medical definition of infertility is the inability to conceive a pregnancy after one year of regular sexual relations without contraception or the inability to carry pregnancy through to a live birth. Prerequisites for fertility weave a complex picture that gains clarity if one understands the basic premises underlying the state of fertility. Simplistically presented, fertility presupposes that the male can produce an adequate number of healthy, mobile sperm, which he is able to discharge on ejaculation from the urethra. In addition, the sperm must be deposited in the female in such a way that penetration of the cervical mucus can be accomplished. The sperm must then ascend through the uterus and reach the fallopian tube at a time in the menstrual cycle when it is possible to fertilize an ovum. Con-

comitantly with all of these steps, the female partner must have produced a normal ovum, capable of being fertilized, that entered the tube within a few hours of the sperm's being deposited and fertilized. This product of conception must then imbed itself into the uterus, implanting in a healthy endometrium capable of nourishing the conceptus, which must accomplish normal growth and development.[18] Each factor, or any variety of combinations of factors, may figure into the etiology of a couple's infertility, the causes of which are obviously innumerable. For the woman, functional causes include endocrine imbalance or failure to ovulate. Significant organic causes are physical defects or injury to the reproductive organs through infection (the leading cause of infertility in women), radiation, or surgery. The woman's fertility is also influenced by such factors as her age, nutritional status, emotional stress, frequency of intercourse, and duration of exposure. Shared factors that may prevent conception are immunologic response to the partner's sperm, lack of knowledge about sexual intercourse, infrequent intercourse, sexual dysfunction, and nonoptimal sexual technique. Regarding the psychologic component of infertility, we have found few studies that gathered research data with any significant degree of breadth or depth.[19–25] The typical treatment in the literature of psychologic effect is that of a vague two-dimensional influence: psychologic factors may cause infertility or infertility may either initiate or deepen psychologic problems, or both.

Considering the large number of male and female components of reproductive physiology and psychology that must interface successfully in order to achieve conception, it is not surprising that at least one of six American couples today find they must confront the problem of infertility. The most frequently quoted statistics claim that 10 per cent of married couples seek medical attention for infertility. However, Hatcher and other experts[26–28] in the field feel that risks to fertility are on the rise and that up to 15 per cent of married couples may be a more current and accurate estimate of the infertile population size. Figures assigning responsibility to male, female, or combined male and female problems for infertility vary, with 35 to 50 per cent female, 30 to 40 per cent male, and 20 to 30 per cent conjoint causation being ranges commonly given. Most agree that 50 per cent of those seeking medical consultation and treatment will eventually conceive.[29-32] It must be noted, however, that pregnancy-risk statistics for this population are higher than in the general population with regard to ectopic pregnancy, spontaneous abortion, and perinatal mortality, all of which effectively reduce the number who will successfully reach biologic parenthood.[33]

ESTABLISHING THE DIAGNOSIS

Hatcher notes that, despite the fact that infertility is a shared problem about 20 per cent of the time, the woman is most often evaluated first, as if female problems were the only causative factors: "It is still too common to find the wife subjected to an operative procedure before it was determined that her husband was azoospermic."[34] A semen analysis is the primary test for male infertility, along with a thorough medical history and physical examination. All of this can often be accomplished in one office visit.

In women, the causes of infertility can be much more complex and may require extensive testing over a long period of time after the initial medical history and physical examination. On the one hand, teaching a woman to do basal body temperature determination often initiates the treatment process and aids in documenting that she does, indeed, ovulate. This simple technique may also be used in pinpointing the best time for intercourse, maximizing the possibility of pregnancy. On the other hand, treatment might be as basic as correcting a woman's understanding of sexual technique, birth control, or douching. Frequently, however, these preliminary steps must be followed by the testing of each of the reproductive organs—cervix, uterus, fallopian tubes, and ovaries. The tests for the proper functioning of each fertility component and the inter-related working of the whole require much time, conscious effort, and dedication from the woman or the couple. She must note her temperature, have intercourse when it is prescribed and in the manner prescribed, watch her diet carefully, present at the physician's office for examination within a set time period of the sexual act, carefully record all aspects of her sexual/menstrual behavior, and undergo tests that are, at best, intrusive and may be painful as well. Although an explanation of infertility may be discovered at any step in the series, a woman would be just as likely to endure the entire process only to be told at the finish that no definitive reason for her infertility was apparent. Despite all of the sophisticated tests now available, determining the cause of infertility continues to be a difficult, tedious, and often impossible task.[35]

STRESS AND INFERTILITY

Some authors[36, 37] feel that infertility may not be a physiologic problem as much as a psychologic one, resulting from some form of anxiety or stress. Stone and Ward[38] noted that in instances when no physical reasons for infertility could be found and a woman became pregnant soon after undergoing testing, the conception was due to a change in the emotional status of the couple. This change was attributed to better acceptance of their situation by the couple, the knowledge that their problem was one shared by many couples, the release of fear and tension, and the relaxation they experienced after unburdening to people skilled in dealing with the problem of infertile couples.[38]

Once the question of inability to reproduce has been raised, what may be a stressful, time-consuming, energy-draining ordeal begins. As one young woman described her experience, "It was so demeaning! To admit that we might have a problem was difficult enough . . . then to have to sit through the doctor's endless, probing questions. Even though I knew it was necessary, it was awful."[39] According to Taymor, the diagnostic and therapeutic regimen required to investigate or to treat infertility is as likely to create psychologic factors as such factors are to create infertility: "It is self-evident that infertility brings feelings of frustration and depression. The tests and treatments engender anxiety and fear. The involvement of a third party in a discussion of private, sexual activity is not without serious implications. These tensions, via the hypothalamic-pituitary pathways, via the autonomic smooth muscle system, or by pathways not yet fully delineated, add their inhibiting weight to whatever organic factors are present."[40] The repeated frustration accompanying conscious plans to conceive and the lack of warmth and spontaneity inherent in coitus-by-prescription lead undeniably to a high level of tension. Investigation and treatment may even result in reactions of anovulatory cycles, impotence, inability to achieve orgasm, and lack of interest in intercourse.[41] Other noted psychologic reactions include anger at unfulfilled plans, guilt, and sadness. In addition, each plan or procedure that fails to achieve conception is experienced as further defeat. Yet, the very lack of concrete data about the etiology of infertility keeps the couple in a state of hopefulness: perhaps, this month.

In group sessions conducted by Wilchins and Park as part of the treatment of five infertile females, the women voiced several common reactions. All of the women expressed feelings of inadequacy and guilt. For some, this included a feeling of being under religious pressure for their inability to fulfill their obligation to reproduce. There was universal difficulty in adapting to the regimentation of fertility studies. Marital problems often grew out of their anxiety and pressured feelings as they vented their feelings on their husband. Husbands were often seen as lacking in empathy and as desiring a child only as living proof of virility.[42]

Kirk studied the psychologic reactions to infertility of 283 couples, finding that involuntary childlessness was experienced as a serious crisis for the women. The men responding to his questionnaire did not use terms with an emergency quality as the women had. They expressed disappointment but felt less deprived than the women did.[43]

Wiehe, in a study of 22 couples conducted soon after the diagnosis of infertility was made, found that subjects tended to evaluate themselves as neutral with regard to their attitude about fertility. Interestingly, on a standardized personality inventory, they characterized themselves as being defensive persons and having little self-awareness and understanding. They further characterized themselves as lacking in introspection, and Wiehe, therefore, questioned their ability to be truly revealing about their psychologic responses to infertility.[44] Another research study that matched a sample of 25 couples seeking infertility therapy with a control group found that those who were infertile interpreted the locus of control over life events to be external to themselves. The infertile women exhibited more neuroticism, anxiety, and emotional disturbance and a marked discrepancy between existing self and ideal self.[45] Schechter also found women to be much more affected by infertility, common reactions in interviews being "I felt different—out of the mainstream of what other women and couples were experiencing" . . . "resentful, bitter—as if God had forgotten me" . . . "freakish" . . . "I just didn't feel like a whole woman."[46]

REACTION TO THE LOSS

A woman's reaction to infertility is more easily comprehended from the perspective of loss, the loss of a vital body function. Menning asserts that there is a predictable, nearly universal syndrome that results from the realization of this loss: a sequence of surprise, denial, isolation, anger, guilt, grief, and resolution. The surprise component results from the common assumption of fertility, the concentration on pregnancy prevention. Denial of infertility is common, and fantasies about pregnancy and children may persist for a very long time. Menning[47] describes this stage of denial as protective, as long as it does not become prolonged, in that it allows a slow, tolerable level of increasing awareness and acceptance. Expectation of what is interpreted as superficial advice such as "just relax . . . don't think about it . . . have a glass of wine before sex . . . hang a maternity dress in your closet . . . " that may follow family and friends' awareness of a couple's infertility can be frustrating and can lead to voluntary isolation. This reaction is very natural in light of the deeply personal nature of the problem area. In her work with a multitude of infertile couples, Menning has repeatedly met those who radically altered their lifestyles in an attempt to avoid all reminders of the childbearing world. Partners may also become alienated from each other as one or the other or both experience feelings of shame, lowered self-esteem, guilt, or loss.[47] Infertility literature speaks repeatedly of the reaction of anger so commonly exhibited either rationally or irrationally.[48-51] Even in the most comfortable doctor-patient relationship, the couple has relinquished virtually all control and may experience anger at the uncomfortable, embarrassing testing regimen. Conversely, anger may be expressed at less rational targets, like teen-age mothers, abortion advocates, larger families, that is, at any possible reminder of the couple's loss. Guilt feelings arise as the couple tries to construct a cause-and-effect relationship, reviewing every minute possibility for an explanation. Menning lists as common guilt producers: premarital sex, birth control, abortion, extramarital sex, venereal disease, masturbation, homosexual thoughts or acts, even sexual pleasure. A common feeling seems to be that if only "the deed" can be pinpointed and atoned for, the person may hold out hope for a pregnancy.[52] By and large, the most frequent response to the knowledge of infertility is grief, felt not only as a reaction to the loss of fertility but to the loss of the "potential, anonymous, idealized child."[53]

A major difficulty in infertility work is the

all-too-often absence of a clear endpoint. The outcome may be unclear—one more test, one untried treatment, re-evaluation later, help from psychotherapy—and thus, the process of grieving is delayed. Kraft[54] believes that resolution depends upon the individual's level of character development and the manner in which past life stresses have been managed. For those with healthy self-identification, this crisis will be handled with positive adaptation through the steps outlined, leading to resignation. As in the mourning related to a death, resolution is often not absolute but may resurface during later, stressful life experiences—but rarely ever to the painful degree of the initial response. Once resolution is achieved, life can finally go on.

Only in recent years have there been organized systems to provide help to individuals and couples facing the traumas that accompany infertility. The best known is a national organization, RESOLVE, founded in 1973 by Barbara Eck Menning. It is through such community-based groups that individuals and couples are able to express their pain and anger in a safe environment with others who will listen and support them as they work toward acceptance of their diagnosis and altered life plans.[55]

PLANNING FOR THE FUTURE

When the couple is ready to make plans for the future, there are questions to be considered. First, whether they wish to parent; and second, if so, whether there are avenues open to them (artificial insemination or adoption) by which they may fulfill this wish.

Artificial Insemination

Nijs and Rouffa in *The Infertile Couple*, argue that before a couple can choose an alternative avenue to parenthood (particularly artificial insemination), the resolution of feelings (anger, guilt, loss) about infertility must be accompanied by new self-definitions without the procreative dimension. Sexuality and procreation have to be separated, and each partner has to affirm the other in this new situation. The need for partners to re-establish a good sexual relationship on this new basis is emphasized. They maintain that "a child has a right to parents and a good parent is primarily, a good partner. Each partner has to place the child in the perspective of his or her relation to the other one." If this new level of intimacy is achieved, artificial insemination is a "technical intervention on a biological plane."[56]

Adoption

Rock and co-workers[57] caution people not to use adoption as a ready remedy but rather to "work through" their feelings about infertility so that there will not be barriers to the process of adaptation. As the body of knowledge concerning the psychologic reactions to infertility has grown, there has been increasing awareness that many couples subscribe to the myth, either consciously or not, that the inability to conceive a child is linked to the inability to parent. Researchers agree that adaptation through grief and resolution to the loss of the biologic function will play a role in determining the ability to assume parenting functions, that emotional reactions to infertility must be experienced and resolved if one's parenting capacities are to be unleashed.[58, 59] Wiehe[60] relates resolution of the infertility crisis to subsequent parenting and notes several studies that report a significant relationship between inability to accept one's infertility and the lack of success as an adoptive parent. When the inability to parent biologically has been confronted and the resultant intrapersonal and interpersonal conflicts have been resolved, confidence in one's ability to parent another's child is enhanced.

It is often remarked that frequently, after adoption of a child, a woman becomes pregnant. Although the relationship between these two events has not been established,[61] Benedek reported that adoption or even the idea of adoption improves the woman's ability to conceive. Often, the experience with an adopted child relaxes the tension that had its roots in feelings of inadequacy, and conception occurs; Benedek assumed that the woman's anxiety regarding motherhood diminished when she was able to love and care for a child.[62]

THE NURSE'S ROLE

The nurse, as counselor/liaison/advocate, has a crucial role to play in the care of the couple seeking medical attention for infertility. As Menning poignantly reminds us, although a 50 per cent eventual pregnancy rate means joy and parenthood for half the country's couples who are in an infertility program, it also means that there is another 50 per cent who must face a final diagnosis of infertility.[63]

Nurses hold a pivotal position with all of these couples. Their major focus is facilitation of the adaptive process. Nurses do this by supportive listening, providing accurate explanations, helping the woman or couple to understand the components and results of testing, and affirming the validity of the wide variety of feelings that they may experience. Nurses are instrumental in referring couples to the appropriate source of help—physician, psychiatrist, or support group. Nurses serve as guides in helping the couple move toward a healthy resolution. It is clear that they are in a position to facilitate the process of adaptation, which will have an influence on all other aspects of subsequent living for the woman or couple.

A CASE STUDY

After five years of marriage and careful contraceptive use, S and W began to plan a healthy pregnancy. They used basal body temperature (BBT) recording and regular intercourse, and she ate a well-balanced diet, exercised regularly, and abstained from alcohol and all medications. The passage of time (18 months) without conception brought with it a deep feeling of frustration and anxiety about S's ability to conceive. Therefore, S and W sought the advice of an infertility specialist.

Thorough physical exams, laboratory testing, and study of their BBT charts led to a diagnosis of anovulatory menstrual cycles and a prescription for the fertility drug, Clomid. After three cycles and no success, S was tired . . . tired of a physician who, she felt, was not giving them straight answers; tired of scheduling intercourse; tired of lying in bed with hips elevated for up to two hours after intercourse in hopes of conceiving; tired of worrying what effects the drug Clomid might have on her body.

At this point, S and W changed specialists, finding a physician in whom they felt confident. He also prescribed Clomid but advised they not attempt conception in the first cycle. Thus, they enjoyed spontaneous intercourse, did not schedule their love-making, drank alcohol occasionally, decided they could be a happy childless couple, and contacted an adoption agency. By the time of the follow-up visit, S and W had conceived.

The couple describe their initial reaction as one of shocked surprise, then fear: fear of miscarriage, of multiple gestation, of parenthood. Being able to share these fears and work through them with their physician and friends brought a degree of relief and sense of support. The pregnancy was uncomplicated, and S gave birth to a 7½ pound baby girl at term. At present, she is happily mothering her six-month-old daughter and looking forward to future pregnancies.

References

1. Deutsch, Helen. *The Psychology of Women*, Vol. II. New York: Grune and Stratton, 1945, p. 23.
2. Fogel, C., and Woods, L. (eds.) *Health Care of Women: A Nursing Perspective*. St. Louis: C. V. Mosby, 1981, p. 263.
3. Ibid., p. 263.
4. Erikson, Erik. *Childhood and Society*. New York: Norton and Co., Inc., 1950, p. 231.
5. Deutsch, Helen, op. cit., pp. 90–91.
6. Kraft, Adrienne, Palombo, Joseph, and Mitchell, Dorena. The psychological dimensions of infertility. *American Journal of Orthopsychiatry*, Vol. 50, October 1980, p. 624.
7. Rossi, Alice S. Transition to parenthood. *Journal of Marriage and the Family*, February 1968, p. 30.
8. Benedek, Therese. Motherhood and nurturing. *In* Anthony, E. J., and Benedek, T. (eds.): *Parenthood: Its Psychology and Psychopathology*. Boston: Little, Brown and Co., 1979, p. 154.
9. Schechter, Marshall. About adoptive parents. *In* Anthony, E. J., and Benedek, T. (eds.): *Parenthood: Its Psychology and Psychopathology*. Boston: Little, Brown and Co., 1970, p. 361.
10. Rainwater, Lee. *Family Design: Marital Sexuality, Family Size and Contraception*. Chicago: Aldine Publishing Co., 1965, p. 118.
11. Fogel and Woods, op. cit., p. 264.
12. Ibid., p. 257.
13. Christie, G. L. The psychological and social management of the infertile couple. *In* Pepperell, R. J., Hudson, B., and Wood, C. (eds.): *The Infertile Couple*. New York: Churchill Livingstone, 1980, p. 230.
14. Kraft, Adrienne, et al., op. cit., p. 613.
15. Kolb, Lawrence. Disturbances of the body-image. *In* Arieti, S. (ed.): *American Handbook of Psychiatry*. New York: Basic Books, 1959, pp. 749–769.
16. Schechter, Marshall, op. cit., p. 360.
17. Menning, Barbara E. Counseling infertile couples. *Contemporary OB/GYN*, Vol. 13, February 1979, p. 104.
18. The American Fertility Society. *How to Organize a Basic Study of the Infertile Couple*. Birmingham, AL., Summer 1971, p. 2.
19. Benedek, Therese, Ham, George, Robbins, Fred, et al. Some emotional factors in infertility. *Psychosomatic Medicine*, Vol. 15, 1953, pp. 485–497.
20. Kraft, Adrienne, et al., op. cit., p. 620.
21. Deutsch, Helen, op. cit., p. 111.
22. Benedek, Therese. Motherhood and nurturing, op. cit., p. 155.
23. Platt, J. J., Ficher, Ilda, and Silver, Maurice. Infertile couples' personality traits and self-ideal concept discrepancies. *Fertility and Sterility*, Vol. 24, December 1973, p. 972.
24. Eisner, Betty. Some psychological differences between fertile and infertile women. *Journal of Clinical Psychology*, Vol. 19, 1963, p. 394.
25. Taymor, M. L. *The Management of Infertility*. Springfield, IL.: Charles C Thomas, 1969, p. 122.
26. Hatcher, Robert, Stewart, Gary, Stewart, Felicia, et al. (eds.): *Contraceptive Technology 1982–1983*, 11th ed. New York: Irvington Pub., Inc., 1982, p. 213.
27. Kraft, Adrienne, et al., op. cit., p. 620.
28. Birnbaum, Stanley, and Westheimer, Olie. Procedures and prognosis for the infertile couple. *Mother's Manual*, July/August 1980, p. 1.
29. Hatcher, Robert, et al., op. cit., pp. 219, 228.
30. Kraft, Adrienne, et al., op. cit., p. 620.
31. Birnbaum and Westheimer, op. cit., p. 1.

32. Menning, Barbara E., op. cit., p. 101.
33. Hatcher, Robert, et al., op. cit., p. 228.
34. Ibid., p. 219.
35. Birnbaum and Westheimer, op. cit., pp. 1–2.
36. Ibid., p. 2.
37. Mai, Francois, Munday, Robert, and Rump, Eric. Psychiatric interview comparisons between infertile and fertile couples. *Psychosomatic Medicine,* Vol. 34, September/October 1972, pp. 431–437.
38. Stone, A., and Ward, M. E. Factors responsible for pregnancy in 500 infertility cases. *Fertility and Sterility,* Vol. 7, 1956, p. 8.
39. Personal communication, anonymous, April 15, 1982.
40. Taymor, M. L., op. cit., p. 122.
41. de Watteville, Hubert. Psychologic factors in the treatment of sterility. *Ferility and Sterility,* Vol. 8, 1957, p. 21.
42. Wilchins, S. A., and Park, R. Use of group "rap sessions" in the adjunctive treatment of five infertile females. *Journal of the Medical Society of New Jersey,* Vol. 71, 1974, p. 951.
43. Kirk, D. *Shared Fate.* New York: Free Press of Glencoe, 1964.
44. Ibid., pp. 29–30.
45. Platt, J. J., et al., op. cit., p. 976.
46. Schechter, Marshall, op. cit., p. 358.
47. Menning, Barbara E., op. cit., pp. 102–106.
48. Christie, G. L., op. cit., p. 243.
49. Menning, Barbara E., op. cit., p. 103.
50. Kraft, Adrienne, et al., op. cit., p. 622.
51. Christie, G. L., op. cit., p. 236.
52. Menning, Barbara E., op. cit., p. 104.
53. Christie, G. L., op. cit., p. 243.
54. Kraft, Adrienne, et al., op. cit., p. 624.
55. Menning, Barbara E., op. cit., pp. 101–106.
56. Christie, G. L., op. cit., pp. 244–245.
57. Rock, John, Tietze, Christopher, and McLaughlin, Helen, Effect of adoption on infertility. *Fertility and Sterility,* Vol. 16, 1965, pp. 305–311, 312.
58. Kraft, G. L., op. cit., p. 627.
59. Christie, G. L., op. cit., p. 244.
60. Wiehe, Vernon, op. cit., pp. 28–29.
61. Rock et al., op. cit., pp. 311–312.
62. Benedek, Therese, op. cit., p. 494.
63. Menning, Barbara E., op. cit., p. 101.

17

EATING DISORDERS AND WOMEN

MARCEA KJERVIK

Marcea Kjervik's chapter on eating disorders includes discussions of anorexia nervosa, bulimia, and obesity. The characteristics of these conditions and their treatment, including nursing interventions, are identified.

Most people have at times been concerned about their weight but not to the pathologic degree that will be dealt with in this chapter. Our western society praises slenderness, particularly for women. Some individuals misuse eating in their efforts to cope with problems of living. Food has been used not only to satisfy a biologic need but also to reflect the cultural and political climate of the day. Therefore, eating disorders in women are not strictly a psychiatric problem but also a problem of female socialization.[1]

The goal in this chapter is to illustrate how many factors and influences interact in the development of abnormal eating patterns and how they can be corrected. Anorexia nervosa, bulimia and obesity are defined; demographic data are reviewed, characteristics amplified, and treatment discussed.

ANOREXIA NERVOSA

Definition

Anorexia means "the lack of appetite."[2] The patient suffers from a severe loss of weight that is caused by purposely limiting her food intake.[3] In general, then, anorexia nervosa occurs in persons who deliberately starve themselves by avoidance of food, resulting in weight loss that causes physical, emotional, and behavioral changes.[4] The course of the disease leads to clinical starvation, severe cachexia, and eventual death.[5] The incidence of anorexia is 5 per cent in the general popula-tion, age of onset ranges from 12 to 18 years of age, and it is found mostly in women.[6]

Anorexics are usually the youngest daughters in small families with older parents and often no brothers.[7] Prognosis is poorest for patients who are anorexic and then become bulimic.

Characteristics

Physical findings for the anorexic include amenorrhea; dehydration with signs and symptoms such as vomiting, cold intolerance, polyuria, lanugo hair, and hypotension; bradycardia; hematologic abnormalities; EEG abnormalities; low basal metabolic rate; and sleep disturbances characterized by hyperactivity.[8] The weight loss is usually 15 to 25 per cent of normal body weight. Mortality rates are based on fluid and electrolyte imbalance, starvation, suicide, tuberculosis, or gastric dilatation.[9]

Psychologically, anorexics ruminate about food and their fear of gaining weight, are narcissistically self-absorbed, tend to regress to an infantile behavior pattern, and have a history of being compliant at home and overachievers in school.[10] They suppress and then deny feelings of hunger, fatigue, and personal ineffectiveness; and they deny their thinness.[11] They also are introverted, conscientious, anxious, and have obsessive-compulsive traits.[12]

Normal maturation is interpreted by anorexics as "fatness." They deny their illness by failing to recognize their nutritional needs. Yet

175

they hoard food, seem to enjoy losing weight as a means of controlling their environment, and have a distorted body image.[13] Infertility may result from their long-standing lack of appetite. Whatever the outward criticism of their bodies, the deeper anxiety is with their growing up and having to be independent.[14] Their entire lives have been geared to living up to their families' expectations, and this results in feeling as if they are disappointing failures.[15] Outwardly, they appear to come from "harmonious" homes.[16]

Anorexics are usually neat, intelligent, and obedient, and they tend to reject feminine maturation and to resist the traditional passive-receptive females roles that their mothers accepted. Often, their mothers are subservient and overprotective, their fathers are seen as heroes who praise their daughters' appearance. Together, they do not encourage their daughter to be self-reliant, expressive, independent, or assertive. Anorexics establish their identity from social approval. In other words, they have an external locus of control, and when they feel rejected, they blame their bodies.[17] Parents often refuse to be blamed and expect the anorexic to feel guilty for causing unhappiness and worry at home.

The process of emancipation is thwarted because of a life change event—the family moving or the arrival of a new baby who does not become involved in the enmeshment of the family. Finding closeness and friendship outside the family becomes difficult, especially because of misperceptions and self-deceptions that are used to cover anxiety. This in turn only increases anorexics' feelings of helplessness because of the influence of their internal urges and external demands and their overall fear of being incapable of leading their own lives. So, what started in response to their ravenous hunger for love and attention has become a way of relieving generalized tension and anxiety.[18] In general, they grow up confused about themselves and are unable to develop a healthy identity, autonomy, or control.[19]

CASE STUDY

"Carey," a 15-year-old white, single, 85-pound female student, accompanied by her mother after being referred by her local physician, came to a mental health center after losing 30 pounds within the last year. She made it clear that she had no problem but was only pacifying her mother. During the previous year, she had begun voluntarily to lose weight, when she babysat for a family who barely had food enough to eat. Gradually, she enjoyed the control she had over herself and others by telling herself her body was "spongy" and receiving attention when she refused to eat. When her teachers complained of her weight loss, her mother took her to their local physician, who immediately sent her to the local mental health center.

Carey is the youngest of three children, having two older sisters. They bitterly complained of her "ordering" them around. Her father is an alcoholic who verbally abused his wife routinely. He, however, is a successful executive in a nationally known corporation. This information was discovered when Carey divulged that she idealized him and disparaged her "servant-like" mother. Her mother is passive, especially in conflict situations. Carey repeated several times that she would never end up like her mother, that is, give up her career as a ballet instructor, have children, and be a "servant."

At the initial visit, Carey was resistant to any therapy for herself. She didn't view herself as emaciated. She had amenorrhea, swam 3 miles daily, was an overachiever in school, and was preoccupied by food. She cooked all the meals at home.

Carey was seen individually on several occasions, before the family came for a treatment interview. An assessment was then made regarding the family members' observations of the patient. The parents were seen for couples counseling whenever the father was in town. The focus was on making communication more overt rather than covert. Carey was working on making lists of her self-imposed obligations regarding eating patterns, noting her thoughts when she refused to eat, and monitoring her fantasies.

The therapist occasionally ate with the family. Carey's mother made comments about her needing to eat more, and her father commented on how nice she looked. Most of the conversation, however, focused on the other siblings' activities in school, Carey's father's next trip, or gossip about neighbors.

Carey was negative and stubborn in her compliance with family interactions. She had been very active with others at school but lost her best friend to a "boy," and she was emphatic that she would never do that to a friend. She then began to isolate herself from others, even her acquaintances, but continued to participate even more strenuously in her first love, swimming. When she began to lose speed in competition because of her lack of strength, she swam more miles. It was her swimming instructor who prompted her to strive for the Olympics but reported to Carey's mother that she wouldn't make the team unless she had more strength.

Carey became as vigorous about making lists and increasing her swimming schedule as she was about avoiding eating and communicating. She lost 10 more pounds, and the therapist had her placed in the hospital against her wishes. This "betrayal" by the therapist caused their relationship to be strained during the early days of her hospitalization. A controlled high-carbohydrate protein diet was indicated, and if she didn't comply, tube feedings were used. Family sessions continued, with the focus on decreasing the aura of "normalcy." The family members in general were unable to express feelings, especially anger. When conflicts were brought to the surface, they were clarified and then negotiated. The parents were seen conjointly for several sessions; there was much resistance on both sides, that is, the mother not wanting to give up her role and the father avoiding his responsibility. The individual work with Carey focused on her saying whatever she felt like saying. She was encouraged not to try to please the therapist. The therapist wanted to get to know her, her actions, thoughts, and feelings. This approach was interrupted by her hospitalization, but she was able to again explore her fears of what would happen if she allowed herself to grow up.

Carey wanted to get out of the hospital and get well. She left the hospital two months after admission. She continued to be obsessed about her need to avoid certain foods and other "musts" but gradually became less rigid as she developed a healthy relationship with her therapist. Her fantasies were usually of a sexual nature, and since they were handled with sensitivity by her therapist, she was less frightened to talk about them. She continued in individual therapy, which terminated several years later. She did come back periodically, whenever she felt stressed again by another life change. She thought of gorging and purging when she entered college and found other young women relieving their anxieties in that manner. She took it upon herself to monitor her behavior, thoughts, and feelings and ask for an appointment with the therapist. She is now 20 years old, is doing well academically, continues to swim, although not competitively, and enjoys the company of young men.

Her parents continue in their old modes of behavior. Her mother, however, has begun to involve herself in civic activities. No change has occurred in her father. Her other sister is single and bulimic. Her older sister is happily married.

Nursing Interventions

Treatment for the anorexic patient may include individual, family, and group therapies, with behavioral management and medical maintenance. The personality of the anorexic determines which type of therapy will be most effective. A combination of therapies is sometimes necessary during the course of treatment.

Individual treatment focuses on correction of faulty self-perception or distorted body image, strengthening of the ego, and promotion of an insight into the social factors that condition women to be passive and to value their bodies only to conform with cultural standards.[20] It should be kept in mind that the typical anorexic patient has a delusional disturbance in body image, a disturbance of perception or interpretation (or both) of stimuli arising within her body, and a paralyzing sense of ineffectiveness. Perfectionism and obsessionality are ways she tries to repair her low self-esteem. The need to be perfect is a defense to cover the intense emptiness and loneliness. She generally does everything her parents tell her to do, but that is not the way to develop identity. Depression and anger accompany a dependent position, while fear and panic accompany an independent one. Losing weight accompanies a pervasive fear of growing up, which includes a fear of love relationships. Weight loss is the one area in which the anorexic patient can be herself and be autonomous, when every other area of her life is dependent. Hyperactivity results from her empty sense of self. Depression is caused by rigid expectations that can never be met and by her feeling dependent once again. Acquiring a sensitivity to her internal resources rather than depending on externals for gratification will lead to successful treatment.

Family therapy is used to re-establish positive object relationships and an internal locus of control.[21] Learning to communicate openly rather than covertly regarding all aspects of living leads to the negotiation of conflicts.[22] Enmeshment or overinvolvement, overprotectiveness, rigidity, and poor conflict resolution are problems of interaction that need exploration. The anorexic patient has a particular role in the family's pattern of interaction and conflict avoidance. She may become triangled between her parents, build an alliance with one of her parents, or be detoured by her parents' blaming her for the family problems. Therefore, it is necessary to reframe the problems that emphasize and clarify interpersonal difficulties, with the emphasis on developmental tasks. The therapist should work to make the distribution of power age appropriate and should check to see whether the family can give emotional nurturance.[23]

Behavioral treatments involve operant conditioning using reinforcement on an intermittent schedule, intrinsic reinforcers, and encouragement of the patient to take responsibility for her biologic maturity and to deal with family conflicts. It is hoped that these treatments will lead to the patient's desire to become well and get out of the hospital. Weight gain, mouthfuls eaten, meal size, or number of meals within a restricted period of time are rewarded by verbal reinforcement, attainment of privileges, permitted physical activity, and material and mental rewards. Cognitive therapy involves challenging erroneous assumptions and attitudes. Social skills are taught in order for the patient to develop effective interpersonal interactions and assertive behaviors. Encouragement of other levels of activity and alternative sources of pleasure need to be investigated. General stress management, problem solving, and emancipation from the family are essential for long-term change.[24]

Medical approaches deal with the signs and symptoms of physical and physiologic abnormalities. Hormone treatment, drugs to stimulate appetite, and neuroleptics of the phenothiazine group have been used.[25]

The aims of treatment are (1) to help resolve psychologic conflicts, and (2) to admit the patient to a psychiatric unit with good nursing care in order to increase the patient's weight to a normal level and return her to a normal menstrual pattern.

BULIMIA

Definition

Bulimia is defined as "ox hunger," or voracious hunger.[26] Bulimarexia combines starving with gorging and purging through vomiting or use of laxatives, or both, in order to start the cycle anew.[27] Actually, bulimics have "hunger pangs" as we know them but claim that they're always hungry; and the bulimarexic denies hunger at times but acts out her conflict at other times by gorging. This episodic binge eating is accompanied by the awareness that this is an abnormal eating pattern, then by the fear of being unable to control eating, and finally by feelings of depression and self-depreciation after the binges.[28] Other terms used for this disorder are bulimarexia, bulimia nervosa, dysorexia, and dietary chaos syndrome.[29]

Statistics

The incidence of bulimia, as with anorexia, is about 5 per cent in the general population. Usually, the age of onset is 16 to 20 years of age.[30] Bulimia is seen more frequently in females, but because bulimia has been identified only in the last 10 years, male college students are now noted to be affected as well.[31]

Bulimics usually have attended college and have had some heterosexual experience.[32] These persons usually binge at least weekly in the evenings, taking in about 4800 calories of carbohydrates (starches and sugars) and some salts, with an expenditure of about $10 per binge.[33] Their sexual, social, vocational, and financial functioning is negatively affected when they are actively bulimic. As stated earlier, prognosis is poorest for patients who are anorexic and then become bulimic. Almost 50 per cent of anorexics become bulimic. Forty to 60 per cent of bulimics recover.[34] The mortality rate for anorexics and bulimics together is 20 per cent.[35]

Characteristics

Bulimics tend to have many physical complaints such as weakness; lethargy; sore throat; signs and symptoms resulting from exposure to acidic gastric contents, such as caries, inflammation of parotid glands, and ulcers; menstrual irregularities; dehydration due to vomiting, laxative use, and diuretic use; elevated BUN; urinary infections and renal failure; epileptic seizures; tetany; and EEG abnormalities.[36]

Psychologically, bulimics suffer from overwhelming urges to overeat, avoid the effects of the food they do eat by vomiting or using purgatives or both, and live in morbid fear of becoming fat.[37] Therefore, they experience a vicious cycle of anxiety.[38]

Most bulimics express an exaggerated fear of becoming fat, and most view themselves as overweight. In reality, most are of normal weight or underweight. From the onset of their symptoms of bulimia, they usually experience marked fluctuations in their weight (10 pounds or more). Before an episode of binging, they crave food, have an uncontrollable appetite, and feel depressed. Afterward, they feel full, guilty, and worried about their lack of control.[39]

Often, bulimics begin the binging/purging cycle after having dieted. Life-change events such as returning to school or changing jobs may precipitate their new eating style.[40] Food is their all-consuming preoccupation. Their overeating is described as an involuntary, almost unconscious habit that results from feelings quite different from normal hunger. Their focus is on not gaining weight. Their deeper anxiety revolves around their perfectionism, all-or-nothing way of thinking, and passive/aggressive tendencies in dealing with their anger. They often avoid social interactions, fearing conflicts or rejection or both. They hide their uncontrollable eating. Bulimics tend to avoid cooking and eating experiences so as not to lose control, especially in front of others. They believe that they are controlled by their environment and fear losing control at any time.[41] When depressed, they lose sleep, become anxious, feel guilty, and are interpersonally sensitive. Poor impulse control is reported, as evidenced by kleptomania and chemical abuse.[42] They tend to be extroverted and hysterical yet nonassertive and use an external locus of control that leads them back to their interpersonal difficulties.[43]

Bulimics usually describe their childhoods as unhappy, and they remember crying easily, feeling dependent on others, and fighting with their peers. There often are numerous arguments between their parents. Their mothers are usually depressed, hostile, dissatisfied with family relationships, and not very nurturing. Their fathers are impulsive, have a low frustration tolerance, are excitable, also are not satisfied at home, and often are alcoholic. Families generally experience much conflict, lack of cohesiveness, and lack of structure despite their rigidity.[44]

A bulimic obsessed with her size and appetite may be expressing her anxiety over her conflict between her "appetites" and the necessity to control them.[45]

CASE STUDY

"Judy," a 30-year-old white, single, employed, slightly overweight, self-referred woman, came to a mental health clinic complaining of her bouts of binging and purging for three months and of her long-standing depression. One year prior to this Judy had gone to her family doctor to obtain a diet to lose weight. She had followed the directions to the letter and after three months had lost the weight she had wanted to lose. She was happy with herself and enjoyed others' company more than in the past. Three months later, she began to regain weight pound by pound and she became depressed and started to binge. She worried more when she started using laxatives.

At her initial visit, she admitted to being preoccupied with food and her weight, had vegetative signs of depression, and isolated herself from others but continued to see her family. Judy is the youngest of three, having an older sister and brother. Both were described by Judy as "obese and insecure." She described herself as "intelligent, and well-disciplined at work, superficially outgoing, insecure, having a good sense of humor, verbal, a people pleaser, rigid in my attitudes about myself and others, harsh, shyer than I let on, extremely depressed, lonely and terrified about gaining weight." She claimed that

she was never close to her mother until Judy bought a house and they worked on it together. She views her mother as the healthiest in the family because of her ability to set her mind to some task and complete it. She, however, is uncomfortable dealing with feelings. Her father is a retired researcher. He was described by Judy as "educated, intelligent, insecure, depressed, lonely, unable to deal with feelings, having numerous physical problems, pessimistic, and I see a lot of myself in him." She admitted to being intimidated by her father's and sister's intelligence. She used to be close to her sister before her sister's unsuccessful gastrojejunostomy surgery several years ago. She remembers herself as always being overweight like her family members. She was an achiever, did well in school, but dropped out in college because of a "fear of succeeding." She felt that her parents were aligned with her other siblings and that she was the "extra" and so was left to her own devices. She had no long-term heterosexual relationships, but she had many woman friends. She was socially active in group settings.

Initially, she was seen only for individual psychotherapy but a group setting was added several months later. At first, she focused on her underlying depression. When she began to explore her present behavior, thoughts, feelings, and their relationship to her role in her family, she was able to make more connections about her conflicts. In the group therapy, at first she hid her depression but admitted to her bulimia. Appearing strong to others and being a perfectionist caused her much pain. She acted as if she was superior to others but in reality she thought less of herself than others did. She began to take risks by telling others her feelings regarding her anger about herself, about not completing school or anything in her estimation. She tended to be a workaholic but gave herself no credit for her accomplishments. Whenever she felt lonely or depressed, she ran to her parents' house. Gradually, she began to explore her lack of intimate relationships.

After first venturing to interact with homosexual males, she began to take more risks with heterosexual males with whom she might be able to establish a relationship. Her depression lifted, her bulimia was fairly inactive, she used her family's house less as a refuge, continued to carry on her work, and generally felt better when she was assertive in asking for what she wanted for herself.

Nursing Intervention

The most successful modes of therapy for bulimics are individual psychodynamic psychotherapy and the use of cognitive/behavioral techniques.[46] Having the patient track her automatic thoughts, basic food beliefs, and in general monitor her behaviors, thoughts, and feelings assists her in staying present oriented rather than global. It is important for the therapist not to encourage or discourage dieting but rather to examine the patient's food beliefs.

The patient's monitoring of her behaviors, thoughts, and feelings that occur before, during, and after the binging and purging cycle is of prime significance. When connections, similarities, and differences during this cycle are noted, the patient gains an understanding of herself and regains the belief that she has control over her life. This is done by use of self-monitoring her daily activity schedule and by the use of the mastery, mood, and pleasure technique.[47] This information is collected by her, she becomes interested in her own data, and she then establishes trust and control at her own rate.

Gradually, the patient will produce rational responses to her automatic thoughts, correct errors in her food beliefs, and come to realize that she can control her behavior by identifying critical times and the coping behaviors that have helped her in the past.

Therefore, she needs first to monitor the frequency of her binge-eating and vomiting, to determine antecedents (situational, social, emotional, cognitive, and/or physiologic cues), and to note the consequences of binge-eating. Second, the bulimic must analyze the antecedent factors, and consequences. Finally, she should design an intervention program which includes changing eating behavior, manipulation of antecedent factors, learning of adaptive skills and manipulation of consequences.[48]

If the patient has difficulty using the preceding tools (behavioral/cognitive treatment), psychodynamic therapy begins. There are no "goods" or "bads" but rather an adaptation that may lead to the patient's wanting to change. It is of value to set goals, to give the patient articles to read in order for her to learn about her disorder, to use group treatment so that she learns that others have similar problems, to use assertiveness training to help her say what she wants, and to use relapse training (what to do if she slips) to help her accept herself.

When families are involved, it is useful for the patient to have a distraction such as involvement in another project or activity so that she does not focus all of her time on her eating disorder. Many of these patients have difficulties in separation and the developmental tasks of antonomy and individuation. Food seems to be a mood-altering chemical, resulting in rage, alienation, need to inflict pain, or tension reduction. The binge fills a nurturant need and the syndrome, an identity need. The purge seems to reduce tension and appears to be a thought-out act and an autonomous statement after "giving in" to nurturant needs. Environmental events—specifically, developmental challenge—lead to highly individualized mental events and mental conflict. The misuse of food is an attempt to deal with this conflict.[49] Learning that it is permissible to depend on others sometimes also helps the bulimic to be more self-acceptant.[50]

In supportive group treatment, imaging (placing oneself somewhere else in one's own mind), writing therapy, food poetry, prioritizing components of personal wellness, having the favorite food around at all times, fantasy chaining, and "letting go" in order to see what happens are all techniques that can be directed by an effective therapy leader to enable the patient to learn particularly about her food beliefs.[51]

Psychodynamically, once the bulimic believes she has some control over her eating disorder, she then can focus on thoughts and feelings that have caused her obsession about food. Depression, insecurity, dependency, anxiety, shame control, perfectionism, all-or-nothing thinking, the passive-aggressive response to anger, fear of competition—all are areas of concern that need to be explored for understanding and, perhaps for a change in behavior. Correcting misperceptions is essential for growth and change.

Medical treatment involves relieving the symptoms of dehydration, ulcers, tooth decay, and electrolyte imbalance. Because bulimic patients usually are desperate for help, they will follow the treatment guidelines set for them.[52]

The aims of treatment are (1) to teach patients that they have control over their eating and (2) to resolve underlying intrapsychic problems.

If the bulimic patient also has anorexia, the initial aim of treatment is medical intervention. Most associated deaths are the result of a patient with anorexia as well as bulimia.

OBESITY

Definition

Being obese is defined as being "fat, corpulent or overweight."[53] Most people become obese as adults rather than as children, with the incidence increasing with age. The prevalence of obesity reaches a peak at age 40, when 35 per cent of men and 40 per cent of women meet the requirements of being overweight, according to weight/height charts. Obesity is most frequently found in the lower class and in large families. Obesity has an adverse effect on morbidity and mortality rates, with cardiovascular disease being the major cause of death. Compared with adult-onset obesity, juvenile-onset obesity tends to be more severe and more resistant to treatment.[54]

Characteristics

Endogenous (primary) obesity is caused by genetic or metabolic difficulties, whereas exogenous (secondary) obesity is caused by overeating.[55] An increase in adipose tissue mass can lead to an increase in fat cell size (hypertrophic) or result from an increase in fat cell number (hyperplastic), or both. Obesity is also attributed to the amount of physical activity expended; the more sedentary the person, the greater that person's weight.[56]

Physical abnormalities as a result of obesity may include dyspnea, orthopedic problems, menstrual problems, skin disorders, blood-pressure elevations, hyperuricemia, impaired glucose tolerance, and plasma-lipid elevations.[57]

In general, there are two groups in which obesity is related to psychologic problems: (1) when obesity is intrinsically interwoven with the whole personality development, and (2) when obesity is a reaction to some traumatic event.[58] A uniform picture for all obese patients is difficult to find. Some general observations, however, can be made. Physical inactivity is a consistent contributing factor. Obese children are often oversensitive and sulky, tending to isolate themselves from others except when bullying smaller children. They have an exaggerated interest in and enjoyment of food, with a preference for starchy food. In many cases, obese children are unaware of their own hunger or satiation.[59]

Obese children may be shy, dependent, and compliant, usually having an intense relationship with one of their parents. They fear being teased, for fear of being rejected. They gradually withdraw from others, and then from life in general. They suffer from basic emotional insecurity. They disassociate their feelings, resulting in an inability to adjust to new situations. They are in conflict with their need for power and affection, which results in either passive helplessness or passive aggressiveness.[60]

The family of an obese child is often food oriented, in order to satisfy emotional needs. The mother is frequently in conflict regarding her own femininity and tends to be domineering, overprotective, and indulgent with food. According to the mother's perceptions, the father is weak and incompetent in dealing with the world. In reality, he may be competent in his profession and often is the parent who gives warmth and nourishment to his daughter. As the daughter learns her mother's perceptions of men, she habitually has a deep-seated fear of the "masculine," which leads to a tendency toward confusion in the gender role and sometimes to an intense father-daughter bond. The mother often rejects the daughter as an individual and projects her own dreams onto her. If the daughter is forced into the maternal role too early, she frequently rejects her mature maternal role and prefers to remain a child.[61]

The more serious the disturbance of body image, the poorer the outcome in treatment.[62] It has been found that obese adolescents are unaware of how to be self-directed in controlling their body stimuli and are unable to clarify their requirements for finding satisfactory responses. They have an external locus of control, weak ego boundaries, identity confusion, and lack of willpower.[63] Depressive reactions, suicidal preoccupations, and severe social isolation lead to a functional disorder.[64]

CASE STUDY

"Sara" was a 31-year-old, white, single, unemployed woman weighing about 250 pounds, who was referred from her local physician. She came in feeling "angry and depressed" after recently being fired from her job. She had a history of having problems communicating with her supervisors.

Sara came from a disturbed family background. Her childhood was spent moving from place to place because of her father's construction jobs. She was physically and sexually abused by her father and older brothers. Despite her mother's knowledge of this information, Sara received no support from her. Her mother was physically and emotionally absent from the home most of Sara's formative years.

Sara was quite close to her mother, who had had a stroke and needed much physical care. Her father died when she was young, and her brothers give minimal financial support to help their mother. Because Sara views her mother as a burden, both she and her mother tend to interact in quite passive-aggressive ways toward each other.

Sara worried and was very introspective and passively dependent. She admitted to feeling insecure and nervous and often had personality conflicts with others. She never had a chemical problem or attempted suicide.

Several individual psychotherapy sessions were scheduled and kept before Sara was encouraged to become involved in group treatment. Because she had been seen in therapy before, had some insight, and had the tendency to use projections exclusively, group treatment was the treatment of choice.

While Sara was in group therapy, she was verbal about her anger toward her mother, family, and past employers. She was articulate in describing herself. Other group members commented on their own conflicts in dealing with obese people. Although Sara then became defensive, this stimulated her to become more socially active outside of the group, so as to prove that not everyone avoided her because of her obesity. Her obesity had become a problem for her in adolescence when her mother was unavailable to her and she was placed in various foster homes. Her mother's sudden disappearance from the home occurred after she witnessed an unlawful act.

Sara did not talk about her eating habits but insisted that she had tried numerous diets with few results. She claimed that she had primary obesity but that it was never diagnosed. She tended to have rigid control of her feelings. Although she gave the external appearance of being calm, Sara raised her voice and used more hand motions when upset.

Sara was unaware of her fear of her own femininity and how that fear related to her fear of rejection. She used the group to clarify her distortions in her interactions with others. She also needed support during her frustrations in looking for another job.

Once she became aware of her internal conflicts, she was ready to seek medical clarification for dieting and behavioral support groups for diet and exercise. She was fortunate in that she had developed no physical problems from her long-standing obesity.

Nursing Intervention

The treatments that usually are most successful in dealing with obesity are behavioral support groups and medical management through diet, surgery, or both. Other focuses of treatment are relaxation techniques to decrease anxiety, assertiveness training to help the patient learn to express what she wants, and development of self-awareness to help her discover that her internal life does not need so much protection as represented by her layers of fat.

The aims for treatment depend on what the obese woman views as her top priority (for example, redirection or acceptance of her present self). Goal setting is essential. Questions that a therapist might keep in mind are:

1. Does the patient experience herself and her body as one?
2. Can she recognize her bodily functions?
3. Are her frustrations alleviated by eating?
4. If she lost weight, would she have to be good, strong, successful, feminine, and attractive?
5. Is she concealing her lack of self-confidence by her large body, which gives her a feeling of strength?[66]

CONCLUSION

Women with anorexia, bulimia, or obesity have distorted perceptions of themselves. They put food into their mouths or starve themselves rather than let their anger out. Clinging dependency was encouraged in their families without permitting them to become individuals in their own right. Gradually, they were unable to recognize normal hunger and other bodily sensations. Depressed emotions through the use of control helped them survive in their families but caused them difficulties in differentiating themselves from their families, in letting go, and in growing up. They generally suffer loneliness.

Treatment is directed toward helping the patient achieve emotional stability and maturity and develop and maintain normal physiologic functioning. To rule out an underlying medical condition, routine laboratory tests for electrolytes, renal and liver amylose, and thyroid functions need to be performed. Therefore, a physical and neurologic examination and a dental referral are essential.

In the obese patient's family, she learns whether she belongs; and in the world, she learns that she is separate. Identity develops from the interaction of her developmentally learning a sense of belonging and a sense of autonomy, by trying out her own ideas in the world. If she adopts a rigid style of functioning, rather than being spontaneous, she will remain the child and not fulfill her potential.[67]

It is most important that the nurse remember to be aware of his or her own values regarding eating disorders while working with these patients. The patient needs to set her own goals and progress at her own rate of development, yet she needs to be provoked to change her thoughts and eventually her behaviors. Her feelings toward herself will change in response to her opening herself up to her internal motivations, letting go of her perfectionism, and becoming spontaneous and thus acceptant of all aspects of herself. She then will be able to say more consistently what she wants and will more often be heard.

References

1. Hawkins, Raymond, C., II, and Clement, Pamela F. Development and construct validation of a self-report measure of binge eating tendencies. *Additive Behaviors,* Vol. 5, 1980, p. 220.
2. Bruch, Hilde. *The Golden Cage.* New York: Vintage Books, 1978, p. x.
3. Tolstrup, Kai. The Treatment of Anorexia Nervosa in Childhood and Adolescence. *Journal of Child Psychology and Psychiatry,* Vol. 16, 1975, p. 75.
4. Bemis, Kelly M. Current approaches to the etiology and treatment of anorexia nervosa. *Psychological Bulletin,* Vol. 85, 1978, p. 593.
5. Sours, John A. The primary anorexia nervosa syndrome. *In* Noshpitz, J. D. (ed.). *Basic Handbook of Child Psychiatry,* Vol. II. New York: Basic Books, Inc., 1979, p. 568.
6. Finck, Karen, and Comeau, Deborah. Anorexia and bulimia: Starving for perfection. Papers presented through Health Counseling Services, Minneapolis, February 4, 1982.
7. Hilde, Bruch, *Golden Cage,* p. 25.
8. Bemis, Kelly M., op cit., pp. 594–595.
9. Finck and Comeau, op. cit.
10. Bruch, Hilde, p. 9.
11. Anyan, Walter R. *Adolescent Medicine in Primary Care.* New York: John Wiley and Sons, 1978, p. 320.
12. Bemis, Kelly M., op. cit., p. 596.
13. *Diagnostic and Statistical Manual of Mental Disorders,* 3rd ed. (DSM-III). Washington, DC: Division of Public Affairs, American Psychiatric Association, 1980, pp. 67–68.
14. Bruch, Hilde, *Golden Cage,* p. 65.
15. Ibid., p. 24.
16. Ibid., p. 29.
17. Woodman, Marian. *The Owl Was A Baker's Daughter.* Toronto, Canada: Inner City Books, 1980, p. 39.
18. Bruch, Hilde, *Golden Cage,* pp. 83, 89.
19. Ibid., p. 41.
20. Bemis, Kelly M., op. cit., p. 611.
21. Rollins, Nancy, and Blackwell, Amelia. The treatment of anorexia nervosa in children and adolescents: Stage I. *Journal of Child Psychology Psychiatry,* Vol. 9, 1968, p. 90.
22. Sours, John A., op. cit., p. 579.
23. Bemis, Kelly M., op cit., p. 601.
24. Ibid., p. 603.
25. Tolstrup, Kai, op. cit., p. 76.
26. Casper, Regina C., et al. Bulimia. *Archives of General Psychiatry,* Vol. 37, September 1980, p. 1030.
27. Pogrebin, Letty Cottin. *Growing Up Free—Raising Your Child in the 80's.* New York: McGraw-Hill, 1980, p. 69.
28. *DSM-III,* op. cit., pp. 69–71.
29. Rosen, James C., and Lietenberg, Harold. Bulimia nervosa: Treatment with exposure and response prevention. *Behavior Therapy,* Vol. 13, 1982, p. 117.
30. Hampton, Anna C., et al. Bulimia: Research and treatment. Papers Presented at the Homm Clinic, Minneapolis, June 14, 1982.
31. Pyle, Richard, et al. Bulimia: A report of 34 cases. *Journal of Clinical Psychiatry,* Vol. 42, February 1981, p. 61.
32. Casper, Regina C., et al., op. cit., p. 1032.
33. Hampton, Anna C., et al., op. cit.
34. Pyle, Richard, et al., op. cit., pp. 60–62.
35. Pogrebin, Letty C., op. cit., p. 69.
36. Pyle, Richard, et al., op. cit., p. 63.
37. Russell, Gerald. Bulimia nervosa: An ominous variant of anorexia nervosa. *Psychological Medicine,* Vol. 9, 1979, p. 445.
38. Rosen, James C., op. cit., p. 117.
39. Hampton, Anna C., et al., op. cit., Bulimia papers, 1982.
40. Pyle, Richard, et al., op. cit., p. 61.
41. Hampton, Anna C., et al., op. cit.
42. Casper, Regina C., et al., op. cit., p. 1030.
43. Hawkins and Clement, op. cit., p. 224.
44. Hampton, Anna C., et al., op. cit.
45. Chernin, Kim. *The Obsession. Reflections on the Tyranny of Slenderness.* New York: Harper and Row, Publishers, 1981, p. 2.
46. Finck and Comeau, op. cit.
47. Beck, A. T. *Cognitive Therapy and the Emotional Disorders.* New York: International Universities Press, 1976.
48. Hampton, Anna C., et al., op. cit.
49. Garner, D. M., Garfinkel, P. E., et al. A multidimensional psychotherapy for anorexia nervosa. *International Journal of Eating Disorders,* Vol. 1, 1982, pp. 3–46.
50. Bruch, Hilde. *Eating Disorders: Obesity, Anorexia Nervosa, and the Person Within.* New York: Basic Books, Inc., 1973, p. 124.
51. Lockard, Melinda. Compulsive eater. Paper presented at a conference on Being Fat in America at the Earle Brown Center, March 13, 1982.
52. Hampton, Anna C., et al., op. cit.
53. *The Random House College Dictionary.* New York: Random House, Inc., p. 916.
54. Stunkard, Albert J. Obesity. *In* Arieti, Silvana, and Brodie H. Keith (eds.) *American Handbooks of Psychiatry,* Vol. VII. New York: Basic Books, Inc., 1981, pp. 455–456.
55. Woodman, Marian, op. cit., p. 11.
56. Stunkard, Albert J., op. cit., pp. 461–462.
57. Ibid., pp. 464–465.
58. Bruch, Hilde, *Eating Disorders.*
59. Bruch, Hilde, *Eating Disorders,* pp. 136–139.
60. Woodman, Marian, op. cit., pp. 50–51.
61. Woodman, Marian, op. cit., p. 39.
62. Bruch, Hilde, *Eating Disorders,* p. 147.
63. Ibid., pp. 154–155.
64. Stunkard, Albert J., op. cit., p. 466.
65. Ibid., p. 473.
66. Bruch, Hilde, *Eating Disorders,* pp. 325–327.
67. Ibid.

Suggested Readings

Anyan, Walter R. *Adolescent Medicine in Primary Care.* New York: John Wiley and Sons, 1978.
Beck, A. T. *Cognitive Therapy and the Emotional Disorders.* New York: International Universities Press, 1976.

Bemis, Kelly M. Current approaches to the etiology and treatment of anorexia nervosa. *Psychological Bulletin,* Vol. 85, 1978, pp. 593–617.

Boshind-Lodahl, M. Cinderella's step-sisters: A feminist perspective on anorexia nervosa and bulimia. *Signs: Journal of Women in Culture and Society,* Vol. 2, 1976, pp. 342–356.

Bruch, Hilde. *Eating Disorders: Obesity, Anorexia Nervosa, and the Person Within.* New York: Basic Books, Inc., 1973.

Bruch, Hilde. The Golden Cage. New York: Vintage Books, 1978.

Casper, Regina C., et al. Bulimia. *Archives of General Psychiatry,* Vol. 37, September 1980, pp. 1030–1035.

Chernin, Kim. *The Obsession. Reflections on the Tyranny of Slenderness.* New York: Harper and Row, 1981.

Crisp, A. H. *Anorexia Nervosa: Let Me Be.* New York: Grune and Stratton, 1980.

Dally, Peter, Gomez, Joan, and Issacs, A. J. *Anorexia Nervosa.* London: William Heinemann Medical Books, Ltd., 1979.

Dutta, D., Goswami, P., and Phookan, H. R. A case history of a 11-year old girl with voracious and perverted appetite. *Child Psychiatry Quarterly,* Vol. 10, July 1977, pp. 12–14.

Echert, E., Goldberg, S. C., Halmi, K. A., Casper, R. C., and Davis, J. M. Behavior therapy in anorexia nervosa. *British Journal of Psychiatry,* Vol. 134, 1979, pp. 55–59.

Fairburn, C. G. Self-induced vomiting. *Journal of Psychosomatic Research,* Vol. 24, 1980, pp. 193–197.

Finck, Karen, and Deborah Comeau. Anorexia and Bulimia: Starving for Perfection. Papers presented through Health Counseling Services, Minneapolis, February 4, 1982.

Garfinkil, P. E., Moldofsky, H., and Garner, D. M. The heterogeneity of anorexia nervosa: Bulimia as a distinct subgroup. *Archives of General Psychiatry,* Vol. 37, 1980, pp. 1036–1040.

Garner, D. M., Garfinkel, P. E., and Bemis, K. M. A multidimensional psychotherapy for anorexia nervosa. *International Journal of Eating Disorders,* Vol. 1, 1982, pp. 3–46.

Hampton, Anna C., Johnson, Craig, and Wallace, Marcie. Bulemia: Research and treatment. Papers presented at the Hamm Clinic, Minneapolis, June 14, 1982.

Hawkins, Raymond C., and Clement, Pamela. Development and construct validation of a self-report measure of binge eating tendencies. *Addictive Behavior,* Vol. 5, 1980, pp. 219–226.

Kintner, Martha, Boss, Pauline G., and Johnson, Nancy. The relationship between dysfunctional family environments and family member food intake. *Journal of Marriage and the Family,* Vol. 43, August, 1981, pp. 633–641.

Laube, Janet Johnson, and Weiland, Ronnye. The binging/purging syndrome. Papers presented at a conference on Empowering Women for Survival and Change at the National Association of Social Workers, Minneapolis, May 15, 1982.

Leckie, E. U., and Withers, R. F. J. Obesity and depression. *Journal of Psychosomatic Research,* Vol. 11, 1967, pp. 107–115.

Levenkron, Steven. *The Best Little Girl in the World.* Chicago: Contemporary Books, Inc., 1978.

Lockard, Melinda. Compulsive eater. Paper presented at a conference on Being Fat in America at the Earle Brown Center, March 13, 1982.

Loro, A. D., and Orleans, C. S. Binge eating and obesity: Preliminary findings and guidelines for behavioral analysis and treatment. *Addictive Behavior,* Vol. 6, 1981, pp. 155–166.

Minachin, S., Rosman, B. L., et al. *Psychosomatic Families: Anorexia Nervosa in Context.* Cambridge, MA, Harvard University Press, 1978.

Mitchell, James E., Pyle, Richard L., and Eckert, Elke D. Frequency and duration of binge eating episodes in patients with bulimia. *American Journal of Psychiatry,* Vol. 138, June, 1981, pp. 835–836.

Pogrebin, Letty Cottin. *Growing Up Free—Raising Your Child in the 80's.* New York: McGraw-Hill, 1980.

Pyle, Richard, Mitchell, James E., and Eckert, Elke D. Bulimia: A report of 34 cases. *Journal of Clinical Psychiatry,* Vol. 42, 1981, pp. 60–64.

Rao, N. V. S., and Surya, Prakash. Adjustment reaction of childhood. *Child Psychiatry Quarterly,* Vol. 10, January, 1977, pp. 8–26.

Rollins, Nancy, and Blackwell, Amelia. The treatment of anorexia nervosa in children and adolescents: Stage I. *Journal of Child Psychology and Psychiatry,* Vol. 9, 1968, pp. 81–91.

Rosen, James C. Bulimia nervosa: Treatment with exposure and response prevention. *Behavior Therapy,* Vol. 13, 1982, pp. 117–124.

Russell, Gerald, Bulimia nervosa. *Psychological Medicine,* Vol. 9, 1979, pp, 429–448.

Salkind, M. R., Fincharn, Jill, and Silverstone, Trevor. Is anorexia nervosa a phobic disorder? A psychophysiological enquiry. *Biological Psychiatry,* Vol. 15, 1980, pp. 803–808.

Schwartz, Donald M., and Thompson, Michael G. Do anorectics get well? Current research and future needs. *American Journal of Psychiatry,* Vol. 3, March 1981, pp. 319–323.

Selvini-Polazzoli, M. *Self-Starvation: From Individual to Family Therapy in Treatment of Anorexia Nervosa.* New York: Jason Aronson, 1978.

Sours, John A. The primary anorexia nervosa syndrome. *In* Noshpitz, J. D. (ed.) *Basic Handbook of Child Psychiatry,* Vol. II. New York: Basic Books, Inc., 1979.

Stunkard, Albert J. Obesity. *In* Arieti, Silvano, and Brodie, H. Keith (eds.) *American Handbook of Psychiatry,* Vol. VII. New York: Basic Books, Inc., 1981.

Thomas, A., and Chress, A. *The Dynamics of Psychological Development.* New York: Brunner Mazel, 1980.

Tolstrup, Kai. The treatment of anorexia nervosa in childhood and adolescence. *Journal of Child Psychology and Psychiatry,* Vol. 16, 1975, pp. 75–78.

Vigerski, Robert A. *Anorexia Nervosa.* New York: Raven Press, 1977.

Wardle, J. Dietary restraint and binge-eating. *Behavioral Analysis and Modification,* Vol. 4, 1980, pp. 201–209.

Wilson, G. J. Obesity, binge-eating and behavior therapy: Some clinical observations. *Behavior Therapy,* Vol. 7, 1976, pp. 700–701.

Woodman, Marian. *The Owl Was a Baker's Daughter: Obesity, Anorexia Nervosa, and the Repressed Feminine.* Toronto, Canada: Inner City Books, 1980.

Woodman, Marian. *Addiction to Perfection: The Still Unravished Bride.* Toronto, Canada. Inner City Books, 1982.

18

WOMEN IN PAIN
HOLLY BRANCH

This chapter by Holly Branch about the chronic pain syndrome in women presents the theory base of chronic pain from both the physiologic and psychologic viewpoints. Case studies illustrate the real-life experiences of women in pain. The interaction technique is the intervention presented by the author for serious consideration.

Pain is exciting. That's correct, exciting. Pain is perhaps the most crucial challenge to the nurse; the common denominator of our professional role identity is to provide for the relief of human suffering. The provision of that relief and the actualization of our professional self-image, then, should be approached with great excitement. However, many nurses practicing with persons in pain have quite the opposite feeling. In fact, expressions of inadequacy, anger, and guilt can be heard from nurses who seem to be almost universally frustrated in their attempts to care for those in pain. Perhaps the reason for this frustration is the nature of pain itself. Its subjectivity prevents nurses from achieving true empathy; its lack of physical substance lends a barrier to its eradication; and its complications leave a formidable responsibility for rehabilitation.

Much has been written on nursing management of women in acute pain, such as the pain of childbirth, and on pain associated with terminal illness, as with cancer. Relatively little attention has been paid to the nursing care of women with chronic, intractable pain. It seems almost as if these persons are given up as hopeless and told that they must learn to cope with their situation on their own. Unfortunately, many nurses have no idea how to create a plan of care and implement it to assist in coping with chronic pain. One obvious reason for this lack of understanding is the absence of or a misconstrued conceptual framework for chronic pain, for it can be a disease, whereas

acute and terminal pain are symptoms. The second reason is that many nurses find it difficult to achieve a satisfactory nurse-patient relationship with those in chronic pain because of their feelings about chronicity, chemical dependency, and psychologic dysfunction. These three factors are threatening to nurses, and they may think that they lack the necessary psychosocial skills needed to deal with them.

To provide effective and appropriate nursing care, one needs mastery of two areas, which can be described as theory base and interaction technique. Theory base is the collection and organization of one's academic knowledge into a conceptual framework that is applicable to clinical experience. Interaction technique refers to one's ability to integrate the professional and personal self and present a caring human being to the nurse-patient relationship. Both theory base and interaction technique are integral to the meeting of the pain challenge and are both given due attention in this chapter.

THEORY BASE

What does one need to know about pain? Isn't it enough to know that pain is indicative of human destruction and suffering and that it is the responsibility of nurses to provide for the cessation of the agony by whatever means are delegated to them by physicians, requested of them by the suffering, or seem appropriate on the basis of their professional nursing assessment? No, that is not enough, and that statement is not even necessarily correct. What one does need is a conceptual framework for chronic pain that can account for the many phenomena of that disease and from which appropriate interventions will follow.

To understand phenomena, it is usually logical to begin with a definition. Throughout the literature several authors have defined pain in several ways. Typically, the various disciplines of medicine, psychiatry, ministry, sociology, surgery, psychology, and often nursing have attempted to define pain according to their experiences with pain through their own theory base and social institution constructs. Such definitions demonstrate a rigid and myopic comprehension of pain and its resultant diagnosis and management. I assert that pain simply cannot be defined. No social institution can define a naturally occurring phenomenon such as pain. Pain is subjective and for that reason is not conducive to objective definition. Because of nursing's tradition of viewing the human person as a whole being, it is appropriate at this point to cite nursing's most well-known author in the field of pain, Margo McCaffery. She states that pain is "whatever the experiencing person says it is and exists whenever he says it does."[1] To define pain in that way, as a completely subjective phenomenon, is the only viable alternative for those who deal with persons in pain.

It is necessary to differentiate between pain as a sensory experience and the resultant behaviors that are exhibited as a response to this sensory stimulus. Pain behaviors are indeed open to definition and, to ensure proper assessment and treatment, must be defined accurately and objectively. Pain behaviors consist of any action that can be objectively denoted. These may include verbal manifestations varying from a simple "ouch" to a tirade of complaints and expletives; physiologic manifestations ranging from changes in autonomic functions such as pulse, blood pressure, and diaphoresis to gross behaviors such as limping, limited range of motion, and use of assistive devices such as crutches or braces; and psychosocial pain behaviors such as withdrawal, hostility, agitation, dependency, and social, recreational, and vocational dysfunction. This division between pain the experience and pain the behavior must be kept in mind and will be of great significance for the learning of both the interaction technique and the theory base.

It is appropriate to backstep a bit to provide a historic perspective on the development of theories on pain transmission. Among the first people to talk about pain and pain relief were the ancient Chinese. They believed that the human ear simulated an upside-down fetus and that every part of the human body corresponded to a part of the ear. At that time, when a person complained of pain the physician would locate the part of the ear that corresponded to the part of the body in pain and attempt to relieve the pain by inserting a metal staple or needle into that part of the ear. This technique, called acupuncture, is presently used on peripheral nerves. It is interesting that it was taboo for a physician to look at or touch any part of a woman's body except for her ear.

In early Western medicine, Aristotle made the assertion that pain was an emotion that was the absence of pleasure. Today, we know that pain is not an emotion but rather a bodily sensation. This is not to say, however, that the experience of pain cannot elicit emotional reactions or that emotional states cannot affect the intensity of the pain experience, for surely this is the case.

In the 1600s Descartes' assertions were the forerunners to the theories of pain belonging to this century. Descartes supposed that there were connections or strings connecting every part of the body with the brain. He termed these strings "tendons." When a person stepped on a tack or injured herself or himself, it caused a tugging on the tendon, which traveled up to the brain. Descartes conjectured that the sensation of pain was a result of this tugging on the brain.

Early this century, the specificity theory was developed. The theory stated that there are specialized pain receptors all over the body that are designed to react to noxious stimuli and send pain impulses along specialized nerve fibers to a specific pain center in the brain. Hence, the specificity theory claimed that there is a direct connection between the part of the body that hurts and the pain center in the brain, so that when a person steps on a tack the pain receptors in the foot send messages of pain along the pain nerve pathways directly to the brain, which then allows for the sensation of pain. This concept of pain transmission is most common among the lay patient population and is surprisingly prevalent in the thinking of health professionals.

There are, however, two pieces of evidence that confound the viability of the theory. The first comes from the research of Beecher[2] into the amount of pain perceived by wounded soldiers. According to the classic specificity theory, there should be a direct correlation between the amount of nerve damage and pain perceived, but Beecher found quite the opposite. In fact, he found many soldiers with extensive injuries who were actually unaware of pain. The second piece of evidence comes from clinical exposure to amputees. Phantom limb pain, which is actually sensed in the missing part itself, is initiated by gentle or non-noxious stimuli and can often be agonizing. It is apparent that there cannot be a direct connection between the pain receptors in the hurting part and the pain center in the brain, because the part that hurts is not there. That, along with the fact that the pain receptors in this case are not specific to noxious stimuli, lends to the inadequacy of the specificity theory.

There subsequently followed a group of pain theories known as pattern theories, which stressed the concepts of stimulus intensity, central summation, or input control system. The idea behind stimulus intensity was that all nerve endings are alike, so that pain is a result of the intensity of stimulation as opposed to specificity. Central summation refers to the concept of reverberating circuits of pain in the spinal column that may be triggered by noxious or non-noxious stimuli and are interpreted centrally (in the brain) as pain. This is opposed to the previous opinion that excessive peripheral stimulation was the mechanism for pain and afforded an explanation for phantom limb pain. The input control system proposed that the rapid velocity of certain nonpain nerve fibers inhibited the transmission of impulses in the slower-firing pain fibers. Although each of these theories offered individually valuable concepts, they were too narrowly constructed to account for the overall nature of pain transmission.

In 1965, Melzack and Wall[3] hypothesized the gate control theory. The gate control theory uses certain concepts from both the specificity and pattern theories in addition to some innovations to provide a theory that is generally applicable to clinical findings. Before exploring the intricacies of this theory, it is necessary to diverge and cover some basic neuroanatomy and physiology.

Pain transmission commences with cell destruction, which results in the release of certain proteolytic enzymes. These act on gamma globins to produce a series of polypeptides, which dilate blood vessels and trigger afferent nerve fibers. The pain pathway continues from these afferent fibers to the spinal cord via the dorsal root, up through the reticular brainstem and on to the thalamus, where pain is perceived, and finally to the cortex, where the cognitive, affective, and motor responses are determined.

There are three types of afferent nerve fibers, each responsible for different sensations. Beta fibers are large in diameter, have the fastest conduction velocity and lowest firing threshold, and are responsible for nonpainful or touch sensations. The gamma-delta, or A, fibers have a moderate diameter, conduction velocity, and firing threshold and are responsible for pinprick or knifelike pain, which is often characteristic of acute pain. The C fibers are of small diameter, slow velocity, and high threshold and are responsible for burning and aching, which is usually the nature of prolonged pain.

The gate control theory recognizes the idea of fiber specificity but qualifies it with stimulus intensity. In other words, there are specific fibers for transmission of pain as mentioned above, but smaller fibers are also capable of being triggered by non-noxious stimuli, so that one additional factor in determining whether pain will be sensed is the intensity of the stimulus. The main assertion of the gate control theory is the existence of a gate in the spinal cord which, when open, allows the transmission of pain to the brain for perception and reaction. When the gate is closed, pain messages are not allowed to reach the brain. The gate operates by degree; there are degrees of being open and being closed, as opposed to an either/or situation.

The gate is not any visible structure but rather a complex biochemical reaction. It consists of cells of substantia gelatinosa in the dorsal column of the spinal cord and operates as part of the input control system by collecting and modulating incoming impulses before sending them on to the T cells, whose function is to fire the impulses to the brain. The gate can be opened or closed in response to afferent activity from the body or efferent activity from the brain. One special characteristic of the gate is its relationship to the impulses of the beta, or touch, fibers. When these impulses reach the gate they are able to influence it to close to incoming messages from the A and C, or pain, fibers. The gate is also influenced by the central control trigger of the brain, whose efferent messages about the psychologic status of the individual affect the afferent conduction. The exact mechanism of the central control trigger is not known.

The gate may also be affected by endorphins. Endorphins are chemical substances found in the brain and are thought to provide pain relief through the same mechanism as the opiates, by attaching to receptor sites in the brain. The relationship between endorphins and pain has only recently been discovered and is being widely researched.

To provide a more comprehensive understanding of pain in a clinical sense, the concepts of pain threshold and the pain loop will be introduced. The pain threshold can actually be divided into two areas: the pain perception threshold and the pain reaction threshold. The pain perception threshold is that level or intensity of pain that reaches one's awareness, or perception. Pain perception thresholds are presumably the same for all persons regardless of demographic variables. The pain reaction threshold is the level pain reaches when it produces an observable behavioral response or reaction. This threshold does indeed vary according to age, sex, race, religion, childhood experiences, and many other variables. Hypothetically, then, if one could apply the same pain to a group of individuals, they would all perceive the pain at the same time, but their reactions to it would vary widely in terms of both degree and time.

To best explain the psychosocial aspects of pain, the concept of the pain loop will be used. The pain loop is a theoretical model used to conceptualize the abstract phenomenon of pain. An arbitrary value of 50 points will be assigned to the pain perception threshold, and a value of 75 points will designate the pain reaction threshold. Remember that it is at the level of the gate in the spinal column that these thresholds exist and that messages received by the gate may either come "up" from the body or "down" from the brain. The "points" will denote the quantity and quality of the messages coming to the gate. So at 50 points, the combined messages from the brain and the body reach the pain perception threshold of the gate, and the gate opens to the degree that pain is perceived. Similarly, if the combined messages from the brain and the body accumulate to 75 points, the gate opens to the degree that the person will react to the sensation of pain.

With these things in mind, some examples of various pain situations will be explored. The first three examples will focus on the healthy person, and the latter three will describe chronic pain states. The first example concerns the situation of a healthy woman on an average day (Fig. 18.1). The messages reaching the gate from the brain emanate from the problems and attentions of daily living, such as getting to work on time or sending the children off to school, and perhaps total 25 points. On an average day in this healthy woman's life she steps on a tack, and the messages from that injury bring 35 points to the gate. Thirty-five points from the body and 25 points from the brain total 60 points at the gate. Sixty points surpasses the pain perception threshold, and the gate opens to the degree that the woman will perceive the pain associated with her injury. The gate does not open to the point at which she would react to the pain, the pain reaction threshold. So, after perceiving the

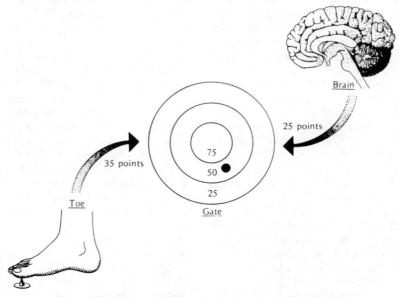

Figure 18.1. Pain in the life of a healthy woman: Example 1.

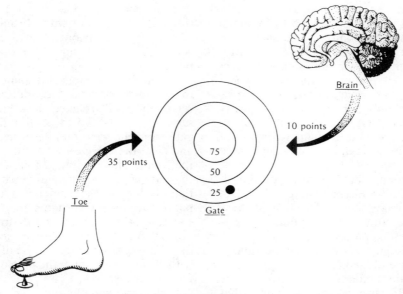

Figure 18.2. Pain in the life of a healthy woman: Example 2.

pain she goes about her daily activities without reacting to her perceptions.

The second example makes reference to the same healthy woman in the first example but under different circumstances (Fig. 18.2). On this particular day she is very relaxed and calm, well rested, and generally satisfied with her life situation. For these reasons the messages from the brain total only 10 points. Stepping on the same tack and receiving the same injury, she again accumulates 35 points from her foot. Ten points from the brain and 35 points from the foot total 45 points at the gate. Forty-five points is under the pain perception threshold, so the gate remains closed and the woman is not aware of the pain from her injury. Certainly, many of us have received bruises and minor cuts and have been unable to explain their origin; the above dynamics were probably in operation during those injuries.

In the third example, the same healthy woman is used but in a third set of circumstances (Fig. 18.3). This time the woman is experiencing a day that is not going particularly well; perhaps the car won't start, or there is a family argument, or performance at work was

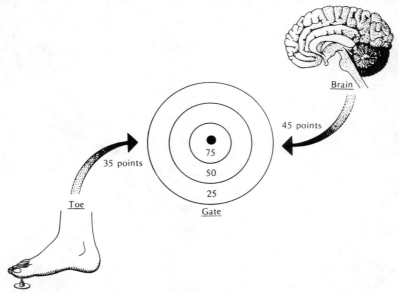

Figure 18.3. Pain in the life of a healthy woman: Example 3.

not satisfactory. The tensions and worries of a day such as this send messages worth 45 points down to the gate. Stepping on that same tack yields the same 35 points from the foot. Forty-five points from the brain and 35 points from the foot total 80 points at the gate, which constitute the pain reaction threshold. This woman will not only perceive the pain in her foot but will react to it with observable behavior that may range from a slight wrinkling of the brow to a loud scream or an exaggerated limp.

Before beginning the last three examples, which deal with chronic pain states, there are some vital issues to clarify. The first of these concerns the amount of organic damage present in the hurting part of the woman with chronic pain. Regardless of medical diagnosis or results from diagnostic testing, there is always a certain amount of damage in the painful part. Because persons in pain either underuse or misuse the affected part, there generally exists some organic damage from atrophied muscle at the very least. As an arbitrary figure, 35 points' worth of damage will be assigned to the hurt part of the woman in chronic pain.

In the fourth example, the woman is suffering from chronic pain of the foot, and this is an average day in her life (Fig. 18.4). On such a day, she is receiving 25 points' worth of average daily tensions at the gate from her brain. Thirty-five points from the chronic foot damage and 25 points from her brain total 60 points. Sixty points surpasses the pain percep-

tion threshold, so that on an average day in the life of a woman with chronic pain she is aware of the pain but able to cope with the activities of daily living without reacting to the pain.

In the fifth example, the same woman with the same chronic foot condition is having a relatively good, relaxed day (Fig. 18.5). The same 35 points' worth of disability reach the gate from the foot, and because she is relaxed and calm there are only 10 points coming from the brain. This combined total of 45 points at the gate is not enough to open the gate, so that on this day the women is not aware of her pain. Although the time period used in this example is one day, it varies from person to person. But generally there are seconds, hours, or even weeks or longer in the life of a woman with chronic pain when the pain does not break into her awareness.

In the last example, the woman with chronic foot pain is receiving the same 35 points from chronic foot damage at the gate in her spinal column (Fig. 18.6). But because she copes less effectively with this chronic disability, several changes occur that create an accumulation of points from the brain. If this woman is used to working she may find that she is no longer able to work. If she has been a housewife she is no longer able to care for the house and children. Social and recreational activities become a thing of the past. Even sexual activities are a source of pain. She loses her ability to plan ahead or structure her time, because her entire time reference becomes oriented around

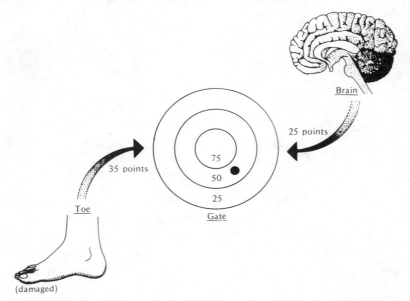

Figure 18.4. Pain in the life of a woman with a chronic foot condition: Example 4.

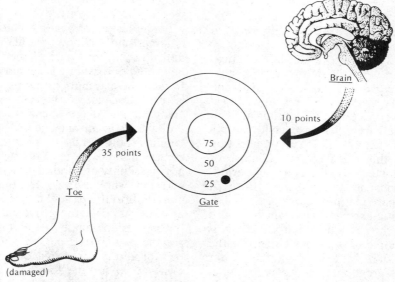

Figure 18.5. Pain in the life of a woman with a chronic foot condition: Example 5.

the pain. When she is in pain she waits for it to stop, and when she is not in pain she fearfully waits for it to appear. Movies, parties, weddings, high school graduations, shopping, picnics, dancing, church services, gardening, and golf have become symbols of hurt. If she starts using narcotics for control of pain she soon notices that they are decreasing in their effect. She fixates on the pills, watching the clock for the hours to tick by until she can take another pill. She is preoccupied with refilling prescriptions and perhaps reaches the point when she can't remember what time she took the last pill or how many she took last time, but she needs them and becomes indiscriminate in their use with this rationalization. Soon there is no evidence in her life that she is productive or worthwhile in any sense that she was used to. Her existence is without meaning or gratification. Depression, anger, anxiety, and fear set in. All of these events, whether they occur on a small scale in one day or accumulate over time, cause 45 points to reach the gate from the brain. Thirty-five points from the chronic foot damage and 45 points from a worried and desperate brain results in 80 points at the gate. These 80 points exceed the pain perception and pain reaction

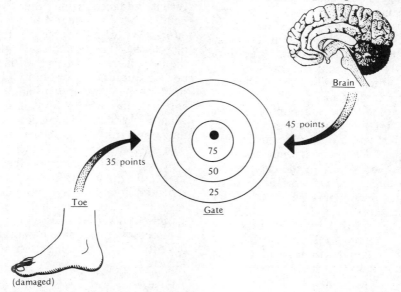

Figure 18.6. Pain in the life of a woman with a chronic foot condition: Example 6.

thresholds, and this woman not only is aware of her pain but reacts to it.

Persons with chronic pain typically react to it in one of two ways, either by underdoing or by overdoing. Those who underdo withdraw, give up, and virtually stop all premorbid activities. They become dependent, passive, and inadequate in their daily responsibilities. Those who overdo tend to dramatically increase their activity level, especially during those periods below the pain perception threshold. All this is an effort to ignore or deny the pain, which usually crops up periodically to an incapacitating degree. Both of these reactions are manifestations of an inability to cope with chronic pain, which is also known as the chronic pain syndrome. This is indeed an example of a vicious circle, for the more this woman reacts to her pain, the greater her tension, depression, and worry become, which operates to allow her to feel the pain even more acutely, leading to an even more exaggerated reaction, and so on.

It is important to note that the value of the points used in the previous examples is arbitrarily chosen but not without consideration. Points coming from either the brain or the rest of the body are always greater than 0 and less than 50, the pain perception threshold. These points are greater than 0, because there is no such thing as an absolute state of health in either the mind or the body. These ideals do not exist in reality. The upper spectrum of the points from the body or the mind does not exceed the pain perception threshold, because pain is a sensory experience composed of input from both the mind and the body. Absolute organic and psychogenic pain are also pure types that do not exist in reality, but between these limits the possible combinations of points from both body and mind are endless and dependent on the individuality of human beings and their environments.

The major point to be made here is that premorbid psychologic dysfunction can never be assumed to be the motive for the acquisition of prolonged pain. This is commonly assumed to be the case, particularly in the case of the woman whose diagnostic testing fails to show organic damage or enough damage to justify her subjective complaints in the diagnostician's opinion. To begin with, there are very few objective data available on the premorbid personality of women in pain. Living with chronic illness, especially pain that has a strong affective component, is generally facilitative of, or concomitant with, personality change. In conclusion, by the time a woman with pain reaches the point of chronicity (medically defined as six months' duration), it is a certainty that she will manifest emotional difficulties. It is simply not important to know whether the psychologic difficulties were a part of the etiology of the pain state or exist as a secondary complication. In fact, the assumption that psychologic illness is the sole cause of the pain state is a tragic error for any diagnostician to make and certainly leads to mismanagement of a case. Such labeling only tends to alienate the patient, create an atmosphere of distrust, and close off any possibility of a therapeutic relationship. In addition, whole areas of treatment options are closed off to the patient as she is ignored while awaiting referral to a psychiatrist. The same mistake can be made by the nurse who fails to see the patient as a person whose existence is painful and is concerned only with "the traction set up for the low back in room 233." Nursing care is ineffectual if it focuses only on physical or psychosocial needs. Whole people become ill and require whole nursing care, which brings us to a consideration of interaction technique.

INTERACTION TECHNIQUE

The interaction technique, as mentioned earlier, is the ability to integrate the professional and personal self to present a caring human being to the nurse-patient relationship. Learning the interaction technique is a delicate matter and deserves lengthy consideration. In many ways it is comparable to learning to ride a bicycle. One can read books and receive verbal guidance from others, which will be helpful, but the integral learning comes from interaction with the bicycle itself. Riding a bicycle is a function of both the person and the machinery, and it is a skill that is learned, not a natural talent or ability. The situation is similar when one is working with women in chronic pain states. Although nurses may read what is written here, which will be helpful, they must ultimately learn to develop their own sklls and style in clinical practice. They may fall down and scrape their knees a few times, but the actual learning must come from repeated interpersonal interaction. It is not easy, but it can be learned. The following is a statement made by a woman in pain, which, it is hoped, will stimulate an appreciation of the importance of learning from patients themselves.

Four years ago I was working on a television documentary, and normally I have a lot of energy; I like to work, keep busy, and am very social. I began not to feel well and as I planned to go away for the winter I decided to have my check-up and pap smear before leaving. I got a letter back saying that my pap test had come back positive, cancer. I was sent to the hospital for a culdoscopy, which was a totally devastating experience. Needless to say, I was terrified of what was going to go on, but the doctor refused to answer my questions when I asked him to please explain what he was going to do so that I could relax. He told me I wouldn't understand it because it was all in medical terms. After he got me into the stirrups set up for the culdoscopy, he brought in a class of interns without even asking my permission. They all took their turns looking. Obviously it really put me on edge. Then the doctor began to do biopsies without giving me an anesthetic or telling me what he was doing. He took 12 slices out of my cervix and then walked out of the room, leaving me bleeding and in a great deal of pain. I then had a long conversation with a doctor, who explained my options: that I had cancer very badly and that if I didn't have something done he didn't know how long I would have to live. He told me I could have surgery right away and possibly live a long time, or I could travel as I had planned and not come back. Of course, I was scared; I really did not know what to do. At that moment I became a very passive person and started to let things happen to me. I let myself get talked into a hysterectomy, which may or may not have been necessary—I still don't know.

I entered the hospital and was taken up to a 10-bed obstetrics-gynecology ward, which I thought was incredible: putting in the same room with mothers someone who was going to have a hysterectomy, although I had already decided I didn't want to have any children. However, when the choice is taken away from you at 28 years of age, it is still kind of devastating, and I hadn't gotten it all straight in my mind. It was hard to be in there with all those mothers; I was pretty anxious.

They took me up to the preoperative room and got me ready. I was talking a mile a minute just because I wanted someone to tell me what was going on. I was scared. The operating room nurse seemed upset by the fact that I wasn't more drugged, so she gave me another preop hypo. I don't remember much after that, but I found out later I was hemorrhaging and almost died because no one had come to check on me or paid any attention when my mother told them something was wrong. It was a hard time for me because it was very painful. I had IV needles in me everywhere, and yet they came and took blood out every hour to check my hemoglobin. I couldn't figure out why they were taking it out in one place and putting it in in another. I tried to be as cooperative as I could, but about the fourth day I broke down and cried because I couldn't deal with the situation. I was discharged early because they told me they needed my bed, but I had nowhere to go except a nursing home.

Finally it was arranged that my parents would drive 500 miles to pick me up and take me back to their home. I was in so much pain that I had to stop at several hospitals along the way for hypos. I was at my parents' house for two days, and I ended up in the hospital there. The doctor was our old family doctor, and he was very upset that I had had the operation. He felt it was unnecessary and had been bungled. He didn't even examine me. All this time I kept trying to tell someone that something was wrong because I still had a lot of pain in my side. Finally, I decided to leave. I just needed to be alone to deal with all of it. It was hard staying with my parents because they expect a great deal of people and have a hard time dealing with illness in their children.

For the next five months I was in an incredible amount of pain but continued to work and be very active, hoping it would go away. Then I began to grow hair on my face, developed severe headaches, and gained 30 pounds, and the pain went on without end. I went back to the hospital, but I couldn't get anyone to listen to me about what was wrong. I knew I was going through menopause. This went on for five days; I went back every day for a pelvic exam and a pap smear. By the fifth day I was furious because I had seen a different doctor every day, had to go through the same story every time, and none of the doctors could imagine why I was going through this, because I was "too young." So the fifth day I got hysterical, screamed and hollered, hit the desk, and things like that. I was at the end of my rope. By this time I was in a severe depression, which frightened me because I've never been depressed. I seriously thought about killing myself, and I just sat for hours alone trying to cope. So the day I had hysterics in the hospital they called in someone from the mental health unit to take me away so that I would not disturb the other patients, which only made me more furious. Finally an endocrinologist came in and told me I was in menopause. He suggested that I seek counseling, as all the doctors seemed to think that my uterus was connected to my personality, even though I could not find that on any anatomy charts. They thought my problem was that I had not accepted my hysterectomy, but to me that was beside the point by that time. I just didn't want to feel so awful. I went to the mental health unit. I took their tests, and I talked with their counselors. The consensus of doctors who saw me was that I was in better shape mentally than most of the people who worked there.

After that I was referred to another hospital for the regulation of my menopause. The doctor there looked at all women as inferior and neurotic, but I was still in my passive state and went along with everything he said. He gave some hormones, a tranquilizer, and some pain pills, as the pain was still there. I finally stopped taking the pain pills because I didn't want to get addicted, and I was determined to lick it on my own. But again, I had totally cut myself off from all my friends, I wasn't seeing anyone, I was in a bad mood all the time, and I refused to talk to anyone. I was in a great deal of pain all the time, and pains were starting in other parts of my body, which really frightened me.

When I tried to tell the doctor about the new pains in my chest and arm, he told me it was all in my head.

One day the pain was so bad that I couldn't breathe so I went to the emergency room, and they told me I had costal chondritis and that the tranquilizer I was on was making it worse. When I told my doctor about this I found that he had not looked at my chest x-ray at the time he prescribed the tranquilizer, and the x-ray already showed evidence of the disease at that time. So I went back to the first hospital and was assigned another doctor, who I thought would be the answer to my prayers—someone who would understand what I was going through, that I did not function solely in a six-by-nine office, that I functioned in the world, and that I was having a hard time dealing with the pain continually and still trying to straighten out things that were the aftermath of my operation.

By last spring I was once again in a desperate situation. I was ready to kill myself, just to end the suffering. I wasn't trying to get even with anyone; I was just tired of hurting. My brother referred me to a nurse-psychotherapist, and I can't say enough about what a help it has been to deal with someone who understands what is going on. I now understand that pain is not all in my head. It comes from my body as well, and when the two meet, a person's tolerance levels change. I'm back to functioning as a normal person, my creativity has come back, I have a lot of energy, I'm becoming more social, and I'm not in pain nearly as much as I was before. I hardly ever have a bad day now. The weather still affects me somewhat, but there are some things you learn to accept, and that's part of it—acceptance. Therapy has done me wonders.

I think it's really good that women are pioneering in this field because I think we know more about pain than anyone. We deal with it more in our lives than men do; we are more willing to acknowledge it, perhaps. The doctor who was seeing me refused to have anything to do with me when I decided to seek counseling. He felt it was a quackery program, particularly because it was run by women and nurses. He also made the comment that he wasn't there to listen to patients; he was there to look at their hearts and lungs. He told me he wasn't a psychiatrist, that he was just concerned about organs. That seems to be a prevailing attitude, particularly in the case of women, because the implication is that everything is tied to your reproductive organs. You are treated as if you have no identity other than that. I think it is important that people in health care begin to work together for the good of the patient and help the patient realize what is going on in his or her life. Doctors and nurses are only human like anyone else. The knowledge you have is the knowledge you have, and how you put it to use is up to you.

Therapy is helping me deal with the stresses in my life, pain being the biggest stress, although it is now somewhat eliminated. Also, my resentment toward how I felt and how I was treated is being worked through. I think it is important to have this kind of counseling available, because it is essential to vent resentful feelings; otherwise you magnify them all out of proportion and you make yourself sicker. Men and women are the cause of their own disease in the first place, which is a pretty hard thing to realize. We would like to blame it on some almighty power, but we've done it to ourselves. The hardest thing to realize is that you are in charge; that is very frightening. But then you realize you are also in charge of making things better, and that is good because you are only as strong as you want to be. If you want to be strong you can fix it. And I want to be, and I am fixing it.

This woman has indeed lived painfully. She has experienced the acute and chronic pain of physical illness; she has suffered the psychologic pain of depression, anger, and fear; she has encountered that spiritual pain involved with accountability; and she has coped with the cultural or sociologic pain that plagues women seeking assistance in a male-dominated health care system.

How have health professionals compounded the pain in the lives of persons such as this woman? This can best be understood by looking at the development of the "pain career" and the role that health professionals play in that development. As mentioned earlier, it is inherent in the role identity of health care professionals that they are dedicated to providing relief for human pain and suffering. Their first contact with the woman in pain is obviously after the onset of the initial pain symptoms, the acute phase. Following their role's script, they make every effort to alleviate both the pain and what appears to be the source of that pain. Seemingly, the most appropriate approach during this acute phase is to directly treat the pain with rest and medication. The problems arise somewhere between the acute and chronic phases of pain, which is a rather nebulous time span since, according to medical definition, pain does not achieve chronicity until it is of six months' duration. Use of the treatment approaches for acute pain generally produces iatrogenic complications after prolonged application. Specifically, three such iatrogenic situations will be discussed.

Persons in pain who are advised to rest or to exercise or work until they feel pain can learn more pain—and pain can be learned. This is called a work-to-tolerance prescription and operates according to the following diagram:

Activity ⟶ pain ⟶ rest ⟶ (+R)

The person is active until she experiences pain, and then she is allowed to rest. Rest (R), then, assumes the characteristics of a positive reinforcer that increases the likelihood of pain occurring again because it is rewarded by rest. This kind of biologic learning occurs in the patient at a subconscious level. In addition to reinforcing pain, prolonged periods of rest reduce self-worth by eliminating sources of worth such as the performance of daily responsibilities and social interaction. Such situations are breeding grounds for depression, fear, anxiety, and dependency.

Similarly, medications used for acute pain are frequently extended beyond the acute phase and into the chronic. The use of pain medications, particularly narcotics, operates like rest as a positive reinforcement to the reappearance of pain:

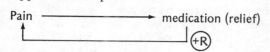

Iatrogenic chemical dependence and its ramifications are often a part of chronic pain states.

There is a third aspect of this acute care approach that is confounding when used beyond the acute stage, and that is the concept of direct intervention to the hurting part. During the acute phase, efforts are geared toward diagnosis and treatment of the affected part. After this point diagnosis is no longer engaged in, for it generally shows no organic damage, a healed injury, or intractable damage for which there is no appropriate direct intervention. The patient is then told that she must learn to live with her condition, without any clue as to how to go about doing it. In addition, another factor begins to operate. By this time the patient is a threat to health professionals because she is failing to be relieved of her pain, which indicates that they are failing to fulfill their professional role identity. When faced with such a threat, health professionals may resort to many tactics to alleviate or reduce the threat. Among the most common is labeling the patient as one who has imaginary pain solely to resolve neurotic conflict, obtain narcotics to maintain an addiction, or secure financial secondary gain through litigation or compensation. Although such factors may be influential, they are rarely a conscious motivation, and such attitudes and behaviors on the part of health care professionals promote distrust and resentment on the part of the patient and lay the foundation for a nonproductive relationship.

So what can be done in a positive sense? The most important factor in the rehabilitation of the woman with chronic pain is the establishment of a therapeutic nurse-patient relationship. The most important component of a therapeutic nurse-patient relationship is trust. Such trust emanates from understanding of and belief in each other. That kind of trust, understanding, and belief is impossible to achieve if the nurse is preoccupied with determining whether the patient's pain is real or imaginary and, if it is imaginary, what the payoff is. This kind of preoccupation is nonproductive. Unless the nurse can come to accept the ideology that all pain is a real sensory experience with both psychologic and physical components, the nursing care will be ineffective. It is fairly common to hear nurses say that they know psychogenic pain feels real to the patient, but even this type of thinking is not functional for it still propagates the concept of dualism. All pain is real, or all pain is imaginary, whichever way is easiest to conceptualize, but pain simply *is*. Unless this frame of reference is adopted, the nurse's energies will be misdirected toward direct intervention of the pain itself, which is inappropriate in a chronic situation. When the existence of pain is accepted as a given, the nurse then becomes more free to direct healing energy toward a more appropriate focus—the patient as a person. The patient as a person has suffered physical, emotional, spiritual, vocational, recreational, social, and familial dysfunction as a result of living in pain. In chronic pain states it is these dysfunctions that demand the attention of the nurse. Even though the patient is usually aware of the dysfunctional lifestyle, it is a pattern that she has grown used to and is generally resistant to change. She operates on the misconception that the pain must be eradicated before she can return to a state of health. It is only with the support of the therapeutic nurse-patient relationship that the patient can begin to risk changing despite the pain.

While keeping in mind the concept of the pain loop, the nursing plan of care must be designed to reduce the incoming points from both the body and the mind, to provide whole nursing care for an entirely ill individual. The expected outcome of such a plan is to assist the patient to achieve control over her situation so that she is able to maintain herself below the pain reaction threshold. A section will be devoted to nursing guidelines for intervention in each of these two areas.

In the physical realm is the concern of chemical dependency, although this also contributes points from the brain. Many nurses are blatantly angry about having to give narcotics to addicted patients, yet many also feel hesitant to bring these concerns to the attention of the physicians who are responsible for that delegation. It is indeed the nurse's professional responsibility to bring her opinions about possible addiction to the attention of the physician, for the nurse is in a position to have more information on patient status because more time is spent in patient contact. If the physician chooses not to withdraw narcotics from the patient, the nurse still has the right to refuse to give that medication if he or she believes it is detrimental to the patient. It may be an inconvenience or an increased risk to one's reputation, but it is imperative to be assertive with professional convictions. For the nurse who is willing to give narcotic medications there is always the problem of the patient requesting medication before it can be given. This can be frustrating to a busy nurse and create irritation toward the patient. One way to alleviate this situation, as well as foster independence and responsibility in the patient, is to provide her with a pen, a blank medication record, and a clock. A contract is then arranged between the nurse and the patient. The patient is to keep track of her medication intake for her own record and not request medication until it can be given, and the nurse will follow through with prompt and unquestioning administration of the drug. This kind of contract can avoid the power struggles that often exist between the nurse and the patient over the administration of pain medication. Such a record can also be a way of making the patient more aware of her chemical intake and possible dependency.

If the doctor is agreeable to a withdrawal from narcotics, this record can be used by the patient to assist in setting up the withdrawal schedule, for surely the patient should be consulted so as to provide her with a sense of control and motivation. The first step in setting up a withdrawal schedule is to establish a fixed rather than PRN routine of medication intake. A fixed intake refers to setting up regular times for giving the medication, regardless of whether the patient requests it. This avoids the learning situation described earlier in which taking pain medication in response to pain positively reinforces the pain. The next step is to eliminate one time of administration

per day so that, if a patient is taking a certain pain medication 10 times per day, she will be withdrawn in 10 days. The use of major tranquilizers and antidepressants as an adjunct to withdrawal is often appropriate to assist with relaxation. At no time should placebos be used, for they are dishonest and rob the patient of integrity and independence. Remember that chemical dependency is a disease of delusion, and intervention is highly frustrating, for both the patient and the health care professional. But until the patient is able to function with a mind and body free of narcotics she will be unable to take the remaining steps toward overcoming the disability of her pain.

Another aspect of the physical component of the disability is the deteriorated condition of the muscles in the affected part, as well as overall lowered resistance. Depending, of course, on the privileges of the patient, the nurse should encourage the patient to be as active as possible. Activity should be prescribed according to a work-to-quota program as opposed to the work-to-tolerance program mentioned earlier. In a work-to-quota program the baseline activity level of the patient is assessed, and daily goals of improvement in all areas are set up. The patient then is expected to achieve these daily goals regardless of her pain level. In this way, rest is a positive reinforcer to activity, and pain is not a meaningful variable. In addition to strengthening atrophied muscles and improving general stamina, a program of progressive muscle relaxation and deep breathing can be taught to the patient. Exercising tight, spastic muscles can be destructive, and such a relaxation program can potentiate the effects of increased activity. Also, this relaxation helps to reduce the points of tension coming from the brain.

The therapeutic use of touch, heat, and cold should also be considered in this category of intervention. Stimulation of the beta, or touch, fibers will affect the gate's reception of the pain impulses and possibly reduce the points from the body, so that the gate will close below the pain reaction threshold. Frequent touching of the patient and use of cold packs, ice applications, heating pads, and warm showers and baths are possible alternatives.

At the other end of the spectrum is the challenge of reducing points reaching the gate from the mind. One needn't be a certified psychoanalyst to intervene here; as mentioned earlier, the most important prerequisite is a trusting therapeutic relationship with the patient. One common roadblock to the establishment of this relationship is frequent complaining of pain by the patient. To many nurses this behavior is irritating and lends to their feeling of inadequacy. Patients usually operate on the assumption that nurses need to know every aspect of their pain, and they have grown used to communication with others through their pain. One way to alleviate this confusion is again by the use of a contract. The nurse should explain that because the situation is chronic, there is no reason for the patient to continually refer to the pain and that the nurse is aware of and believes in its presence but is unable to do anything directly to make it go away. The nurse should indicate an interest in knowing more about the patient as a person. This is likely to be a new and threatening idea to the patient; so she is likely to continue with the pattern she is used to—relating through pain. When this happens the nurse should state that he or she will leave the room because the patient is talking about pain but will return in 15 minutes or whatever time period is convenient. It is important that the nurse be warm but firm in this respect so that the patient knows that she is not being personally rejected but that this pain behavior is unacceptable. It is also important to return to the patient after the time period stated. Remaining consistent with this approach will lead the patient to believe that she is of value as a person, not just as a pain patient, and will add considerably to her self-worth. In time, with consistency and support, the pain-legitimating behavior of complaining should cease.

One topic of great concern to nursing is assessment, and this is valid, for without assessment, formulation of a plan of care becomes an impossibility. But without the open honesty and trust of a therapeutic nurse-patient relationship the assessment will most likely be incomplete and heavily focused on physical detail, which is the safest and most familiar material for the patient to reveal. Once the relationship is begun, the nurse should also explore the areas of social and recreational activities, family functioning, vocation, finances, emotional status, spirituality, self-image, plans for the future, and sexuality. One framework for this type of assessment is to ask the patient what has changed in each of these areas in her life from premorbid status to present. This outlining of change will give the nurse a clue as to the areas needing special focus so that an individualized plan of care can be created. The importance of using the other members of the health care team cannot be understated. Occupational therapy, recreational therapy, physical therapy, social work, psychology, chaplaincy, vocational rehabilitation, and chemical dependency consultation should be readily available.

Finally, we approach the most crucial aspect of the nursing plan of care: facilitation of coping and acceptance. The structure most adaptable to this task is the grief process outlined by Kübler-Ross.[4] Indeed, with chronic pain, the patient undergoes a multitude of changes in all areas of her life. Concomitant with change is loss. The patient with chronic pain must deal with the grief of her many losses if she is to learn to accept and cope with the pain. But, unlike the patient with terminal illness, there is no resolution with death. Meaning must be defined for life, not death. The patient with chronic pain is faced with new losses every day, loss of opportunity, loss of chance, and loss of freedom of becoming. Because of this, the chronic pain patient never reaches an ultimate and final acceptance. The stages of denial, depression, anger, bargaining, and acceptance resurface continually throughout this person's life. It is the task of nurses to educate persons in pain with everything they know about the disease. Cognitive clarity is one positive step toward resolution of any dilemma. Nurses must inform these patients of the signs and symptoms of depression, anger, fear, anxiety, dependency, and denial so that they can learn to recognize these feelings and behaviors in themselves. Beyond this, nurses must teach patients how to resolve these states, how to deal with them, and how to move ever forward to acceptance. There is no single correct way to do this, but reference to psychiatric nursing texts can offer specific guidelines for specific behavioral patterns. As the patient gains skill in this area, the stages of acceptance can become longer in duration and be achieved more quickly.

When a patient reaches acceptance, she knows the reality of her situation. This does not mean she has given up. On the contrary, acceptance requires hard work for its maintenance. Acceptance implies a meaningful, productive lifestyle within the reality of the patient's context. Acceptance does not necessarily show itself through undaunted joy but rather through a sense of security in knowing one's past and present and having faith in one's ability to deal with the future. Disability is ultimately only a state of mind.

Nursing care can be the most effective treatment modality for the woman suffering from chronic pain if the focus remains on the woman as a person.

References

1. McGaffery, Margo. *Nursing Management of the Patient with Pain*. Philadelphia: J. B. Lippincott, 1972, p. 8.
2. Beecher, H. The subjective response and reaction to sensation. *American Journal of Medicine*, vol. 10, 1956, p. 107; The psychological and cultural influences on the reaction to pain. *Nursing Forum*, vol. 7, 1968, p. 262.
3. Melzack, R., and Wall, P. Pain mechanisms: A new theory. *Science*, vol. 150, 1965, p. 971.
4. Kübler-Ross, Elisabeth. *On Death and Dying*. New York: Macmillan, 1972.

Selected Readings

J. Blaylock. The psychological and cultural influrences on the reaction to pain. *Nursing Forum*, vol. 7, 1968, p 262.
K. Casey. The neurophysiological basis of pain. *Postgraduate Medicine,* vol. 53, May, 1965, p. 58.
R. Sternbach. *Pain: A Psychophysiological Analysis*. New York: Academic, 1968.
R. Sternbach. *Pain Patients: Traits and Treatment*. New York: Academic, 1968.
M. Zborowski. *People in Pain*. San Francisco: Jossey-Baas, Inc., 1969.

IV

LOSS

This section deals with the experience and effects of loss on women, beginning with a chapter on the potential health crisis of hysterectomy, and continuing with the losses generated by menopause, divorce, depression, and widowhood, and concluding with the tragic loss of a child.

19

THE POTENTIAL HEALTH CARE CRISIS OF HYSTERECTOMY

KAREN FINCK

Karen Finck's chapter on the hysterectomy experience includes the rationale for surgery and its effects. This is followed by a detailed presentation of nursing interventions, including both affective aspects and object relations.

There has always been a consistent pattern of change in the functioning of the female reproductive system. The uterus is the center of the changing process in which the biologic functions of the body are manifested. The actualization of the biologic functions of the female body begins at puberty with the onset of menstruation. For some women the biologic functions are realized with the birth of a child. In the lives of other women, physiology, situation, or choice intercedes and the realization does not occur. When the potential childbearing years end, the biologic functions of the female body terminate in the natural process of menopause.

In recent years this pattern of consistent change has gained the possibility of alteration. With the advancement of medical technology, two surgical procedures that cause the termination of the biologic functions of the female body have been developed and perfected to the extent of increasingly widespread usage. These procedures, hysterectomy and tubal ligation, alter the pattern in such a way that the termination of the childbearing functions no longer necessarily coincides with the natural process of menopause.

Alteration in the pattern of biologic functioning does not in itself constitute a health care crisis. As the surgical procedures themselves are examined, it becomes apparent that one procedure has far-reaching consequences

and contains a strong possibility of constituting a health care crisis for women. The other procedure involves a much higher rate of successful adaptation, with generally only very minimal psychologic disturbance.

Tubal ligation is a surgical procedure specifically executed for the purpose of terminating the childbearing capacity of a woman. It is well designed, creating only minor alteration in the anatomic structure of the female body and causing only negligible effects on the processes of menstruation and menopause. The decision to perform tubal ligation is based solely on the desire of the woman to alter her pattern of reproductive functioning so that the termination of her childbearing capacity occurs before the onset of menopause. The combination of these factors promotes a response to tubal ligation that is generally very satisfactory and rarely constitutes a health care crisis.

Conversely, hysterectomy is not designed and executed solely for the purpose of terminating the childbearing capacity of a woman. Reasons for the performance of this surgery are varied, and resultant changes in the female anatomic structure are more pronounced. Unlike tubal ligation, hysterectomy involves not only alteration in the pattern of biologic functioning but also removal of an organ from the female body and the concurrent termination of the functions of that organ. Thus, physiologic and psychologic effects of hysterectomy are more extensive and provide for wide variations in women's response to the procedure. These variations in response coupled with the incidence of and reasons for performance of the procedure give credence to the view of the hysterectomy experience as a potential health care crisis and provide broad implications in the nursing management of this crisis.

Before examining the components of the hysterectomy experience, it is necessary to clarify terminology and discuss the incidence of the surgery.

TERMINOLOGY OF THE SURGICAL PROCEDURE

The term "hysterectomy" indicates the surgical removal of the uterus. In previous years, only the body of the uterus was removed. This was referred to as a partial or subtotal hysterectomy. More commonly performed at present is a total hysterectomy involving removal of the entire uterus. A radical hysterectomy is the removal of the entire uterus plus lymph nodes and surrounding ligaments.[1]

There are two surgical methods used to remove the uterus. In an abdominal hysterectomy a 4- to 6-inch incision is made in the lower abdomen through which the uterus is removed. In a vaginal hysterectomy, the uterus is removed through the vagina, and there is no visible scar. This is generally the method of choice when uterine prolapse, cystoceles, or rectoceles are present.[2]

Although a hysterectomy does not include the removal of the adnexa, in certain conditions these are removed at the same time. This often causes confusion in the terminology for the lay population. In some literature, removal of the uterus and the ovaries is referred to as a panhysterectomy or complete hysterectomy. This is often confused with total hysterectomy, which does not involve removal of the adnexa. This is more readily understood when the adnexa to be removed are specified. Thus, removal of the ovaries is referred to as a bilateral oophorectomy, and removal of the fallopian tubes is known as a salpingectomy. Therefore, a woman who has had her entire uterus, fallopian tubes, and ovaries removed abdominally is referred to as having had a total abdominal hysterectomy and bilateral salpino-oophorectomy.

There also appears to be another frame of reference for the terminology of hysterectomy. Although it does not appear to be in widespread usage, there is no doubt of its existence.

Some medical professionals have referred to hysterectomy as "having the works out" or have told women that "they were rotten inside" or that it was "no good having your tubes tied; your womb would only go bad like a dead tooth without a nerve and you would have to have it out later."[3] I was told by a young woman that her physician referred to her impending hysterectomy as "taking that old gray bag out." She tearfully stated that this statement made her feel "like an old cow." Another woman reported that her gynecologist stated, "We are taking out the cradle, but we are leaving in the playpen." Further indication of the trauma that this terminology can cause is exemplified in the case of a woman who was told by her physician that she was "all cleaned out" after her hysterectomy because she had been "in a terrible mess and all rotten inside." The woman never felt "clean" again and developed a compulsive need to constantly discuss the surgery.[4] It is clear that this type of terminology is dehumanizing, sexist, and detrimental to the health care recipient and therefore should not be tolerated.

Later, as we investigate the real and imagined effects of changes in female anatomy after hysterectomy on various aspects of women's lives, it will become even more apparent why correct use of terminology is essential.

INCIDENCE OF PERFORMANCE OF HYSTERECTOMY

The surgical removal of the uterus has recently become the most commonly performed major surgery in the United States. There was a 25 per cent increase in the number of hysterectomies performed in the United States from 1970 to 1975.[5] It is reported that the trend to perform hysterectomies is increasing. Statistics indicate that in 1975 there were 725,000 hysterectomies performed in this country compared with 658,000 tonsillectomies, the previously most commonly performed major surgery. By 1978, the number dropped to 644,000.[5a] It is estimated that almost half of all American women over the age of 40 will be advised to have a hysterectomy.[6]

These statistics indicate that alteration in the biologic functioning of the female body by hysterectomy is not only a possibility but, for a vast number of women, also a reality.

THEORETICAL FRAMEWORK

The basis for the woman's response to the hysterectomy experience is determined by the

HYSTERECTOMY

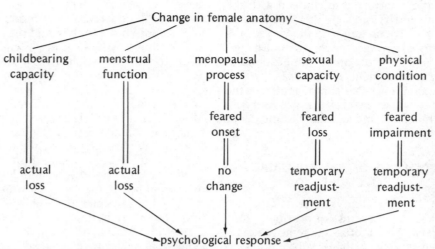

Figure 19.1. Theoretical framework for the relationships among variables and the areas related to hysterectomy.

woman's concept of her uterine anatomy and physiology. The formulation of this concept includes the woman's knowledge about the actual functions of her uterus and her personal perceptions of uterine anatomy and physiology which are derived from her individual developmental experiences.[7] Realistic and imaginary functions attributed to the uterus intermingle to produce a psychologic response to hysterectomy that is unique to every woman.

However, the literature on hysterectomy reveals frequently held perceptions of various functions attributed to the uterus. These perceptions can be categorized into the related areas of childbearing capacity, menstrual functioning, menopausal process, sexual capacity, and physical condition. Identification of the effects of hysterectomy on each area will assist in delineating the areas in which actual loss is incurred, the areas that involve feared loss or change, and the areas that require temporary readjustment. The complex network of relationships among the variables can then be explored and comprehended. The categorization of the areas and the comprehension of the relationships among the variables are key factors that enable a theoretical framework to be devised. This theoretical framework will afford a more comprehensive view of the hysterectomy experience. The structure of the theoretical framework is conceptualized in Figure 19.1.

The theoretical framework can be used to identify areas in which nursing interventions can be made. The focus of nursing intervention

in each area can be derived from the description of the potential hysterectomy crisis along pertinent ego-function parameters. These parameters include affective aspects, defensive aspects, cognitive aspects, reality aspects, and object relations.[8] The three parameters of cognitive aspects, affective aspects, and object relations can be used as the focus of nursing interventions. A description of nursing interventions focused on the three ego-function parameters will enable the nurse to identify nursing interventions in each area and then to individualize the interventions to meet the needs of specific health care recipients.

Nursing Interventions Focusing on Cognitive Aspects

Nursing intervention in this area consists primarily of providing information to health care recipients. This education is provided by the hospital nursing staff to facilitate recovery at home after discharge.[8a] Patient teaching has long been recognized as a nursing responsibility.

The research of Johnson and colleagues[9] has revealed the significance of providing information to health care recipients.

These investigators demonstrated in a study that presenting knowledge to patients affects the patients' responses to a given procedure. Patients who were given knowledge about either the technical detail of the procedure or the sensations patients frequently experience during the procedure required less sedation than control patients.[9] Johnson states in further research that "preparatory information may reduce emotional response to procedures which are an unavoidable part of health care, for example, diagnostic examinations, injections, dental procedures, and surgery."[10]

Researchers working in the area of hysterectomy seem to concur with this concept. They suggest that presenting information to a woman undergoing hysterectomy can affect her psychologic response to the procedure by reducing the reactions of anxiety, fright, and shock. When concealed anxieties can be brought into the woman's awareness through discussion of the implications of hysterectomy, the postoperative psychiatric complications may be lessened.[11] An explanation of the procedure to be performed can help to prevent fright neurosis, which is often a major factor in the response to hysterectomy.[12] Psychologic shock followed by feelings of deprivation and resentment, which occurs in many women after they are told they need a hysterectomy, can be alleviated if information regarding the reasons for the effects of the procedure is provided.[13]

Research reveals to us the importance women who have had hysterectomies place on information. When information is provided, most women find it very helpful and, when information is not given, many women feel it to be a definitely unmet need.[14]

Although it is clear that education in this area is of primary importance, it is equally clear when reviewing literature on hysterectomy that education is often not provided. In an attempt to discover what knowledge women possess about the reasons for and effects of hysterectomy, I examined hysterectomy literature for reported misconceptions and devised a test that measured selected knowledge women had about hysterectomy. The results of this study (referred to as the "Hysterectomy Knowledge Study") are discussed wherever applicable in this chapter. It will provide the nurse with baseline information on what a specific group of women knows about hysterectomy.

Since it deals only with a specific group of women, population characteristics must be discussed. There were 186 women who participated in the study. The age range was equally distributed (except for a smaller percentage of women under 25 and over 65 years old). Most women in the study were white (98 per cent) and either Protestant (58 per cent) or Catholic (31 per cent). They were usually married (91 per cent), with children (88 per cent). Almost all of the women had completed high school (95 per cent), and over half of the women either attended or completed college. About one half of the women were employed. Twenty per cent had had a hysterectomy.

The reader must be cautioned that, although the "Hysterectomy Knowledge Study" will provide useful information about one group of women, this must not be generalized to all women. Williams has demonstrated that there is a strong indication of cultural patterning of the feminine role.[15] This implies that different cultural groups of women possess different knowledge in the area of hysterectomy, as do women of different educational backgrounds. Therefore, the information presented from the "Hysterectomy Knowledge Study" will provide only general guidelines for assessing the knowledge individual women possess about hysterectomy.

Nursing Interventions Focusing on Affective Aspects

Nursing interventions in this area concentrate on accepting, understanding, and providing support for expression of feelings women experience as related to hysterectomy.

Raphael, in a study investigating the perception of the crisis of hysterectomy, found that over half of the study sample perceived the opportunity to discuss their feelings about the surgery as being helpful. None of the women felt that the opportunity to express their feelings was unhelpful. One third of the women who did not have the opportunity to express their feelings felt that this was an unmet need.[16] Thus it is extremely important in terms of quality health care for women to be afforded the opportunity to express their feelings about hysterectomy.

In order for this to be accomplished in an atmosphere of acceptance, it is necessary for the nurse to comprehend the possible implications of loss of the uterus. If the woman views this loss as significant, the nurse must be prepared to support and encourage expression of the grieving process. As the woman begins a redefinition of her role as a female, the nurse can facilitate the examination of role and identity and provide support and encouragement. With an overall goal of using the individual's strengths to promote healthy long-term adaptation to hysterectomy rather than of elimination of psychologic pain, the nurse can help the woman to view this time in her life as a redefinition of her role as a woman, similar to that which occurs during menopause.

Nursing Interventions Focusing on Object Relations

Object relations will be confined to those significant persons on whom the health care recipient is emotionally dependent. Nursing interventions will be limited to involvement with those significant persons who can help provide psychologic support for the expression of needs by the health care recipient. The focus of interventions in object relations will be on the motivation of significant persons to be accepting and supportive of expression of feelings by the woman as she undergoes the experience of hysterectomy. The nurse can help to motivate significant persons by encouraging direct communication, giving them information, and accepting the direct expression of their needs and feelings.

A woman tends to develop a diffuse body image and self-concept, which are linked, through dependency, to her evaluation by others. A woman's self-esteem is dependent largely on the expressed feelings of acceptance and appreciation from others.[17] Therefore, as a woman faces hysterectomy, which may be perceived as a threat to her self-esteem, body image, and identity, her needs for acceptance and reassurance of love by significant persons increase greatly. Psychologic adjustment to hysterectomy is eased when the response from the woman's environment is not unduly negative.[18] Conversely, rejection by significant others often precipitates posthysterectomy depression.[19] The value of nursing interventions focusing on object relations is further emphasized by a study in which women viewed relationships that encouraged expression of their feelings about hysterectomy as helpful. When these relationships did not exist, women felt this to be an unmet need, an area in which their social network failed them.[20]

INDICATIONS FOR HYSTERECTOMY

Physical Conditions

Benign Uterine Disease. Fibromyomata (commonly referred to as fibroids) constitute the most frequent indication for hysterectomy. Fibroids are benign tumors of the uterus. They are generally slow in growth and painless except when pressure is applied. The presence of fibroids in the uterus is common, occurring in 40 per cent of all women over 40 years of age.[21] Often fibroids are asymptomatic and require no treatment. If symptoms appear and are not severe, treatment may be deferred until after menopause, at which point fibroid tumors tend to regress in size naturally, thus possibly eliminating the need for treatment.

Sarcomatous degeneration of fibroids is rare, malignant change being found in only 0.1 to 0.5 per cent of patients operated on for fibromyomata. When symptoms of abnormal uterine bleeding, pelvic pressure, pressure on contiguous organs, and/or abdominal distention occur, treatment may be necessary. Treatment involves myomectomy (removal of the tumors) or hysterectomy.[22]

Adenomyosis is a condition involving enlargement of the uterus caused by the invasion of the myometrium by the endometrium. Symptoms are acquired dysmenorrhea and menorrhagia. If curettage fails to eliminate the symptoms and if the woman's childbearing needs are over, hysterectomy is recommended.[23]

Dysfunctional uterine bleeding of menopause is another frequent indication for hysterectomy. Often hysterectomy is chosen as the treatment of choice if there are concurrent changes in the endometrium. The alternative treatment of curettage alleviates the dysfunctional bleeding in 60 per cent of the cases the first time it is performed. Curettage performed for the second time alleviates 70 to 75 per cent of the dysfunctional bleeding until menopause supervenes.[24]

Malignant Uterine Disease. Twenty per cent of all hysterectomies are performed to alleviate malignancies of the cervix, the body of the uterus, or adjacent organs. The diagnosis is based on the results of the Pap smear, dilatation and curettage, or aspiration curettage.[25] Treatment for all types of cancer of the uterus is generally surgical removal of the uterus. In some instances, irradiation or chemical therapy is used conjunctively with surgery. The presence of precancerous lesions (cell changes that may indicate impending malignancy) may also necessitate hysterectomy.[26]

Removal of the Normal Uterus. There are other conditions that may necessitate the removal of the uterus, even if the uterus is not diseased. Established indicators for the removal of the normal uterus are as follows: the presence of ovarian, oviduct, and vaginal cancer; chronic pelvic inflammation; and genital prolapse.

Removal of the normal uterus involves much that is subjective and philosophical; thus, there are differences of opinion as to the necessity of this surgery. This is more clearly shown by the relative indicators for the removal of the normal uterus, which include mental retardation, ectopic pregnancy, familial history of cancer, pelvic pain, hydatidiform mole, postirradiation of the uterus, benign ovarian disease, pelvic tuberculosis, postpartum hemorrhage, and dysfunctional bleeding.[27]

Although sterilization has been considered a relative indicator for hysterectomy in the past, many physicians now believe that hysterectomy as an alternative to tubal sterilization is unacceptable.[27a] However, studies indicate that hysterectomy sterilizations are increasing in number.[27b]

Psychologic Conditions

The uterus is sometimes removed for the psychiatric conditions of phobias (especially cancerophobia) and hypochondriasis. Hysterectomy, in these cases, rarely removes the phobia or lessens hypochondriac thinking.[28]

On a more general basis, the relationship between the functioning of the female reproductive system and the emotions is close and complex. Psychologic factors may influence the development and course of gynecologic disease or symptoms.[29] Or the uterus may become the conversion focus for many psychoemotional ills of women.[30]

The concept that either the emotional status of a woman may precipitate the need for hysterectomy (owing to increased gynecologic symptoms) or a woman may displace emotional problems onto her reproductive functioning seems credible, although there have been few studies performed to substantiate this.

Unnecessary Hysterectomies

Research indicates that of all hysterectomies performed, from 32 per cent[31] to 39 per cent[32] may be unnecessary. These statistics include those cases in which less extensive alternative treatment could have been sufficient and the few cases in which hysterectomy was later determined to be contraindicated.

In general, all physical and psychologic conditions, with the exception of malignant disease, may lead to an unnecessary hysterectomy.

Nursing Interventions

Difficulty in understanding and accepting the need for surgery correlates strongly with poor outcome of hysterectomy.[33] This finding provides clear evidence of the importance of satisfactorily explaining the reasons for surgery.

The results of the "Hysterectomy Knowledge Study" indicate that 65 per cent of the women knew that the most frequent reason for removal of the uterus is the presence of fibroids. However, 19 per cent of the women believed that most hysterectomies are performed because the woman has cancer, and 16 per cent believed that most hysterectomies are performed unnecessarily.

If the woman believes that most hysterectomies are performed because cancer is present, she probably feels that there is a large possibility of cancer being present in her body. The fear of uterine cancer is experienced by many women,[34] and the fear becomes more pronounced as the woman gets older.[35] This fear of cancer has long been the pretext of proponents of performing hysterectomy for fibroids, by both physicians and patients alike.[36] The magnitude of this fear and the actual percentage of cancerous degeneration of fibroids do not correlate.

The variation in the magnitude of the fear of cancer compared with the rate of cancerous degeneration of fibroids and the percentage of hysterectomies performed for cancer may be a large factor in the woman's decision to have a hysterectomy, regardless of the preoperative diagnosis. The fear of cancer may be a component of preoperative distress. Fear of cancer may also increase the woman's need for reassurance postoperatively.

Recent magazine articles have brought into public awareness the occurrence of unnecessary hysterectomies.[37, 38] Women should be aware of their right to obtain a second medical opinion before deciding to have a hysterectomy. Increased efforts in public education may reduce the percentage of unnecessary hysterectomies and help women to make more educated health care decisions. Nursing involvement in public education can help to ensure that women are provided information in all areas of the issue.

There are reports in the literature of women who believe that the need for hysterectomy is directly caused by excessive sexual activity.[39, 40] There are also reports that hysterectomy is viewed by some women as a punishment for real or imagined "sins," generally sexual in nature (including sexual promiscuity, sexual enjoyment, masturbation, and abortion).[41-43] If these are a woman's perceptions, it is imperative that the beliefs of her sexual partner be assessed to ascertain whether he supports these perceptions. The couple should then be provided with a clear explanation of reproductive functioning and referred for therapy if necessary.

A complete history should be taken from all women before a decision to perform hysterectomy is made. (This is especially necessary for the woman who presents vague, ill-defined complaints.) The history should include physical and emotional components, and present stress-related problems should be explored.[44] If the woman is currently experiencing many stress-related situations, perhaps elective hysterectomy should be postponed. If the stress is severe, psychotherapy may be more appropriate than hysterectomy.

If the woman exhibits an obvious psychiatric disorder, consultation with a psychiatrist or therapist before surgery is recommended. If the hysterectomy is elective, it may be decided against.[45] If the hysterectomy is not elective, the therapist may help the nurse or physician or both to anticipate postoperative problems more accurately.

More nursing research is needed to identify how psychologic stress is related to the functioning of the female reproductive system. Increased research in this area could help to ensure that women are not treated surgically for psychologic problems.

CHANGES IN ANATOMY PRODUCED BY HYSTERECTOMY

The uterus is a hollow, thick-walled, muscular organ shaped somewhat like a pear. In a mature woman, its size at the top measures approximately 2.5 by 2 inches. It narrows to a diameter of about 1 inch at the cervix and is about 3 inches long. The functions of the uterus are those of childbearing and menstruation.[46] Each month the uterine walls become thickened with a lining of blood. If conception has occurred, the uterus will become the nurturing place of growth for the fetus.

Hysterectomy removes this organ, thus eliminating its functions. When the uterus is removed from the body, fluid and the slight readjustment of other organs displace the resultant gap. The ligaments that held the uterus in place are attached to the vaginal walls.[47] Thus, with the exception of the absence of the uterus, the interior anatomic structure after hysterectomy appears similar to that before hysterectomy. The external anatomic structure appears exactly the same pre- and postsurgically, with the exception of the presence of an abdominal scar if the abdominal surgical technique is used.

The two ovaries are almond shaped and measure about 1.25 inches long. Ovaries are connected to the lateral border of the uterus by the ovarian ligament.[48] The functions of the ovaries are the monthly release of ova (eggs) and the production of hormones.[49]

Removal of the uterus may cause a temporary hormonal imbalance. However, the ovaries continue to function and will continue to function normally until the onset of menopause.[50, 51]

If an oophorectomy is performed concurrently with hysterectomy, the ovaries are removed and their functions are terminated. Especially if the woman is young, hormonal replacement therapy may be indicated to prevent the onset of surgical menopause.[52]

Nursing Interventions

Many women are ignorant about the anatomy of their sexual and reproductive organs.[53] The functions of the uterus and ovaries are very often confusing to women. When they are asked to identify these functions, general answers like babies, sex, hormones, and regulating are offered.[54] The "Hysterectomy Knowledge Study" results indicate the level of this confusion. Women's responses, when asked to select the functions of the uterus and ovaries, are shown in Table 19.1.

Only 38 per cent of the women answered the question of the functions of the uterus totally correctly, selecting both menstrual and childbearing functions, and only 37 per cent of the women indicated that both the release of eggs and production of hormones were the correct responses to the question of ovarian functioning. Thus, it seems well established that more education is needed in the area of the female reproductive system.

As the changes in anatomy after hysterec-

Table 19.1. **Women's Responses in "Hysterectomy Knowledge Study"**

Functions of Uterus	Functions of Ovaries
Holds menstrual blood, 49%	Hold menstrual blood, 6%
Place where sexual intercourse occurs, 3%	Produce hormones, 54%
Produces hormones, 8%	Release eggs, 92%
Place where a baby grows, 97%	Control a woman's sex drive, 9%
Controls a woman's sex drive, 1%	Place where sexual intercourse occurs, 1%

tomy are explored it is discovered that "women's understanding about what actually happens when they have a hysterectomy is extremely variable and rarely adequate in terms of the degree of understanding they would like to have about what is being done to their bodies."[55] Women often have only a crude understanding of what the surgeon has done to their anatomy,[56] knowing only that their "womb" has been removed.[57] Often women do not even know whether they have had an oophorectomy along with the hysterectomy.[58]

Reports in the literature indicate that some women think they have a hole inside after the uterus is removed.[59] One fourth of the women in the "Hysterectomy Knowledge Study" thought there would be an empty space where the uterus had originally been. This is an important concept to correct, because it leads to speculation and concern by women who wonder if things will pass through the hole or whether something was left behind in surgery to fill the hole.[60]

Women are also confused about the functioning of their ovaries after hysterectomy. Of the women in the "Hysterectomy Knowledge Study," 56 per cent knew the ovaries would continue to function, 14 per cent thought ovaries functioned at a reduced rate, and 30 per cent thought the ovaries no longer functioned at all after hysterectomy.

Obviously, patient education will eliminate many of these misconceptions. Nursing intervention appears to be simple and concise in this area. However, there are factors that complicate the transfer of information from the nurse to the patient. Unformulated personal beliefs about anatomy and physiology of reproductive organs may come into awareness only when the organs are diseased.[61] As one woman stated, "You just don't think about things like your womanly organs until they give you trouble."[62] When the woman is faced with surgery she may have an emotional response that is limiting her awareness. Thus, it may not occur to her to ask questions. Other women may be so confused about the functions of their organs that they have difficulty formulating questions. Some women don't want to show a lack of knowledge or be embarrassed, so they don't ask questions.[63] Other women are not given the opportunity to ask questions.[64]

In providing quality patient care, a nurse cannot afford to wait for the woman to ask questions. The woman may never ask them,

or she may ask these questions of people who cannot provide the correct answers.[65]

EFFECTS OF HYSTERECTOMY ON CHILDBEARING CAPACITY

Hysterectomy affects a woman with total and irreversible loss of childbearing capacity. This loss of the biologic functions of a woman's body is reported by many authors to be of great significance in the emotional response to the surgery.[66-69]

Removal of the uterus and the resultant loss of the ability to bear children have potential psychologic consequences for all women.[70] This can be understood only when there is clear differentiation between the ability to bear children and the desire for children. Ability to bear children is the crucial factor, not desire to bear children or desire to bear more children. This concept is evidenced by the findings that wanting more children versus not wanting more children does not correlate with outcome of hysterectomy,[71] nor does having children versus not having children.[72]

The ability to bear children serves a wide variety of needs and functions in the life of a woman. This ability is of significance in the self-image of a woman.[73] The multifaceted relationship between the ability to bear children and the self-image of a woman can be defined in various ways. For many women "the biologic ability to reproduce is intimately connected with the adjustment of women as a feminine figure."[74] For some women childbearing provides a sense of achievement and fulfillment[75] or sense of completeness.[76] For other women it represents a sense of power, with resultant loss of the ability to bear children representing an extreme form of powerlessness.[77]

In the literature, women have defined their sense of self in relation to their ability to have children. Some state that having children is expected of them[78] and is therefore their duty. Other women have defined this in terms of being useful[79] or being a proper woman,[80] and yet others have defined the ability to have children as the reason for their existence on earth[81] and even as their total identification as a woman.[82]

The degree to which a woman defines her sense of self in terms of the biologic functions of her body seems to be a crucial factor in the extent of her sense of loss over the cessation of childbearing capacity after hysterectomy. This is probably related in some degree to cultural patterning of the feminine role[83] and the trends of society in general.

In viewing the extensive connections between the self-image of a woman and the ability to bear children, the sense of loss that occurs with the removal of the uterus can be comprehended. However, some women do not appear to experience an extensive sense of loss and perhaps even feel no sense of loss. Many women feel indifferent or delighted about their resultant sterility after hysterectomy,[84] and the relief from fear of pregnancy may be a major factor in the good outcome after hysterectomy for some women.[85] Still other women have hysterectomies for the sole purpose of sterilization. Thus, the response to the loss of childbearing capacity ranges from devastation to delight.

Nursing Interventions

There are isolated reports in the literature that indicate that some women do not know that hysterectomy causes cessation of the childbearing capacity.[86, 87] In the "Hysterectomy Knowledge Study" almost 4 per cent of the women did not correctly answer the question regarding ability to give birth after hysterectomy. Thus, it cannot be assumed that women know that after a hysterectomy they can no longer give birth to a child.

Comprehension of the meaning of losing the ability to bear children occurs readily when the women is young, married, and desires to have children. The young woman's sense of loss is easily accepted and even expected by her family, friends, and medical personnel. Although the response of a premenopausal woman with fewer than two children has been found to be more severe in all gynecologic surgery,[88] this does not mean that other women who are not in positions or do not desire to have children will not experience loss. Unless there is a conscious awareness by the nurse that the issue is the ability to bear children (not the feasibility of bearing children), the loss of the unmarried woman, the woman who by choice does not desire children, and the homosexual woman will not be understood.

The inability to differentiate between the ability to have children and the desire to have children may be a factor in the reports of women who express concern and anger that they were not prepared for the sense of loss they felt at the termination of their childbearing capacities after hysterectomy.[89] The "Hysterectomy Knowledge Study" results tend to confirm that women are not aware that the ability to bear children is the crucial issue. Although only 8 per cent of the women did not believe that being able to have children is an important part of the way women see themselves, 14 per cent believed that, if a woman has all the children she wants, a hysterectomy will have no emotional effect on her. Eleven per cent of the women believed that, if a woman is unmarried and does not want children, a hysterectomy will have no emotional effect on her; and 30 per cent believed that a hysterectomy performed after a woman has gone through menopause will have no emotional effect on her. It can be seen from these data why women are not prepared for the sense of loss.

Even though it would seem likely that the menopausal woman would not be subjected to psychologic stress from loss of her childbearing capacity, this is not necessarily the case. Menopause occurs during the climacteric and the climacteric is a time when old doubts and insecurities may emerge, because it is a time of change in a woman's life. Thus, increased psychologic stress may occur from a hysterectomy performed at this time.[90] The menopausal process involves the cessation of the ability to bear children, and this carries with it the process of psychologic readjustment. When the resolution of psychologic components of the climacteric is incomplete, it can be speculated that even the postmenopausal woman may become subject to emotional stress owing to re-emergence of the sense of loss of her childbearing capacity. It can also be speculated that at the age of menopause, if the women has had children, the children are generally adults. If the children have not fulfilled the mother's expectations by this point, the woman may see herself as having failed in her role of mothering. Menopause and hysterectomy are obvious indications that the woman will have no further chances to re-establish herself in a mothering role. She may express this in excessive concern about her children or in bitterness about the way they "turned out."

Women can be encouraged to verbalize their feelings about the significance of their ability to bear children. Older women, women with many children, or women in situations that are not conducive to childbearing may be embarrassed to discuss their feelings about childbearing ability. The nurse can help to minimize embarrassment by helping the woman to talk about the basis for her identity. Whether the woman sees herself as primarily a caregiver, a wife, a professional, and so forth, the nurse can offer support and help the woman to realistically explore changes that hysterectomy may bring to her life. If the loss is felt to be significant to the woman, the nurse, by accepting the woman's expression of feelings, will be assisting her to complete the grieving process.

If the woman wants to be sterilized, this can also be supported by the nurse. However, the performance of hysterectomy solely for sterilization purposes generally should not be supported by the nurse. Tubal ligation is a much more appropriate procedure for sterilization. Standard morbidity of hysterectomy ranges from 42 to 45 per cent. Morbidity of tubal ligations ranges from 1.5 to 20 per cent.[91] Thus, physical distress from hysterectomy is much greater, as is psychologic distress. Tubal ligation has a much higher rate of positive long-term response than does hysterectomy.[92]

Hysterectomies for sterilization purposes only are being labeled more often as unnecessary hysterectomies because of the increased risks of psychologic and physical morbidity compared with the less-extensive procedure of tubal ligations. One reason for the performance of hysterectomy for sterilization purposes may be that women do not know of the greater risks hysterectomy entails. The results of the "Hysterectomy Knowledge Study" indicate that almost 30 per cent of the women thought that women have the same emotional response to hysterectomy as they do to tubal ligation. Almost half of the women thought that hysterectomies are as medically safe as tubal ligations. These findings indicate that increased efforts should be made in the area of public education.

EFFECTS OF HYSTERECTOMY ON MENSTRUAL FUNCTION

Hysterectomy causes the complete cessation of menstruation. Hormones continue to maintain their cyclic pattern, but the accompanying menstrual bleeding no longer occurs. Thus, a hysterectomy will alleviate dysfunctional bleeding, for example, but will not alleviate symptoms associated with menstruation, such as tension, headaches, water retention, and irritability.[93]

To understand the potential sense of loss experienced by the woman with the cessation of menstruation, it is necessary to examine how the woman views the experience of menstruation and to identify what functions she attributes to the process of menstruation.

Drellich and Bieber report that the majority of women have positive feelings toward the menstrual function and that many women feel a loss of this valued process when menstrual function is terminated. However, they also report frequent negative attitudes expressed by many women toward the symptoms that accompany menstruation.[94] Thus, it appears that, in order to recognize positive feelings about menstruation, menstruation must be distinguished from the often distressful symptoms that accompany it. The inability to differentiate between the symptoms and the process of menstruation could provide an explanation of the variation in the findings of Drellich and Bieber (in which women viewed the loss of menstruation with sadness) and those of another researcher, who found the vast majority of his study sample to be pleased or unconcerned about the loss of menstrual function after hysterectomy.[95]

The functions women attribute to menstruation also give an indication of their responses to the loss of this process. Some women appear to view menstruation as a cleaning or excretory function. These women seem to associate their menstrual blood with their body wastes. They consider menstruation to be a healthy process that removes "bad blood" or "noxious waste" from the body. Loss of menstrual function causes them to become concerned about what will happen to them if they don't get rid of the waste.[96, 97]

Other women view menstruation as a regulatory function. For these women monthly periods provide a predictability to their daily living and serve to regulate their activities. This "rhythm of life" provides a pattern, and some women attribute variations in emotion, strength, and vitality to this pattern.[98]

Menstruation is the outward manifestation of the ability to bear children.[99] With each monthly bleeding comes the reminder that the uterus is capable of nurturing life. When menstruation ceases, the woman is faced with evidence that she can no longer bear children. This in turn accentuates an inability that may be vital to the woman's identity.

Nursing Interventions

There are reports in the literature that indicate that not all women know that a hysterectomy causes cessation of menstruation.[100] Thus, a nurse cannot assume that the woman who has had a hysterectomy knows she will no longer menstruate. This is further evidenced by the "Hysterectomy Knowledge Study," in which over 5 per cent of the participants believed that after hysterectomy the menstrual period either did not stop but became irregular, or continued to occur as it did before the hysterectomy.

Twenty-two per cent of the participants in the "Hysterectomy Knowledge Study" believed that hysterectomies would cure premenstrual tension. By increased involvement of nurses in public education programs regarding hysterectomy, the number of hysterectomies performed to alleviate premenstrual tension can be reduced and women who expect that premenstrual tension will disappear with hysterectomy can be spared distress and disappointment.

In responding to a woman who has lost the ability to menstruate, the nurse must remember that feelings about menstruation are dependent on many factors, such as symptoms accompanying menstruation, what the woman believes to be the functions of menstruation, the woman's adolescent experiences involving the onset of menstruation, and cultural attitudes about menstruation. Menstruation is often an emotionally laden process. Some women refer to menstruation as "the curse," and many women feel this terminology is accurate. Other women have positive feelings about this female function and view its termination as a loss. In order to provide an attitude of acceptance of the woman's positive or negative feelings about the cessation of her menstruation after hysterectomy, the nurse may find it necessary to explore her own personal feelings about the menstrual process.

EFFECTS OF HYSTERECTOMY ON MENOPAUSAL PROCESS

Hysterectomy does not induce menopause, nor does it prevent the process of menopause.[101] There are three aspects of menopause: cessation of the menses, psychologic adjustment to the termination of childbearing capacity, and permanent reduction of hormonal (estrogen) level. After hysterectomy the woman experiences cessation of the menses and begins psychologic adjustment to the loss of childbearing capacity. However, she does not experience permanent reduction of hormonal levels, and this factor is the qualifying determinant of menopause.

The relation of hysterectomy to menopause becomes increasingly confusing as one examines literature that indicates that, although permanent reduction of hormonal levels does not occur after hysterectomy, a temporary hormonal imbalance often occurs, causing some premenopausal women to experience hot flashes, a symptom commonly associated with menopause.[102] It should be stressed that this condition is temporary, can occur at any age, and generally disappears naturally or can be treated by hormonal replacement.[103]

Therefore, a premenopausal woman who has a hysterectomy may or may not experience some temporary hot flashes after her surgery. Hot flashes in this instance are not indicative of menopause. The woman's ovaries are still functioning and will continue to function until her natural menopause. Masters and Johnson suggest that the only correlation between hysterectomy and menopause is that the young woman who has a hysterectomy may experience menopause a few years sooner than women who had not had hysterectomies.[104]

Hysterectomy with bilateral oophorectomy does induce surgical menopause in the premenopausal woman.[105] In this instance, the woman, again, may or may not experience menopausal symptoms. Although the symptoms of surgical menopause do not appear to be more severe than the symptoms of natural menopause, the suddenness of the surgical menopause can be psychologically distressing. To minimize the distress and lessen the physical discomforts of surgical menopause, estrogen therapy replacement is usually recommended.[106]

Nursing Interventions

The high level of confusion regarding the relationship between hysterectomy and menopause can be seen clearly in the responses of the women who participated in the "Hysterectomy Knowledge Study." Only 52 per cent of the women knew that, after a hysterectomy, menopause would occur at the normal time. Over 36 per cent thought that menopause would be brought on by hysterectomy; and just under 12 per cent thought menopause could be prevented by hysterectomy.

There are also reports in the literature of women who, not understanding the relationship between hysterectomy and menopause, fear that changes in their physical appearances associated with menopause will occur, such as dry, wrinkled skin, rapid aging, and grey hair or that they will acquire masculine characteristics such as facial hair and a deeper voice.[107-109] Approximately 5 per cent of the women in the "Hysterectomy Knowledge Study" believed this to be true. Education can help to alleviate these misconceptions.

The premenopausal woman facing hysterectomy with bilateral oophorectomy should be told she will be experiencing surgical menopause. The menopausal symptoms she may experience should be discussed along with an explanation of estrogen replacement therapy if necessary.

The woman facing hysterectomy may be frightened and most probably will be confused about the relationship between hysterectomy and menopause. She may not ask questions; she may not even be able to formulate questions in her mind about a subject that is extremely confusing to her. The nurse can be most helpful in reducing the stressful fear and confusion the woman may be experiencing by providing information, encouraging the woman to discuss her fears, and accepting the woman's needs for reassurance.

EFFECTS OF HYSTERECTOMY ON SEXUAL CAPACITY

Hysterectomy affects sexual functioning minimally in the areas of sexual ability and libido, generally requiring only a short period of readjustment.

In most cases, sexual intercourse can be cautiously resumed about six weeks after the hysterectomy has been performed. Initial intercourse should be gentle because the woman's abdomen may feel tender. It may take three to four months before normal coital pressure becomes comfortable to the woman. This period of adjustment appears to be the same for either vaginal or abdominal hysterectomy.[110]

During this period of readjustment the couple may experience difficulty with intromission, dryness in the vagina, dyspareunia (painful coitus), or bleeding.[111] Frank bleeding and dyspareunia should be brought immediately to the attention of the physician. Dyspareunia generally can be treated and relieved.[112] The majority of women find that sexual intercourse is the same or better after hysterectomy.[113]

The woman's ability to achieve orgasm may diminish for a short time after the surgery, owing to stress.[114] This is only a temporary condition; there have been only very isolated cases in the literature in which the woman's ability to achieve orgasm was diminished for a great length of time.[115] In general, women retain orgasmic ability.[116]

The woman's desire for sex may decrease for a period of time after hysterectomy.[117] In one study women reported a lack of libido so frequently that the researcher concluded the lack of libido must be considered a normal condition after hysterectomy.[118] Conversely, other studies report that lack of libido is much less frequent[119] or not related to hysterectomy.[120] Although it appears that many women do experience a decrease in desire for sexual activity, it is generally only very temporary. Libido is based on many psychologic factors. This is evidenced in the finding that other women report an increase in libido after hysterectomy.[121] This increase may occur because the woman feels relief from the distressing physical symptoms that prompted her hysterectomy or because she experiences relief from the fear of pregnancy.

Hysterectomy with oophorectomy does not end a woman's desire for sexual activity. A woman's sex drive often does not diminish even when the ovaries are surgically removed.[122] A woman's desire for sexual intimacy, it appears, is based more extensively on psychologic factors than on basic physiology. Thus (regardless of whether an oophorectomy has been performed), the majority of women experience comparable libido and sexual relationships before and after hysterectomy.[123]

Nursing Interventions

Hysterectomy literature abounds with reported fears and misconceptions women have about the effects of hysterectomy on sexual ability and desire. Women fear they will no longer desire sexual intercourse,[124] that sexual intercourse will no longer be a satisfactory experience for their husbands,[125] and that they will no longer be physically able to have sexual intercourse.[126] There are even reports of women and their sexual partners who fear that sexual activity caused the condition that made removal of the uterus necessary and that resumption of sexual intercourse would cause resumption of the disease.[127] There are also reports of men who fear that penile injury will occur if they have coitus with a woman who has had a hysterectomy[128] or that they will contract cancer by having intercourse with a woman who has had her uterus removed because of the presence of cancer.[129] Until recent years, sex was not considered a proper topic of discussion, and it appears that this cultural taboo was also experienced by members of the health care professions.

The "Hysterectomy Knowledge Study" shows a decline in the acceptance of this cultural taboo. Over 99 per cent of the women in the study knew that hysterectomy did not end a woman's desire for sex. Just over 96 per cent knew that a woman could have sexual intercourse and that it would feel the same to her after hysterectomy. Ninety-three per cent felt that a woman could have an orgasm after hysterectomy if she had experienced it before the surgery. Ninety-six per cent of the women thought that a woman's desire for sex would remain the same or increase after hysterectomy; and the same percentage knew that sexual intercourse would feel the same to the woman's sexual partner after hysterectomy. It appears that articles in women's magazines about sexual functioning after hysterectomy[130, 131] along with other media presentations have provided education regarding sexual functioning to the public.

These encouraging statistics, however, do not eliminate the need for informative discussions about the effects of hysterectomy on sexual functioning. It must be remembered that women of various cultural and educational backgrounds will probably display variations of knowledge in this area.

In a study by Krueger and colleagues, over half of the women who had hysterectomies indicated that they would like nurses to provide information regarding sexual adjustment after surgery. Less than one sixth of these women stated that a nurse had been most valuable in providing them with this information.[131a]

If women are not informed that resumption of sexual intercourse will require a time of readjustment and that they may experience initial difficulties, the experience of sexual intercourse after hysterectomy may be painful, negative, and fear producing. These factors tend to have adverse effects on a woman's libido, thus increasing the possibility of sexual impairment. If women are informed about possible initial difficulties before their first experience with sexual intercourse after hysterectomy, along with methods to alleviate difficulties, the anxiety level can be reduced, which in turn can help make intercourse more pleasurable. If the woman experiences initial dryness in the vagina, the use of water-soluble lubricating jelly can be suggested, or it can be recommended that the couple prolong lovemaking before intercourse. Gentle intercourse will be more pleasurable to the woman. The occurrence of pain during intercourse should be brought to the physician's attention so that treatment can be provided.

The response of the woman's sexual partner is crucial in the sexual adjustment after hysterectomy.[132] He should be included in discussions on sexual functioning and encouraged to ask questions. If he is given information and supported in expressing concerns or fears, he may be better able to support the woman, thus making the sexual adjustment period easier for both of them. This would be true for a homosexual partner as well.

Discussions on sexual functioning are difficult and embarrassing for some people. Many women are uncomfortable asking a male physician questions that are sexual in nature.[133] Such questions as "When will I be healed properly?" are often indicators of a need to discuss when sexual functioning can be resumed.[134] When the nurse is alert to directly and indirectly expressed needs of the health care recipient and takes the initiative to discuss sexual response to hysterectomy, more helpful interventions can be made and the quality of health care will improve.

EFFECTS OF HYSTERECTOMY ON PHYSICAL CONDITION

Physical effects of hysterectomy include the mortality rate of the surgery, frequently occurring physical symptoms experienced after the surgery, and the characteristics of the recovery period.

The surgical procedure itself is relatively safe in terms of mortality. In recent years, estimates of mortality range from one death per 1000 surgeries performed to one death per 4000 surgeries.[135]

The necessity for blood transfusions during and following surgery has been reduced by the use of progestogens and iron prior to surgery. However, studies continue to report blood transfusions for 7 to 15 per cent of hysterectomy cases.[27a]

Postoperative urinary tract infections occur frequently, especially after vaginal hysterectomies. In one series of studies, urinary tract infection occurred in approximately 20 to 25 per cent of the women.[136]

Headache is another physical symptom that seems to occur frequently after hysterectomy. Richards reports that half of his sample population of women who had hysterectomies complained of headaches postoperatively.[137] (Less than one sixth of these women had complained of headaches preoperatively.)

Weight gain also appears to occur frequently after hysterectomy. Dodds and co-workers found that approximately one half of the women in their study sample gained under 10 pounds; the other half gained from 10 to 30 pounds after hysterectomy.[138]

Hot flashes after hysterectomy are experienced by approximately 50 to 60 per cent of women.[139, 140] These hot flashes occur regardless of the age of the woman and whether or not she has had an oophorectomy along with the hysterectomy. Hot flashes appear to be a temporary symptom, usually subsiding within six months.

Studies dealing with the recovery period of hysterectomy report that, for about one half of the women studied, this period is characterized by extreme fatigue and weakness.[141] Generally, most women can resume their normal activities within six weeks to three months after hysterectomy,[142] although there are instances of some women taking up to six months to resume normal activities.[143]

The length of the recovery period from hysterectomy varies. Williams found that the recovery period (time from hospital discharge until the person felt fully recovered) was an average of two months. However, she states that the range was from two weeks to six months and that some women did not feel well at the six-month interview.[144] Richards found the average time for the women in his study to feel fully recovered after hysterectomy was 11.9 months (compared with three months for women in the control group who had other surgeries).[145] The wide variation reported in the length of the recovery time is difficult to understand.

Nursing Interventions

Some women express fears about physical symptoms after hysterectomy that are extreme and occur very rarely, such as permanently losing bowel and bladder control and never being as physically strong or healthy after hysterectomy. The "Hysterectomy Knowledge Study" indicates that these extreme fears about hysterectomy are not as prevalent at present. Under 3 per cent of the women in the study thought that a woman would never be as physically strong or healthy after hysterectomy. Only 1 per cent thought that many women permanently lost control of bowel and bladder after hysterectomy.

However, results from the "Hysterectomy Knowledge Study" indicate that many women know little about physical symptoms that actually do occur after hysterectomy. Just less than 50 per cent of the women knew that temporary urinary problems could occur, that hot flashes were a possible physical symptom, and that weight gain could occur. Less than 20 per cent thought headaches were a possible physical symptom.

The nurse can provide women with the information that these symptoms may occur. Women should be told the symptoms of urinary tract infection, so that if it does occur it can be treated promptly. Knowing that headaches may occur and that she may experience hot flashes can alleviate the possible anxiety that may accompany these symptoms if the woman is not prepared for their possible occurrence. If weight gain after hysterectomy would be distressing to the woman, she can be placed on a moderate diet to prevent this. This information can be presented to the woman in a manner that does not imply that she will experience these symptoms but that indicates that these symptoms are experienced by some women.

In the "Hysterectomy Knowledge Study" most women (97 per cent) knew that after hysterectomy women could return to work or household duties six to eight weeks after surgery. Most women (89 per cent) thought recovery time was six to 12 weeks after surgery. The remaining 11 per cent thought that the recovery time was generally one year or that women never fully recovered.

It appears that when recovery time takes longer than three months (it is often assumed that recovery time for major surgery is one to three months),[146] the woman is probably not prepared for this occurrence. Anxiety may be alleviated if the woman understands in advance that wide variations in the length of recovery time from hysterectomy do occur.

An overview of the goals of nursing interventions in the area of physical effects of hysterectomy includes alleviating extreme anxiety about the physical effects of the surgery, bringing into public awareness that hysterectomy contains risks of mortality and physical morbidity, and preparing health care recipients for possible physical symptoms they may experience after hysterectomy.

PSYCHOLOGIC RESPONSE TO HYSTERECTOMY

The psychologic response to hysterectomy has been the focus of many studies. Studies performed to determine the psychologic aftermath of hysterectomy, using the criterion of admission to a mental hospital or psychiatric institute, do not prove (either because statistical significance is not established or because of poor study design) that hysterectomy leads to psychiatric disability requiring admission to a psychiatric institute.[147-151] However, studies that use referral to a psychiatrist as the criterion for emotional distress produced by hysterectomy indicate that referral to a psychiatrist after hysterectomy occurs 2.5 times more often than referral after other surgeries.[152] Similarly, studies examining the incidence of psychiatric symptoms after hysterectomy do provide evidence of intense psychologic response after hysterectomy.[153-159]

The most common response to hysterectomy is depression. The reported incidence ranges from 4 per cent[160] of the women studied to 70 per cent,[161] with an average of approximately 30 per cent. This depression may or may not be accompanied by agitation.

These studies indicate the level of intensity of the emotional response. Apparently, an adverse response to hysterectomy does not generally necessitate admission to a psychiatric institute. Depression is a common psychologic response for which some women may seek treatment by a therapist. Other women may experience depression and not seek such treatment.

The identification of women at risk for poor outcome after hysterectomy has also been the focus of studies. Factors that correlate with intense, distressing psychologic response have been identified. Poor outcome correlates with women who have a high general anxiety level, are highly neurotic, have a small number of siblings, have a high ordinal position within the family, have a poor relationship with their own mothers, exhibit extensive concern over the effects of the operation on future sexual relationships, and have difficulty understanding and accepting the need for the surgery.[162] Previous history of depression[163] or previous emotional breakdown correlates strongly with poor outcome of hysterectomy.[164] The factor that one researcher found to correlate most significantly with unfavorable outcome was the degree of "unhelpfulness" experienced by the woman from her social network.[165] It has also been discovered that the immediate postoperative recovery from anesthesia is indicative of the course of the hospital convalescence.[166]

Nursing Interventions

Previous discussions of nursing interventions have been focused on reducing the possibility of intense psychologic distress as a response to hysterectomy. The identification of factors that correlate with poor outcome of hysterectomy can assist the nurse in anticipating and preparing for the possible onset of emotional crisis.

The high number of women experiencing posthysterectomy depression is alarming. Some depression (especially as related to the grieving process) may be necessary in order for the woman to make a healthy long-term adaptive response to the loss of her uterus. It is important that nurses recognize symptoms of depression so that they can direct the woman to treatment if indicated.

Common symptoms of depression include a change in sleeping patterns, a change in eating habits, mood swings, excessive crying, emotional lability, lack of energy, and acquired preoccupation with one's physical condition. This may be accompanied by nervousness and agitation.

FUTURE IMPLICATIONS

The future of hysterectomies is unknown. It is based on another unknown—the future of women. If women remain dependent and uneducated, it is likely that a large percentage of unnecessary and undesired hysterectomies will continue to be performed. (Hysterectomy performed on a woman who desires hysterectomy, for whatever reason, and makes a conscious decision to have the surgery is not included in the category of unnecessary hysterectomies.) One explanation for the occurrence of undesired, unnecessary hysterectomies lies in the relationship between the physician and the health care recipient. It has been charged that many women unquestioningly surrender their uterus to the whims of the physician—the superior male healer. Hysterectomy, in such instances, is best described as a "socially sanctioned genital trauma performed on a female by a male."[167]

It has further been charged that the physician often "cons" a woman into the surrender of her uterus. In these instances, the physician tells the woman she must have a hysterectomy, either making the decision himself or not providing the woman with enough information so that she can participate in the decision-making process. A partial explanation for this is that a physician can charge more money for a hysterectomy than for a less extensive procedure such as a tubal ligation or dilatation and curettage. It is often women of low socioeconomic backgrounds, generally of the black culture, who are "talked into" hysterectomy when a less extensive procedure[168] would suffice.

These are angry charges, and it is likely that the strength of this anger will help to reduce the number of undesired, unnecessary hysterectomies. The anger is also felt by physicians who are not involved in these practices. Unification of physicians, nurses, and the lay population over this issue may lead to stronger public education programs and increased accountability of physicians to their peers.

Perhaps by having hysterectomies, some women are making statements about the anger they feel about their position in society. The recognition of this anger may be associated with the women's movement. The lives of many women have been ruled by the fruits of their uteri. Childbearing and childrearing are felt to have kept many women in bondage. It can be speculated that increased involvement of fathers in the responsibilities of raising children may decrease the need for women to express their anger by having a part of their body removed.

The high incidence of hysterectomies may also have a partial explanation in the decreased need for biologic functions to be the focus of a woman's identity. With the advent of oral contraceptives, concern with overpopulation, and the number of women working outside the home, women may be less inclined to place a heavy emphasis on retaining their uteri.

Perhaps, in the future, the women's movement will help women to gain a new positiveness about their bodies and their female functioning. This positiveness, if coupled with increased medical management of distressful symptoms of menstruation and menopause, may cause a reduction in the number of hysterectomies performed. If menstruation becomes a valued, respected body process, then perhaps what one male physician called "birthday hysterectomies" ("let the woman have her family, then at her 35th or 36th birthday have a vaginal hysterectomy and forget her bleeding, anemias, and shots") will not occur.[27b] Efforts made by nurses through research to identify the effects of stress on the functioning of the female reproductive system may help to reduce the incidence of surgical treatment of a psychoemotional problem.

References

1. Cohen, Marcia. Needless hysterectomies. *Ladies Home Journal,* vol. 93, March 1976, p. 88.
2. Curtis, Lindsay R. *After Hysterectomy What?* Bristol, TN: Beecham Laboratories, 1975, pp. 14–16.
3. Raphael, Beverly. The crisis of hysterectomy. *Australian and New Zealand Journal of Psychiatry,* vol. 6, 1972, p. 114.
4. Raphael, Beverly. Psychiatric aspects of hysterectomy. *In* Howells, John G. (ed.) *Modern Perspectives in the Psychiatric Aspects of Surgery.* New York: Brunner/Mazel, 1976, p. 438.
5. Associated Press, *Minneapolis Tribune,* May 10, 1977, Section B, p. 6.
5a. National Center for Health Statistics. U.S. Dept of HEW, Government Printing Office, 1971–1978.
6. Rodgers, Joann. Are this year's 690,000 hysterectomies all necessary? *Women's Network Directory, 1976,* Minneapolis: Women's Network, 1976, p. 136.
7. Drellich, Marvin G., and Bieber, Irving. The psychologic importance of the uterus and its functions. *Journal of Nervous and Mental Disorders,* vol. 126, 1958, pp. 322–336.
8. Raphael, Crisis of hysterectomy, op. cit., pp. 109–111.
8a. Gould, D. Recovery from hysterectomy. *Nursing Times,* vol. 78, October 1982, pp. 1769–1771.
9. Johnson, Jean E., Morrissey, John F., and Leventhal, Howard. Psychological preparation for an endoscopic examination. *Gastrointestinal Endoscopy* 19, no. 4 (1973): 190–192.
10. Johnson, Jean E. Effects of acute expectations about sensations on the sensory and distress components of pain. *Journal of Personality and Social Psychology,* vol. 27, 1973, pp. 273–274.
11. Chafetz, Morris E. Hysterectomy and castration: An emotional look-alike. *Medical Insight,* vol. 3, January 1971, p. 40.
12. Steiner, M., and Aleksandrowicz, D. R. Psychiatric sequence to gynecological operations. *Israel Annals of Psychiatry and Related Disciplines,* vol. 8, 1970, p. 191.
13. Thompson, Valerie M. Sexual life after hysterectomy. (Letter to the editor.) *British Medical Journal,* vol. 3, July 1975, p. 97.
14. Raphael, op. cit., p. 113.
15. Williams, Margaret A. Cultural patterning of the feminine role. *Nursing Forum,* vol. 12, 1973, p. 386.
16. Raphael, Crisis of hysterectomy, op. cit., p. 113.
17. Green, Robert L. Jr. The emotional aspects of hysterectomy. *Southern Medical Journal,* vol. 66, April 1973, pp. 443–444.
18. Ibid.
19. Melody, George F. Depressive reactions following hysterectomy. *American Journal of Obstetrics and Gynecology,* vol. 83, February 1, 1962, p. 413.
20. Raphael, Crisis of hysterectomy, op. cit., p. 114.
21. Gray, Madeline. *The Changing Years: The Menopause without Fear.* New York: Doubleday and Company, 1967, p. 239.
22. Gusberg, S. B. Indications for hysterectomy. *In* Reid, Duncan, and Barton, T. C. (eds.) *Controversy in Obstetrics and Gynecology.* Philadelphia: W. B. Saunders Company, 1969, p. 316.
23. Ibid., p. 317.
24. Ibid, pp. 317–318.
25. Cohen, op. cit., p. 88.
26. Ibid.
27. Foster, Henry W. Removal of the normal uterus. *Southern Medical Journal,* vol. 69, January 1976, pp. 13–15.
27a. Amirikia, H., and Evans, J. N. Ten-year review of hysterectomies: Trends, indications, and risks. *American Journal of Obstetrics and Gynecology,* vol. 134, June 1979, pp. 431–437.
27b. Pratt, J. H. The unnecessary hysterectomy. *South-*

ern Medical Journal, vol. 73, October 1980, pp. 1360–1364.

28. Raphael, Psychiatric aspects of hysterectomy, op. cit., p. 426.

29. Donovan, John C. Some psychosomatic aspects of obstetrics and gynecology. *American Journal of Obstetrics and Gynecology*, vol. 75, January 1958, p. 78.

30. Gusberg, op. cit., p. 315.

31. Miller, Norma. Hysterectomy: Therapeutic necessity or surgical racket? *American Journal of Obstetrics and Gynecology*, vol. 51, 1946, p. 808.

32. Doyle, James C. Unnecessary hysterectomies. *Journal of the American Medical Association*, vol. 151, January 1953, p. 364.

33. Chynoweth, R. Psychological complications of hysterectomy. *Australian and New Zealand Journal of Psychiatry*, vol. 7, 1973, p. 103.

34. Raphael, Psychiatric aspects of hysterectomy, op. cit., p. 425.

35. Payne, Waverly R. Hysterectomy: A problem in public relations. *American Journal of Obstetrics and Gynecology*, vol. 72, December 1956, p. 1167.

36. Doyle, op. cit., p. 364.

37. Ramsey, Judith. The modern woman's health guide to her own body. *Family Circle*, July 1973, pp. 113–120.

38. Cohen, op. cit., p. 88.

39. Raphael, Psychiatric aspects of hysterectomy, op. cit., p. 430.

40. Drellich and Bieber, op. cit., p. 326.

41. Kroger, William S. Hysterectomy: Psychosomatic factors of the pre-operative and post-operative aspects and managements. *Western Journal of Surgery, Obstetrics and Gynecology*, vol. 65, September-October 1957, pp. 317–323.

42. Raphael, Psychiatric aspects of hysterectomy, op. cit., p. 430.

43. Drellich and Bieber, op. cit., pp. 330–331.

44. Lindemann, Erich. Observations on psychiatric sequelae to surgical operations in women. *American Journal of Psychiatry*, vol. 98, 1941, p. 132.

45. Raphael, Psychiatric aspects of hysterectomy. op. cit., p. 426.

46. Taylor, E. Stewart. *Essentials of Gynecology*. Philadelphia: Lea and Febiger, 1969, p. 35.

47. Ibid., p. 545.

48. Ibid., p. 37.

49. Browne, J. C. McClure. *Postgraduate Obstetrics and Gynecology*. London: Butterworths and Co., 1973, p. 38.

50. Richards, D. H. A post-hysterectomy syndrome. *Lancet*, vol. 2, 1974, p. 985.

51. Lewis, T. L. T. The rationale of operative removal of the ovaries at hysterectomy. In Campbell, Stuart (ed.) *The Management of the Menopause*. Baltimore: University Park Press, 1976, pp. 369–370.

52. Hunter, D. J. S. Oophorectomy and the surgical menopause. In Beard, R. J. (ed.) *The Menopause*. Baltimore: University Park Press, 1976, pp. 208–209.

53. Creaturo, Barbara. I had a hysterectomy. *Cosmopolitan*, August 1969, p. 60.

54. Raphael, Psychiatric aspects of hysterectomy. op. cit., p. 433.

55. Ibid., p. 432.

56. Patterson, Ralph, et al. Social and medical characteristics of hysterectomized and non-hysterectomized psychiatric patients. *Obstetrics and Gynecology*, vol. 15, 1960, p. 215.

57. Raphael, Psychiatric aspects of hysterectomy, op. cit., p. 432.

58. Patterson, Ralph, and Craig, James B. Misconceptions concerning the psychological effects of hysterectomy. *American Journal of Obstetrics and Gynecology*, vol. 85, January 1963, p. 107.

59. Raphael, Psychiatric aspects of hysterectomy, op. cit., p. 432.

60. Ibid.

61. Chaftez, op. cit., p. 43.

62. Ibid.

63. Raphael, Psychiatric aspects of hysterectomy, op. cit., p. 434.

64. Ris, Hania W. What do women want? *Journal of American Medical Women's Association*, vol. 29, October 1974, p. 451.

65. Raphael, Psychiatric aspects of hysterectomy, op. cit., p. 434.

66. Donovan, op. cit., p. 78.

67. Hollender, Marc. A study of patients admitted to a psychiatric hospital after pelvic operations. *American Journal of Obstetrics and Gynecology*, vol. 79, March 1960, pp. 500–501.

68. Wolf, Sanford. Emotional reactions to hysterectomy. *Postgraduate Medicine*, vol. 47, May 1970, pp. 165–169.

69. Ellison, R. M. Psychiatric complications following sterilization of women. *Medical Journal of Australia*, vol. 2, October 17, 1964, pp. 627–628.

70. Tunnadine, Prudence. Gynecological illness after sterilization. (Letter to the editor.) *British Medical Journal*, vol. 1, 1972, pp. 748–749.

71. Raphael, Beverly. Parameters of health outcome following hysterectomy. *Bulletin of the Post-Graduate Committee in Medicine, University of Sydney*, vol. 30, December 1974, p. 218.

72. Barker, Montagu G. Psychiatric illness after hysterectomy. *British Medical Journal*, vol. 2, April 1968, p. 94.

73. Hollender, op. cit., pp. 500–501.

74. Donovan, op. cit., p. 78.

75. Ellison, R. M. Psychiatric complications following sterilization of women. *Medical Journal of Australia*, vol. 2, October 1964, p. 627.

76. Drellich and Bieber, op. cit., pp. 323–324.

77. May, Rollo. *Power and Innocence: A Search for the Sources of Violence*. New York: Dell Publishing Co., 1972, p. 82.

78. Drellich and Bieber, op. cit., p. 323.

79. Williams, op. cit., p. 382.

80. Raphael, Psychiatric aspects of hysterectomy, op. cit., p. 430.

81. Drellich and Bieber, op. cit., p. 323.

82. Menzer, Doris, et al. Patterns of emotional recovery from hysterectomy. *Psychosomatic Medicine*, vol. 19, 1957, p. 386.

83. Williams, op. cit., p. 386.

84. Patterson et al., op. cit., p. 215.

85. Raphael, Psychiatric aspects of hysterectomy, op. cit., p. 431.

86. Wengraf, Fritz. Psychoneurotic symptoms following hysterectomy. *American Journal of Obstetrics and Gynecology*, vol. 52, 1946, p. 648.

87. Raphael, Psychiatric aspects of hysterectomy, op. cit., p. 432.

88. Steiner and Aleksandrowicz, op. cit., pp. 186–192.

89. Rodgers, op. cit., p. 136.

90. Donovan, op. cit., pp. 78–79.

91. Laros, Russel K., and Work, Bruce A. Female sterilization: Vaginal hysterectomy. *American Journal of Obstetrics and Gynecology*, vol. 22, July 15, 1975, pp. 695–697.

92. Barglow, Peter, et al. Hysterectomy and tubal liga-

tion: A psychiatric comparison. *Obstetrics and Gynecology*, vol. 25, April 1965, pp. 522–526.

93. Dalton, Katharina. Discussion on the aftermath of hysterectomy and oophorectomy. *Proceedings of the Royal Society of Medicine*, vol. 50, June 1957, p. 418.
94. Drellich and Bieber, op. cit., p. 324.
95. Dodds, D. T., Potgieter, C. R., and Turner, P. J. The physical and emotional results of hysterectomy. *South African Medical Journal*, vol. 35, 1961, p. 54.
96. Drellich and Bieber, op. cit., p. 325.
97. Raphael, Psychiatric aspects of hysterectomy, op. cit., p. 431.
98. Drellich and Bieber, op. cit., p. 324.
99. Donovan, op. cit., pp. 76–78.
100. Williams, op. cit., p. 440.
101. Lewis, op. cit., p. 368.
102. Richards, op. cit., p. 985.
103. Williams, Margaret. Easier convalescence from hysterectomy. *American Journal of Nursing*, vol. 76, March 1976, p. 440.
104. Masters, William H., and Johnson, Virginia E. What young women should know about hysterectomies. *Redbook*, January 1976, pp. 48–50.
105. Gray, op. cit., p. 229.
106. Hunter, op. cit., pp. 208–209.
107. Raphael, Psychiatric aspects of hysterectomy, op. cit., p. 429.
108. Payne, op. cit., p. 1167.
109. Drellich and Bieber, op. cit., p. 329.
110. Amias, A. G. Sexual life after gynaecological operations. I. *British Medical Journal*, vol. 2, June 1975, p. 608.
111. Craig, G. A., and Jackson, P. Sexual life after vaginal hysterectomy. (Letter to the editor.) *British Medical Journal*, vol. 3, July 1975, p. 97.
112. Masters and Johnson, op. cit., p. 49.
113. Huffman, John W. The effect of gynecological surgery on sexual reactions. *American Journal of Obstetrics and Gynecology*, vol. 59, April 1950, p. 917.
114. Gray, op. cit., p. 248.
115. Tunnadine, op. cit., pp. 748–749.
116. Huffman, op. cit., pp. 915–917.
117. Gray, op. cit., p. 248.
118. Dodds, Potgieter, and Turner, op. cit., p. 54.
119. Richards, op. cit., p. 984.
120. Patterson and Craig, op. cit., p. 109.
121. Ibid.
122. McCary, James Leslie. *Human Sexuality*. New York: D. Van Nostrand Company, 1973, p. 259.
123. Kroger, op. cit., p. 317.
124. Drellich and Bieber, op. cit., p. 325.
125. Williams, op. cit., p. 382.
126. Dalton, op. cit., p. 415.
127. Drellich and Bieber, op. cit., p. 326.
128. Melody, op. cit., p. 141.
129. Ibid.

130. Masters and Johnson, op. cit., pp. 48–51.
131. Cohen, op. cit., p. 88.
131a. Krueger, J. C., Hassell, J., Gossins, D. B., et al. Relationship between nurse counseling and sexual adjustment after hysterectomy. *Nursing Research*, vol. 28, May-June 1979, pp. 145–150.
132. Hollender, Marc H. Hysterectomy and feelings of femininity. *Medical Aspects of Human Sexuality*, vol. 3, July 1969, p. 11.
133. Raphael, Psychiatric aspects of hysterectomy, op. cit., p. 434.
134. Ibid.
135. Cohen, op. cit., p. 90.
136. Richards, op. cit., pp. 984–985.
137. Ibid., p. 984.
138. Dodds, Potgieter, and Turner, op. cit., p. 54.
139. Ackner, London B. Emotional aspects of hysterectomy: A follow-up study of fifty patients under the age of forty. *In* Jores, A., and Freyberger, H. (eds.) *Advances in Psychosomatic Medicine*. New York: Robert Brunner, Inc., 1960, p. 251.
140. Richards, op. cit., p. 985.
141. Williams, op. cit., p. 440.
142. Dodds, Potgieter, and Turner, op. cit., p. 53.
143. Williams, op. cit., p. 438.
144. Ibid.
145. Richards, op. cit., pp. 984–985.
146. Ibid., p. 985.
147. Bragg, Robert L. Risk of admission to a mental hospital following hysterectomy or cholecystectomy. *American Journal of Public Health*, vol. 55, September 1965, pp. 1403–1410.
148. Ellison, op. cit., pp. 625–627.
149. Patterson et al., op. cit., pp. 209–215.
150. Patterson and Craig, op. cit., pp. 104–111.
151. Hollender, op. cit., pp. 498–503.
152. Barker, op. cit., p. 94.
153. Ackner, op. cit., pp. 248–251.
154. Dodds, Potgieter, and Turner, op. cit., pp. 53–55.
155. Barglow et al., op. cit., pp. 520–526.
156. Steiner and Aleksandrowicz, op. cit., pp. 186–192.
157. Melody, op. cit., pp. 410–413.
158. Lindeman, op. cit., pp. 132–139.
159. Moore, James T., and Tolley, Dennis H. Depression following hysterectomy. *Psychosomatics*, vol. 17, April-May-June 1976, pp. 86–89.
160. Melody, op. cit., p. 411.
161. Richards, op. cit., p. 983.
162. Chynoweth, op. cit., p. 103.
163. Melody, op. cit., p. 413.
164. Ackner, op. cit., p. 250.
165. Raphael, Parameters of health outcome, op. cit., pp. 218–219.
166. Menzer et al., op. cit., pp. 385–387.
167. Raphael, Psychiatric aspects of hysterectomy, op. cit., p. 439.
168. Rodger, op. cit., p. 138.

20

MENOPAUSE: A CLOSER LOOK FOR NURSES

RUTH DYER

LINDA C. McKEEVER

This chapter by Ruth Dyer and Linda McKeever on the menopause experience for women begins with a historic view of menopause including various definitions necessary for understanding this experience. The cause of menopause is given, with a critical look at the physical signs and sensations. Finally, a close examination of the experience is taken from several women's viewpoints.

Developmental transitions such as menopause are normal, predictable events that require change or growth of the self biologically, psychologically, and socially. Understanding menopause as a normal developmental transition is key, because this process may either present women with opportunities for growth or represent possible threats to their established adjustment to life. Certain strategies for managing, acknowledging, and accepting these changes may enhance the quality of life or may detract from that quality. Because menopause can be expected to occur in the lives of most women, anticipatory planning with regard to what the experience may be like and how the individual might manage certain aspects of the experience is possible.

Any change requires coping, and, although menopause may be perceived as stressful by some women, other women find the changes it creates uneventful and easily managed. Unfortunately, the information available about what the menopausal experience is like for women remains inadequate and has too often been inaccurate. Increasing research interest in menopause has resulted in the beginning steps of developing accurate knowledge about this event. However, women and health professionals need to realize the limitations and tentativeness of present information about menopause. Research is needed so that women and nurses will understand the menopausal transition in order to determine when strengthening, aiding, or exploring options available to menopausal women might be appropriate actions and when intervention is unnecessary.

This chapter describes current views of menopause, the influences that past views have had on current thinking, and the current knowledge of the menopausal experience. Attempts to distinguish commonly held beliefs from those aspects supported by research will also be made.

EARLY VIEW OF MENOPAUSE

For years, the classic picture of menopause presented a woman in physical and emotional turmoil, exhibiting a multitude of signs and symptoms ranging from a bad taste in the mouth to convulsions, and often on the verge of nervous exhaustion. This clinical picture was in keeping with the prevailing view of a woman as a primarily biologic organism whose function was related to attractiveness, childbearing, and childrearing.[1] When menopause took away her capacity to reproduce the human species, it seemed only natural to society that she would have difficulty coping with this impending "uselessness" and "senescence."[2, 3] Helene Deutsch presents a Freudian perspective of menopause that equates the loss of reproductive capacity to the loss of "service to the species."[4] This loss creates an obsolescence that includes a loss of femininity and sexuality. This perspective has permeated society and has influenced women's self-concept and view of menopause in a negative fashion. In fact, it seems that women were almost obligated to respond negatively to this period of life. "She realizes vividly that the beautiful past, the loving and beloved womanhood, is now to be left behind forever, and by this an intelligent and sensitive woman cannot fail to be profoundly affected."[5]

Kaufert identifies a prevailing myth in American society that is based on the knowledge that menopause occurs as a result of decreased estrogen resulting from ovarian atrophy.[6] This myth, rooted in medicine, defines menopause as a hormone-deficiency disease. By defining menopause as a disease, medicine has been able to take control of its diagnosis and treatment. The treatment has been typically to replace the deficient hormone. This disease orientation removes the idea that menopause is a normal event and that the woman herself has some control over her own body. On the other hand, an opposing myth described by Kaufert explains a perspective that defines menopause as a normal event in the lives of women that is completely manageable by the women themselves.[7] Although this view is more positive in its attitude about menopause, it does trivialize the experiences of those women who find menopause a stressful transition.

The Boston Women's Health Book Collective states that women's ideas regarding menopause have been influenced by media advertisements that portray the middle-aged woman as nervous, depressed, old, and in need of medical treatment.[8] Our cultural emphasis on youth, glamour, and beauty has made middle age unattractive and less valued than youth. Also, the linking of sexuality with reproductive ability has equated menopause with being asexual and reflects society's expectation that, after menopause, women should quietly fade into sexless oblivion.

While struggling to overcome this "partial death," this "biologic withering," women were expected to experience feelings of hopeless-ness, sexlessness, purposelessness, and depression. Anxiety, feelings of loss and inferiority, paranoia, urges to have more children, and alterations in sexual desire were said to be common.[9, 10] Interestingly, increased sexual desire was believed to be more distressing for women than were decreased sexual feelings. When experienced by any woman 30 to 60 years old, these feelings and concerns, as well as almost any physical signs and sensations that were not easily explained by other diagnoses, were quickly attributed to approaching menopause. The labels "menopausal syndrome" or "climacteric syndrome" evolved and are still in use today.

The symptoms usually denoted by these labels can be categorized as either physiologic or psychologic. Physiologic symptoms usually include "hot flashes," chills, night sweats, palpitations, vaginal atrophy, headache, dizziness, back pain, abdominal bloating, breast tenderness, sleeplessness, gastrointestinal disturbances, lack of energy, numbness, and limb pain.[11–15] Symptoms of menopause that are often considered psychologic include weakness, fatigue, headache, nervousness, insomnia, depression, forgetfulness, irritability, anxiety, lack of sexual interest or gratification, and melancholia.[11–16] "Hot flashes" are the most common physiologic symptom reported by menopausal women.[17–19] Research describing the signs and symptoms experienced by menopausal women shows that vasomotor symptoms and genital atrophy are unique to menopause but that the severity of symptoms varies from individual to individual. Some women (15 to 20 per cent) have annoying symptoms and seek medical attention, but the vast majority have few or minor symptoms.[20]

The idea of a "menopausal syndrome" has become even more firmly established, perhaps in part owing to such tools as the Blatt Menopausal Index (BMI), a list of 11 symptoms considered most common in menopausal women. A numeric weight has been assigned to each symptom to reflect its prominence and potential for causing distress in women, as judged by the tool developers. This weight is multiplied by a severity factor when the symptom is present in a woman, and the sum obtained from all complaints is the Blatt Menopausal Index.[21] Although the BMI was originally devised to measure the effect of various medical therapies on the symptoms listed, the tool has also been erroneously viewed as a method for judging whether a woman is menopausal. This is unfortunate, as few of the 11 symptoms have been shown to be more likely to occur during menopause than during other times in life, whereas other signs and symptoms not included in the tool might discriminate more appropriately.[22]

LIMITATIONS OF PRESENT KNOWLEDGE

What is actually known about menopause and the experiences surrounding this event? Quite frankly, our knowledge base remains limited. Little research was focused on menopause before 1945. Besides the fact that the lifespan of only a relatively small proportion of women was expected to exceed the age of menopause, societal taboos made the subject of menopause less than desirable as an area of scientific study. Even when researchers did take an interest, their efforts were often frustrated by the unwillingness of women to share this private aspect of their lives.[23, 24]

Current research is limited in both quality and quantity. Most research has been done on women seeking medical care for menopausal complaints. Consequently, we know little about the experience of those women who may not find it necessary to seek medical care. Even the findings based on well women cannot be generalized to all women. Also, many other life events and changes commonly take place in the years of menopause, greatly complicating any attempt to distinguish those experiences attributable to menopause from those commonly occurring during the entire middle stage of life.

A focus that has been completely neglected until recently is the study of the individual's subjective response to menopause. In an attempt to obtain "objective" evidence, researchers have failed to utilize the opportunity to have those women actually experiencing menopause describe this life event in their own words.

Any description of menopause, then, is admittedly sketchy and tentative. However, the information presented here can provide the nurse with some basis for correcting misconceptions and for evolving an accurate base of knowledge as new research findings become available.

Terms such as "menopause," "female climacteric," and "the change of life" have been used interchangeably in both lay and professional literature. Since these terms may refer to a single event or to a continuum of 20 years or more, confusion results. The following definitions are presented to help the nurse be more precise and consistent in discussing menopause and in examining research findings for implications for practice:

Menopause: The actual cessation of menstruation, which can be said to have occurred after a woman has had no menstrual bleeding for at least one year.[25, 26]

Female climacteric: The period of life characterized by morphologic and physiologic changes in the body that accompany the decreasing function of the ovaries,[27] encompassing those events leading up to and following the actual cessation of menstruation. Menopause is then just one physical event in the entire climacteric experience.

Change of life: The time span of the entire climacteric, rather than simply the event of menopause.

Middle years: Generally, the same time span as the climacteric.

Premenopausal: Describes women whose menstrual pattern is similar to what it was in the preceding years.[28–30]

Postmenopausal: Describes women who have ceased to menstruate for one full year or more.[31–34] Research studies have also used this term to describe women who have ceased to menstruate for at least three years.[35] The second definition is used in this chapter.

Perimenopausal: Describes the time period surrounding the natural cessation of menstruation. In previous research and in this chapter, the term refers to women who have at some time in the past 12 months had irregularities in menstrual bleeding, compared with their previous pattern, or who ceased to menstruate one to three years ago.[36, 37]

An overlap in the meanings of "perimenopausal" and "postmenopausal," when the latter denotes menstruation that has not occurred for one year, is acknowledged. Since irregularities in menses may occur two or more years before actual menopause, it would seem reasonable to allow "perimenopausal" to include two or more years after menopause. Also, the physical changes associated with the postmenopausal period are more likely to become evident two or more years after cessation of menstruation. Further research to clearly define experiences and underlying physiology should lead to more meaningful and consistent definitions.

WHEN DOES MENOPAUSE OCCUR?

Age

The precise age at which menstruation will cease for an individual is not predictable. However, 90 per cent of women experience menopause between the ages of 45 and 54 years. In the United States the average age of women at menopause is 49.5 years.[38] Various factors have been said to affect the age of menopause, such as age at menarche, parity, marital status, and geographic location; however, to date, these claims have not been adequately substantiated by research. Also, the notion that average age at menopause has been increasing through the years is a misinterpretation of research findings.[39]

Artificial Menopause

When the influence of both ovaries is obliterated by such interventions as bilateral surgical removal or irradiation, the woman is said to have experienced artificial menopause. When stimulation of potential cancer is not a contraindication, hormone replacement therapy is often prescribed, especially if the woman is not yet of menopausal age.

Signs of Approaching Menopause

The major physical sign of approaching menopause is menstrual irregularity. This can begin several years before complete cessation of menstruation and may be characterized by lengthening or shortening of cycles, decrease or increase of menstrual flow, or combinations of these characteristics. Often several months pass between menstrual bleedings; occasionally menstrual bleeding resumes after a full year's absence, although if this occurs it is wise to investigate for abnormal causes of bleeding. Some women experience menopause without any changes in their usual menstrual pattern before abrupt cessation.

Women have reported that before their menstrual pattern changed, they experienced alteration of mood and emotional lability that they perceived as signs of approaching menopause. However, a correlation has not yet been supported by research.

WHY DOES MENOPAUSE OCCUR?

It is often said that menopause occurs because the aging ovaries stop producing estrogen. This oversimplification can lead to misconceptions. In fact, the event of menopause usually occurs long before the ovaries actually stop producing estrogen. It is more accurate to say that the cessation of menstruation occurs because the aging ovaries lose their capacity to secrete estrogen and progesterone in the rhythmic pattern necessary for cyclic bleeding to occur.[40] It is, however, accurate to assume that progesterone production from the ovaries ceases.

As a woman enters her 40s, the follicles of the ovary begin to function and mature differently and begin to secrete less and less estrogen. This decrease in estrogen releases the negative-feedback inhibition of follicle-stimulating hormone (FSH) and luteinizing hormone (LH) secreted from the pituitary gland. Even in the presence of increased FSH and LH, ovulation often fails to occur, which may be one reason that fertility decreases after age 40. When ovulation does occur, producing a corpus luteum, that structure also functions irregularly, primarily in decreased progesterone secretion. Since estrogen and progesterone are responsible for the cyclic growth and sloughing of the uterine lining, with their decline the usual menstrual pattern is altered.

The frequency of anovulatory cycles increases toward menopause, and a woman is usually considered sterile after menstruation has ceased entirely. However, there is evidence suggesting that, in at least one case, a woman became pregnant 18 months after her final menses.[41] For safety, contraceptive precautions are usually advised for a full year following menopause.[42]

By the time a woman ceases to menstruate, the levels of estrogen and progesterone are usually greatly reduced. The source of circulating estrogens in postmenopausal women has been a subject of debate. While slight amounts of estrogen continue to be secreted by the ovaries, it was thought that the adrenal glands were the major source of circulating estrogens in menopausal and postmenopausal women.[43] However, others have found that androgenic steroids are converted into estrogens at peripheral body sites rather than in the adrenal gland and that the bulk of this conversion takes place in subcutaneous body fat.[44, 45] It is important to realize that estrogen levels usually decrease gradually and that there is still some estrogen circulating in the bloodstream even after menopause. This means that the changes most closely associated with estrogen-deficiency states (the atrophic changes of external and internal reproductive structures) usually do not become evident for years after the cessation of menstruation.

The increased levels of FSH and LH previously mentioned are currently being examined for their influence, if any, on vasomotor stability. Blood levels of FSH and LH begin to rise a year or more before the last menstrual period and reach maximum levels two to three years after menopause, at which time FSH continues at higher than premenopausal levels for 20 to 30 years after menopause for 70 per cent of women.[46] Further research is needed to shed light on the hypothesis that increased FSH and LH levels increase the vasomotor instability responsible for the "hot flashes" and sweating episodes experienced by some women perimenopausally.

PHYSICAL SIGNS AND SENSATIONS EXPERIENCED

Critical Look at the Menopausal Syndrome

Women report a wide variety of physical signs and sensations perimenopausally, and many of these are included in the group of symptoms labeled the "menopausal syndrome." However, whether such a syndrome actually exists has been questioned.[47-50] In fact, the only characteristics shown to be correlated with the perimenopausal period have been the vasomotor symptoms of "hot flashes" and episodes of sweating.[51-54] This is not to claim that the other sensations do not occur. However, there is not yet sufficient evidence that women should expect these to occur around the time of menopause. Actually, there is a good chance that many women will experience few if any of the symptoms commonly attributed to menopause and that, if they do, it may be to a very mild degree. A number of studies have found that significant numbers of the women studied (15 to 40 per cent) had no symptoms or very few symptoms or complaints perimenopausally.[55-58] As many as 50 per cent of those studied viewed menopause as presenting no difficulty even when symptoms occurred,[59] and only about 10 per cent considered their symptoms incapacitating.[60] Table 20.1 contains a summary of research findings related to the "menopausal syndrome."

Other physical signs and sensations that have been reported by perimenopausal women but that have not yet been shown to be related to menopause include the following: the sensation of less hand coordination, swollen ankles, breast soreness, nausea, pelvic pressure sensations, muscle tightness and tension, decreased perimenstrual discomfort when periods do occur, weight gain, shortness of breath, backache, increased or decreased sexual desire and response, bloatedness, vaginal pruritus, and foul-smelling vaginal discharge.[82-88]

"Hot Flashes" and Other Vasomotor Disturbances

"Hot flashes" and sweating episodes are correlated positively to menopause and are the symptoms that compel some menopausal women to seek medical attention. Not all perimenopausal women experience these symptoms, but their occurrence is relatively common. It is estimated that up to 75 per cent of perimenopausal women may experience "hot flashes," and 25 to 40 per cent of women studied have experienced episodes of sweating.[89-94] Why "hot flashes" are severe for some women and mild for others is not yet known. Some writers have claimed that the intensity and frequency of vasomotor symptoms are related to the amount or abruptness of estrogen decrease in the bloodstream.[95-97] However, these claims lack research support.

Episodes of sweating can occur alone but most commonly accompany hot flashes. Sudden perspiration in varying degrees commonly occurs on the upper lip, forehead, or neck, for example. Some women may note only slight moisture on the lip or forehead whereas others describe drenching sweating episodes, often occurring at night, that may necessitate changing the night clothes and linen.[98-101] These episodes are often followed by a chill or a cold sensation, which may be explained by the cooling effects of evaporation of perspiration.

The "hot flash" has been defined by Voda as the "perception of heat within or on the body that has an origin and spread, has variable intensity or severity, has variable duration lasting from a few seconds to many minutes, and may be accompanied by a variety of bodily sensations. It is sometimes accompanied by a hot flush, which is a change in skin color that may range from pink to bright red."[102] Women have described the hot flash as sudden warm, clammy warm, hot, very hot, or burning hot sensations of the skin. These are usually felt above the waist, especially on the neck and face, but sometimes include the entire body. For some women the sensation is progressive, beginning at one level of the body and moving up toward the face, whereas others feel the flash of heat first in the neck and face and then in the extremities.[103-106]

The frequency and duration of "hot flashes" seem to vary greatly, as does the degree of heat sensed. The "hot flash" was not a serious topic of study until 1975, when Molnar conducted a descriptive study of one woman and found her to experience two "hot flashes" during each 2-hour period. The mean duration of the eight flashes was 3.8 minutes, the range was 2.4 to 4.7 minutes.[107] Dyer obtained subjective reports ranging from "momentary warm feelings occurring three to four times over a span of several months" to "burning, drying heat" lasting 3 to 5 minutes and occurring almost every 15 minutes all day and night.[108] Voda also studied the subjective experience of women with "hot flashes." Self-reports and daily records were used to obtain data from 20 women over a two-week period of time. These women recorded a total of 1041 "hot flashes," with an individual range of 2 to 247. The duration of flashes ranged from 5 seconds to 60 minutes, with a mean duration of 3.31 minutes. It was further found that the hot flash did not restrict itself to one area of the body and varied in severity from mild to moderate to severe.[109]

So far, research suggests that women experiencing "hot flashes" feel much hotter than would be expected when compared with the actual temperature of their skin. Molnar found skin temperature increases of up to 5.5°C on the fingers and toes but of only 0.2 to 0.7°C on the cheeks, an area women often describe as feeling the hottest. Internal temperatures and forehead temperatures tended to decrease with the onset of flashes; this was believed to be due to the evaporation of perspiration. It would seem that a "hot flash" is an explosive activation of certain brain areas. This results in subjective heat distress, vasodilation in extremities, increased heart rate, and stimulation of sweat glands and vasodilators of the face.[110]

As mentioned earlier, the physiologic mechanisms underlying the vasomotor symptoms of "hot flashes" and sweating episodes are not yet clearly known, but the disturbance in the balance of the hypothalamic-pituitary-ovarian mechanism seems to affect the autonomic nervous system by dilating the cutaneous blood vessels. Women have reported that conditions of increased environmental temperature or of increased excitement or stress seem to predispose them to experiencing a "hot flash." Stimuli such as a sharp noise, sudden jolt, or a pinprick have at times brought one on.[111-113]

It is commonly known that estrogen replacement can predictably relieve vasomotor symptoms in most cases. The idea of replacing estrogen gained popularity in the 1950's and 1960's, when many women in their early 40s were advised to begin estrogen replacement and to continue it for the rest of their lives to prevent aging, depression, fatigue, and anxiety. In 1975, estrogen replacement as a treat-

Table 20.1. **Research Findings on Symptoms Labeled "Menopausal Syndrome"**

Symptoms[59]	Summary of Research
Flushings; "hot flashes"	Definitely correlated with menopause; 40–75% of women studied experienced it to some degree; most prevalent in perimenopausal group[61-67]
Episodes of perspiration and "night sweats"	Definitely correlated with menopause; usually but not always associated with "hot flashes;" 25–40% of women studied experienced it to some degree; most prevalent in perimenopausal group[68]
Difficulties sleeping	Has been reported, although not clearly related to menopause; seems to be associated with "night sweats;" one study showed higher incidence in postmenopausal group and suggested this was a geriatric rather than a perimenopausal problem[69]
Fatigue	Commonly reported in up to 50% of women studied, although not clearly related to menopause[70]
Dizziness; palpitations	Neither clearly related to menopause; possibly an accompaniment of "hot flashes;" reported in less than 50% of women studied[71, 72]
Irritability; nervousness	Neither clearly related to menopause; study reports vary from 9–90% incidence in perimenopausal women studied[71-74]
Headaches; aches in joints, muscles, bones; tingling in extremities	Not clearly related to menopause; usually reported to occur in less than 50% of perimenopausal women studied, although some results suggest higher[75-77]
Depression, feeling "blue"	Not clearly related to menopause; reported to occur in 17–78% of perimenopausal women studied[78-81]

ment for "hot flashes" became a topic of concern, as a link was made between estrogen replacement and endometrial carcinoma.[114, 115] As a result of this discovery, the indiscriminate prescription of estrogen for middle-aged women was discouraged. Closer monitoring of the need for estrogen, type of estrogen, dosage, and duration of therapy was encouraged. In 1979, it was estimated that less than 7 million women were still receiving estrogen replacement, compared with 20 million in 1975.[116]

Currently, estrogen is supplemented with progesterone for treatment of vasomotor disturbances related to menopause, in what has come to be known as hormone replacement therapy (HRT). The addition of progestogens during the last 10 days of the three-week course of estrogen therapy has been shown to decrease the risk of endometrial cancer.[117–119] Progestogens cause the sloughing of the endometrial lining, decreasing the chance of hyperplasia of the endometrium. HRT is usually given cyclically; for four to seven days per month the woman receives neither hormone. The lowest dose of estrogen that can manage the symptoms is given for three weeks, with progestogen added during the last seven to 10 days of the three-week cycle to stimulate withdrawal bleeding. Although this is the current treatment trend, some researchers have questioned whether progesterone actually does decrease risk of endometrial cancer.[120–121] Also, the long-range effects of progesterone use are not clear. Nurses need to stay up to date on current research in their area to help keep their perimenopausal patients informed.

As women become more aware of potential dangers involved in estrogen therapy, they need more information to make informed decisions. Certain other risks of estrogen therapy need to be discussed with the potential user, as well as contraindications for treatment, estrogen side effects, and the need for follow-up monitoring while receiving HRT. Women have the right to weigh the risks of HRT with the benefits it affords them. Currently, there is a definite lack of alternatives to help women deal with "hot flashes" or sweating episodes, if they are troublesome. Voda has written a self-care pamphlet for perimenopausal women, entitled, "Coping with the Menopausal Hot Flash."[122] This pamphlet is useful to nurses who may need to inform or intervene with perimenopausal women. Other than this, no specific nursing interventions have been discussed in the literature.

It is important to remember that "hot flashes" and sweating episodes should not be assumed to be undesirable experiences. Women have occasionally reported that the sensation of warmth accompanying a "hot flash" was pleasurable.[123–124]

Atrophic Changes

The physical signs and sensations associated with degenerative changes of the vagina and surrounding structures are frequently included in any discussion of the menopause. As previously pointed out, these atrophic changes usually do not become pronounced until years after menopause, and so associated sensations are more likely to occur in postmenopausal rather than in perimenopausal women.

Certain tissues of the urinary tract and the reproductive system are particularly responsive to estrogen and undergo certain changes as this hormone decreases. Atrophy of the urinary meatus may contribute to frequency and burning associated with urination. The vaginal walls become thinner and less elastic, and secretions become scanty and less acidic. This increases the likelihood of vaginitis developing. Perimenopausally, vaginal changes may result in itching or irritation with intercourse, owing to decreased lubrication. As the atrophy becomes more evident in the postmenopausal years, cracking of drying, fragile tissue may cause vaginal bleeding and pain for some women. However, these signs are by no means inevitable; there is evidence that as many as 50 per cent of women may experience no more than mild vaginal atrophy for many years after menopause.[125]

The gradual loss of subcutaneous fat of the vulva and thinning of pubic hair also usually do not result in marked changes until the late postmenopausal years.

Oral estrogen replacement does predictably relieve atrophic vaginitis.[126] Estrogen-containing vaginal creams can also be helpful. The use of lubricants can help reduce irritation during intercourse, and regular sexual intercourse is considered a prime measure for maintaining lubrication and the vagina's ability to expand.[127] Unfortunately, the alternatives available to women for dealing with atrophic symptoms are still limited.

Osteoporosis and Heart Disease

It is well documented that the declining estrogen level is related to the development of osteoporosis, but determination of which women may be at risk for osteoporosis is not easy, and mass treatment to prevent osteoporosis is questionable.[128–129] Although long-term therapy with estrogen may be beneficial to some women, more research is needed to establish preventive alternatives, such as exercise and calcium supplementation, as well as better detection of those women who are at particular risk for osteoporosis.

No conclusive evidence has been presented to link estrogen with the onset of heart disease nor estrogen-replacement therapy with the risk of coronary heart disease.[130] There is concern that high dosages of estrogen may be linked to thromboembolic diseases, as they have been with oral contraceptives, but more research is needed to establish this fact.[131]

Future research may indicate that estrogen actually protects women from these conditions. However, nurses should be aware that at present this supposed protection is inadequate reason to advise long-term estrogen therapy for all perimenopausal women. The long-term effects of estrogen therapy may be more harmful than its supposed benefits. Again, the risk and benefits must be meticulously weighed by the informed patient.

THOUGHTS, FEELINGS, CONCERNS: THE WOMAN'S POINT OF VIEW

Nursing's holistic view of humanity dictates that nurses be concerned with the meaning individuals assign to their total situation; therefore, a focus on the woman's interpretation of her perimenopausal experience seems particularly appropriate for nursing. Unfortunately, the thoughts, feelings, and concerns of women experiencing menopause have received the least research attention. However, the studies reviewed here may provide some additional clues to the nature of the perimenopausal experience and to those aspects that, to be dealt with more effectively, might require a nurse's assistance.

In a study by Neugarten and Kraines,[132] healthy women indicated which of 28 menopausal symptoms listed they had experienced. Of the 40 women who reported menstrual irregularities or recent cessation of menstruation, more than 50 per cent had experienced being irritable, nervous, excitable, forgetful, or depressed, or "blue." Less than 50 per cent reported being unable to concentrate, having crying spells, feeling suffocated, worrying about their body, and feeling fright or panic.

Only 12 per cent indicated they worried about having a nervous breakdown.[132]

Another group of researchers[133] studied the attitudes and responses to menopause of 51 Israeli women. The analysis of semistructured psychiatric interviews revealed 10 major themes that the researchers then judged as either gains or losses. Themes of gain were (1) feelings of freedom from menstruation, (2) feelings of freedom from pregnancy, and (3) a nonspecific sense of liberation. Themes of loss were feelings of (1) loss of fertility, (2) loss of health as a consequence of cessation of menstruation, (3) loss of femininity, (4) the onset of old age, (5) danger of emotional disturbances, (6) danger of somatic disturbances, and (7) menopause coming "too soon."

In this study, gain themes were considered positive expressions of attitude toward menopause. Of the perimenopausal women studied, 29 per cent were judged to be more positive than negative toward menopause, 12 per cent equally positive and negative, and 59 per cent more negative than positive.[133] It is recognized that this method of attitude measurement is crude. Also, it should be noted that many of the women studied were from very traditional cultures that viewed the woman's role as that of childbearer. As women's roles continue to change in the United States, we may see past attitudes about menopause change as well.

A survey conducted by the Boston Women's Health Book Collective[8] gathered information from 484 women aged 25 to over 60 years. Of those women who considered themselves to be menopausal or postmenopausal, about two thirds felt neutral or positive about the changes they experienced and only one third felt negative. These results differ from those in Maoz's study,[133] based on Israeli women. The Collective's survey also showed that 90 per cent of the perimenopausal women polled felt either positive or neutral about the loss of their ability to have a child. Sexual desire was reported as unchanged by approximately 50 per cent of the women. The remaining 50 per cent were evenly divided between those who felt increased and those who felt dereased sexual desire. Other reported feelings and reactions included nervousness and irritation, tearfulness, regret or even rage at aging, feeling "over the hill," a sense of failure, concern over changes in sexual desire, happiness for the end of the childbearing years and contraceptive devices, feeling better in the knowledge that fears of going crazy during menopause were unfounded, and thoughts that the changes were not drastic or were milder than they might have been.[134]

Dyer[135] carried out a study of perimenopausal unmarried women who were employed. The responses of six women varied greatly when they were asked to describe the thoughts, feelings, and concerns they were experiencing about menopause that were different from their usual experience before the occurrence of menstrual irregularities. One woman in the study reported no differences in feelings at all. Another woman reported feeling very fortunate that during this menopausal time she felt so good, so healthy, and so unconcerned. She wondered whether depression, "hot flashes," or feelings of discouragement would accompany menopause and, if so, whether she had passed the time when those symptoms might occur.

All of the remaining four women in the study reported changes in their moods or coping abilities. This is in accordance with other studies that report irritable or emotionally labile states. The feelings reported were "crabbiness" and vulnerability; a tendency to overreact or to react by crying; feelings of frustration, anger, and nonacceptance of self for crying behavior; and depression and inability to concentrate.

Three of these four women shared thoughts or concerns related to the effect their mood changes had on relationships with others; they thought others must be perturbed or angry at their moods or behavior, felt a need to compensate for touchiness or a desire to withdraw by making an effort to show caring, and did not want moods to negatively affect others. Other feelings expressed about relationships included new awareness of needing other people and their understanding, feeling anger toward those who failed to be understanding of their moods and behavior, increased need to know that family and friends are close, and feeling a greater capacity to have warm feelings toward others.

Two of the women in the study expressed thoughts related to their sexuality, a theme commonly mentioned in other research. As nuns, these women had made early career commitments that precluded marriage and having children. Both women experienced increased sexual desire or attraction for others at this time and more often wondered what it might have been like to be married and have children. One woman expressed a desire to become more accepting of her own feelings but not to the point that she would dwell on them. The other woman expressed feelings of guilt and fear at sexual arousal and concern over coping with these feelings in the presence of men. One reason sexual feelings at this time were not acceptable to these women might be their religious commitment.

Feelings associated with personal identity were reported by two women in the study: awareness of feeling more capable and more loving, a self-sense that their identities included more than the work they produced, and, in contrast, a loss of identity resulting from decreased work productivity.

Other comments were related specifically to menopause: feeling relief and happiness that menopause is happening, feeling anxious for the complete cessation of periods, wondering why others get so upset about menopause and aging, wondering what is still to come with menopause, looking forward to the pace and pressures of life decreasing, and concern over losing sleep at night as the result of "hot flashes" and sweating episodes.[135]

Little can be concluded from the studies just discussed. Obviously, the thoughts, feelings, and concerns experienced by perimenopausal women vary greatly. Some women find parts of the experience unpleasant or bothersome, while others have positive responses to this life event. What makes the menopausal experience stressful to some women and uneventful to others remains unclear.

WHAT INFLUENCES THE PERIMENOPAUSAL EXPERIENCE?

The influence of a multitude of factors on the nature of the perimenopausal experience has been implied but not adequately supported by research.

Estrogen

The relation of estrogen to atrophic vaginal changes and vasomotor symptoms of "hot flashes" and sweating episodes has previously been discussed. The effect of estrogen on other aspects of the perimenopausal experience is still unknown. Claims have been made that estrogen therapy can relieve all the symptoms and distressing feelings associated with the "menopausal syndrome" and can increase a woman's general sense of well-being.[136, 137] The relief of distressing vasomotor or atrophic symptoms by estrogen could very likely result in an overall increase in peace of mind. However, research as yet does not support a clear relationship between estrogen levels and psychologic states during menopause.[138–141] Science has only begun to learn of the scope of influence hormones exert over our lives. It is possible that the hormonal shifts accompanying menopause will be found to physiologically alter emotional lability.

Emotional Stability

At one time, if a woman experienced severe physical symptoms or became upset perimenopausally it was considered an indication of limited personality and emotional strength.[142, 143] There is some indication that women who experience true depressive reactions and psychoneuroses around menopause are those who have exhibited psychiatric disorders previously.[144, 145] However, no correlation has been shown between severity of physical symptoms and emotional stability.[146]

Marriage and Children

Marital status, particularly when associated with the presence or absence of children in the home, is suggested as a factor affecting the perimenopausal experience. A study by the International Health Foundation[34] concluded that the presence of children in the home "buffered" women from experiencing what they labeled "climacteric complaints," compared with women whose children had left the home.[147] A similar conclusion may be inferred from some findings of Jaszmann, van Lith, and Zaat.[148] A problem arises from responses that may be associated with the departure of the youngest child from the home, sometimes referred to as "the empty nest syndrome."[149] Since most research on menopause has involved married women who have had children, this is a significant confounding factor. Single women in study populations have had fewer complaints than have married women.[150, 151]

Cultural Differences

Research suggests cultural differences in menopausal attitudes and experience, apparently mediated by the prevailing beliefs about women and their role in the family and society.

Dowty and co-workers[151] compared the responses to menopausal changes of 54 Israeli women from three different subcultures. These subcultures represented three points on a hypothetic continuum between traditionalism and modernity. Increased centrality of the childbearing role and a subservient position for women in the family characterized the more traditional subcultures. Diminished importance of the role of wife and mother and increased participation in the labor force were considered characteristics of the more modern subcultures.

Those women of the most traditional subculture studied tended to have a negative view of menopause. They had no regrets over the cessation of menstruation but still entertained thoughts of becoming pregnant yet another time, perhaps reflecting the belief that this was their prime function.

The second group of women represented a subculture that was basically traditional but less so than the first group. These women tended to have a more positive view of menopause, feeling great relief that childbearing years were over. They did, however, express concerns over regular menses ceasing, because they viewed this as a health-giving phenomenon.

The women of the most modern subculture studied tended to have a negative view of menopause. In contrast with the focus of traditional women on the effects of menopause involving childbearing and menstruation, these more modern women were more often concerned with changes related to their personality, family, and social environment.[151]

Weideger[152] discussed at length what she considers to be the American culture's "menstrual taboo" and commented on the impact this may have on the perimenopausal experience. Not only is menopause considered "unspeakable," "mysterious," and generally of little significance to anyone but women, it is also seen as an ending of womanhood rather than the beginning that menarche represents. This investigator feels that the prevailing negative social attitudes prevent all but the most extraordinary woman from experiencing pleasure rather than discomfort from physical sensations that may accompany menopause.[153]

Middle Years Experience

In recent years, increased attention has been given to adult developmental processes and the characteristics of the middle years—the 40s through the 60s.[154] Adjustments are demanded by the many events occurring during this time of life. In order to realize the potential for growth presented by these demands, individuals must make an accurate midlife assessment of where they are and have been so that they can more realistically and meaningfully choose how to spend their remaining personal resources, which, they are now beginning to realize, may be limited.[155, 156] For some individuals this task poses no major difficulty, but for others it constitutes a major crisis.[157]

In her book *Passages*, Sheehy described some interesting characteristics of this midlife assessment.[158] The individuals she studied most often faced this reassessment between the ages of 35 and 45. Those who ignored the opportunities for reassessment during this decade were more likely to experience a crisis in their late 40s or 50s. It is interesting to ponder whether the women who accomplish their midlife assessments between the ages of 35 and 45 are better able to cope with the changes of menopause, which usually occur in the late 40s. Could that be a reason few women find menopause a crisis?

MENOPAUSE IN PERSPECTIVE

Any discussion of menopause must finally put that event into proper perspective as but one aspect of the adult woman's growth and development. The influence of events in the middle years on the perimenopausal experience was mentioned, but, more importantly, nurses and female patients as well must realize that the changes occurring perimenopausally are just a single portion of the challenge to be faced at this midlife stage of development.

It is hoped that nurses will use the information presented here to appropriately modify their knowledge base and their interventions with women who will experience menopause. With increased awareness of the limited knowledge in this area, nurses may be stimulated to increase efforts not only to keep abreast of research findings but also to study the perimenopausal experience themselves, whether as nurse-researchers, nurses working with middle-aged female patients, or nurses experiencing menopause themselves.

References

1. Osofsky, H. J., and Seidenberg, R. Is female menopausal depression inevitable? *Obstetrics and Gynecology*, vol. 36, October 1970, pp. 611–615.
2. Kisch, E. H. *The Sexual Life of Woman in its Physiological and Hygienic Aspect*. New York: Allied Book Company, 1916.
3. Hoskins, R. G. The psychological treatment of the menopause. *Journal of Clinical Endocrinology*, vol. 4, 1944, pp. 605–610.
4. Deutsch, H. *The Psychology of Women: Vol. II Motherhood*. New York: Grune & Stratton, 1945.
5. Kisch, op. cit., p. 344.
6. Kaufert, P. Myth and the menopause. *Sociology of Health and Illness*, vol. 4, July 1982, pp. 141–165.
7. Ibid.
8. Boston Women's Health Book Collective. *Our Bodies, Ourselves: A Book by and for Women*, ed. 2. New York: Simon and Schuster, 1979.
9. Kisch, op. cit., p. 344.
10. Deutsch, op. cit.
11. Novak, E. R., Jones, G. S., and Jones, H. W. Management of the menopause. In *Novak's Textbook of Gynecology*, 8th ed. Baltimore: Williams & Wilkins, 1970.
12. Martin, L. L. *Health Care of Women*. Philadelphia: J. B. Lippincott, 1978.
13. Neugarten, B. L., and Kraines, R. J. Menopausal symptoms in women of various ages. *Psychosomatic Medicine*, vol. 27, 1965, pp. 266–273.
14. Kupperman, H. S., Wetchler, B. B., and Blatt, M. H. G. Contemporary therapy of the menopausal syndrome. *Journal of the American Medical Association*, vol. 171, November 1959, pp. 1627–1637.
15. Timiras, P. S., and Meisami, E. Changes in gonadal function. *In* Timiras, P. S. (ed.) *Developmental Physiology and Aging*. New York: MacMillan, 1972.
16. Crawford, M. P., and Hooper, D. Menopause, ageing, and family. *Social Science and Medicine*, vol. 7, 1973, pp. 469–482.
17. Flint, M. The menopause: Reward or punishment. *Psychosomatics*, vol. 16, 1975, pp. 161–163.
18. Novak et al., op. cit.
19. Tucker, S. J. The menopause: How much soma and how much psyche? *Journal of Obstetrics and Gynecological Nursing*, vol. 6, September/October 1977, pp. 40–48.
20. McGuire, L. S., and Sorley, A. K. Understanding and preventing the menopausal crisis. *Nurse Practitioner*, July/August 1978, pp. 15–18.
21. Kupperman, Wetchler, and Blatt, op. cit.
22. Neugarten and Kraines, op. cit.
23. Hannan, J. H. *The Flushings of the Menopause*. London: Bailliere, Tindall & Cox, 1927.
24. Molnar, G. W. Body temperatures during menopausal hot flashes. *Journal of Applied Physiology*, vol. 3, March 1975, pp. 499–503.
25. Timiras and Meisami, op. cit.
26. Treloar, A. E. Menarche, menopause, and intervening fecundability. *Human Biology*, vol. 46, February 1974, pp. 89–107.
27. Timiras and Meisami, op. cit.
28. Jaszmann, L., van Lith, N. D., and Zaat, J. C. A. The perimenopausal symptoms. *Medical and Gynaecologic Sociology*, vol. 4, 1969, pp. 268–277.
29. Jaszmann, L. Epidemiology of climacteric and post-climacteric complaints. *Frontiers of Hormone Research*, vol. 2, 1973, pp. 22–34.
30. van Keep, P. A., and Kellerhals, J. The aging woman. *Frontiers of Hormone Research*, vol. 2, 1973, pp. 160–173.
31. Jaszmann, van Lith, and Zaat, op. cit.
32. Jaszmann, op. cit.
33. van Keep and Kellerhals, op. cit.
34. Kellerhals, P. A. *The Mature Woman: A First Analysis of a Psychosocial Study of Chronological and Menstrual Ageing*. Geneva: International Health Foundation, 1973.
35. Jaszmann, van Lith, and Zaat, op. cit.
36. Ibid.
37. Dyer, R. A. M. A descriptive study of the nature of the subjective perimenopausal experience of single women. Unpublished paper, University of Minnesota, 1977.
38. Treloar, A. E., op. cit.

39. McKinlay, S., Jefferys, M., and Thompson, B. An investigation of the age at menopause. *Journal of Biosocial Science*, vol. 4, 1972, pp. 161–173.

40. Botella-Llusia, Jose. *Endocrinology of Woman*. Philadelphia: W. B. Saunders, 1973.

41. Sharman, A. The menopause. *In* Zuckerman, S. (ed.) *The Ovary*, vol. 1. New York: Academic Press, 1962, p. 539.

42. Curtis, L. R. *The Menopause*. Bristol, TN: S. E. Massengill Company, 1969.

43. Timiras and Meisami, op. cit.

44. Grodin, J. M., Siiteri, P. K., and MacDonald, P. C. Source of estrogen production in postmenopausal women. *Journal of Clinical Endocrinology and Metabolism*, vol. 36, 1973, pp. 207–214.

45. Siiteri, P. K., and MacDonald, P. C. Role of extraglandular estrogen in human endocrinology. *In* Greep, R. O., and Astwood, E. B. (eds.) *Handbook of Physiology*. Section 7, Vol. II, Pt. 1. American Physiologic Society. Baltimore: Williams and Wilkins, 1973.

46. Chakravarti, S., Collins, W. P., Forecast, J. D., et al. Hormonal profiles after the menopause. *British Medical Journal*, vol. 2, October 2, 1976, pp. 784–787.

47. McKinlay, S. M., and McKinlay, J. B. Selected studies of the menopause. *Journal of Biosocial Science*, vol. 5, October 1973, pp. 533–555.

48. Greenhill, M. H. A psychosomatic evaluation of the psychiatric and endocrinological factors in menopause. *Southern Medical Journal*, vol. 39, October 1946, pp. 787–793.

49. Crawford, M. H., and Hooper, D. Menopause, ageing and family. *Social Science and Medicine*, vol. 7, 1973, pp. 469–482.

50. Donovan, J. C. The menopausal syndrome: A study of case histories. *American Journal of Obstetrics and Gynecology*, vol. 62, December 1951, pp. 1281–1291.

51. Jaszmann, van Lith, and Zaat, op. cit.

52. Donovan, J. C. An investigation of the menopause in one thousand women. *Lancet*, vol. 1, pp. 106–108.

53. Thompson, B., Hart, S. A., and Durno, D. Menopausal age and symptomatology in general practice. *Journal of Biosocial Science*, vol. 5, 1973, pp. 71–82.

54. Feeley, E., and Pyne, H. The menopause: Facts and misconceptions. *Nursing Forum*, vol. 14, 1975, pp. 74–86.

55. Jaszmann, van Lith, and Zaat, op. cit.

56. Crawford and Hooper, op. cit.

57. Donovan, Investigation of menopause, op. cit.

58. Thompson, Hart, and Durno, op. cit.

59. Neugarten and Kraines, op. cit.

60. Donovan, Investigation of menopause, op. cit.

61. Kupperman, Wetchler, and Blatt, op. cit.

62. Neugarten and Kraines, op. cit.

63. Jaszmann, van Lith, and Zaat, op. cit.

64. Donovan, Investigation of menopause, op. cit.

65. Thompson, Hart, and Durno, op. cit.

66. Feeley and Pyne, op. cit.

67. Utian, W. H. The true clinical features of postmenopause and oophorectomy, and their response to oestrogen therapy. *South African Medical Journal*, vol. 46, June 3, 1972, pp. 732–737.

68. Thompson, Hart and Durno, op. cit.

69. Jaszmann, op. cit.

70. Jaszmann, van Lith, and Zaat, op. cit.

71. Neugarten and Kraines, op. cit.

72. Jaszmann, van Lith, and Zaat, op. cit.

73. Crawford and Hooper, op. cit.

74. Donovan, Investigation of menopause, op. cit.

75. Neugarten and Kraines, op. cit.

76. Jaszmann, van Lith, and Zaat, op. cit.

77. Donovan, Investigation of menopause, op. cit.

78. Neugarten and Kraines, op. cit.

79. Jaszmann, van Lith, and Zaat, op. cit.

80. Crawford and Hooper, op. cit.

81. Thompson, Hart, and Durno, op. cit.

82. Neugarten and Kraines, op. cit.

83. Jaszmann, van Lith, and Zaat, op. cit.

84. Dyer, op. cit.

85. Donovan, Investigation of menopause, op. cit.

86. Thompson, Hart, and Durno, op. cit.

87. Feely and Pyne, op. cit.

88. Stern, K., and Prados, M. Personality studies in menopausal women. *American Journal of Psychiatry*, vol. 103, 1946, pp. 358–368.

89. Neugarten and Kraines, op. cit.

90. Jaszmann, van Lith, and Zaat, op. cit.

91. Donovan, Investigation of menopause, op. cit.

92. Thompson, Hart, and Durno, op. cit.

93. Feely and Pyne, op. cit.

94. Berger, P. C., and Norsigian, J. Menopause. *In* Boston Women's Health Book Collective *Our Bodies, Our Selves*, ed. 2. New York: Simon and Schuster, 1976.

95. Kisch, op. cit.

96. Hannan, op. cit.

97. Weideger, Paula. *Menstruation and Menopause: The Physiology and Psychology, the Myth and the Reality*. New York: Alfred A. Knopf, 1976.

98. Thompson, Hart, and Durno, op. cit.

99. Dyer, op. cit.

100. Lincoln, Miriam. *You'll Live Through It: Facts About the Menopause*. New York: Harper and Row, 1961.

101. Rogers, J. The menopause. *New England Journal of Medicine*, vol. 254, April 12, 1956, pp. 697–704.

102. Voda, A. M. Coping with the menopausal hot flash. *Patient Counseling and Health Education*, vol. 4, 1982, p. 81.

103. Hannan, op. cit.

104. Molnar, op. cit.

105. Dyer, op. cit.

106. Rogers, op. cit.

107. Molnar, op. cit.

108. Dyer, op. cit.

109. Voda, op. cit.

110. Molnar, op. cit.

111. Ibid.

112. Hannan, op. cit.

113. Dyer, op. cit.

114. Ziel, H. K., and Finkle, W. D. Increased risk of endometrial carcinoma among users of conjugated estrogens. *New England Journal of Medicine*, vol. 293, 1975, pp. 1167–1170.

115. Smith, D., Prentice, R., Thompson, D., and Herrman, W. Association of exogenous estrogen and endometrial carcinoma. *New England Journal of Medicine*, vol. 293, 1975, p. 1164.

116. Elliot, J. Little consensus on prescribing of estrogens for postmenopausal women. *Journal of the American Medical Association*, vol. 242, 1979, p. 1951.

117. Notelovitz, M. When and how to use estrogen therapy in women over 60. *Geriatrics*, vol. 35, 1980, p. 113.

118. King, R. J. Effect of estrogen and progestin treatment on endometria from postmenopausal women. *Cancer Research*, vol. 39, 1979, p. 1094.

119. Schiff, I., Tulchinsky, D., Cramer. D., et al. Oral

medroxyprogesterone in the treatment of postmenopausal symptoms. *Journal of the American Medical Association*, vol. 244, 1980, pp. 1443–1445.

120. Elliot, op. cit.
121. Landau, R. L. What you should know about estrogens. *Journal of the American Medical Association*, vol. 241, 1979, p. 47.
122. Voda, op. cit.
123. Hannan, op. cit.
124. Weideger, op. cit.
125. Botella-Llusia, J., and van Keep, P. A. Vaginal cytology in the postmenopause: A study into some correlates. *Acta Cytologica*, vol. 21, January-February 1977, pp. 18–21.
126. Utian, op. cit.
127. Dresen, S. E. The sexually active middle adult. *American Journal of Nursing*, vol. 75, June 1975, pp. 1001–1005.
128. Gorrie, T. Postmenopausal osteoporosis. *Journal of Obstetrics and Gynecological Nursing*, vol. 11, 1982, pp. 214–219.
129. Lindsay, R., Hart, D. M., Aitken, J. M., et al. Longterm prevention of postmenopausal osteoporosis by estrogen: Evidence for an increased bone mass after delayed onset of estrogen treatment. *Lancet*, vol. 1, 1976, pp. 1038–1041.
130. Mosher, B., and Whelan, E. Postmenopausal estrogen therapy: A review. *Obstetrics and Gynecology Survey*, vol. 36, 1981, pp. 467–475.
131. Tartaglione, T. A., Doering, P. L., Araujo, O. E., et al. Estrogen Therapy in postmenopausal women. *U.S. Pharmacist*, vol. 6, 1981, pp. 62, 64, 66, 68, 70–71.
132. Neugarten and Kraines, op. cit.
133. Maoz, B., et al. Female attitudes to menopause. *Social Psychiatry*, vol. 5, 1970, pp. 35–40.
134. Berger and Norsigian, op. cit.
135. Dyer, op. cit.
136. Curtis, op. cit.
137. Achte, K. Menopause from the psychiatrist's point of view. *Acta Obstetrica et Gynecologica Scandinavica*, vol. 49, 1970, pp. 3–17.
138. Greenhill, op. cit.
139. Utian, op. cit.
140. Stern and Prados, op. cit.
141. Rogers, op. cit.
142. Deutsch, op. cit.
143. Achte, op. cit.
144. Greenhill, op. cit.
145. Stern and Prados, op. cit.
146. Ibid.
147. van Keep and Kellerhals, op. cit.
148. Jaszmann, van Lith, and Zaat, op. cit.
149. Lowenthal, M. F., and Chiriboga, D. Transition to the empty nest. *Archives of General Psychiatry*, vol. 26, January 1972, pp. 8–14.
150. Jaszmann, van Lith, and Zaat, op. cit.
151. Dowty, N., Maoz, B., Antonovsky, A., et al. Climacterium in three cultural contexts. *Tropical and Geographical Medicine*, vol. 22, 1970, pp. 77–86.
152. Weideger, op. cit.
153. Diekelmann, N., and Galloway, K. A time of change. *American Journal of Nursing*, vol. 75, June 1975, pp. 994–996.
154. Sheehy, Gail. *Passages*. New York: E. P. Dutton & Co., 1976.
155. Greenleigh, L. Facing the challenge of changes in middle age. *Geriatrics*, vol. 29, November 1974, pp. 61–68.
156. Sheehy, op. cit.
157. Peplau, H. Mid-life crises. *American Journal of Nursing*, vol. 75, October 1975, pp. 1761–1765.
158. Sheehy, op. cit.

21

DIVORCE AND DEPRESSION IN WOMEN

VERONA C. GORDON

Attitudes are changing toward divorce; and research literature reviews women's reactions to divorce. The impact of divorce on women under various conditions such as poverty and old age is stressed by author Verona Gordon. The interventions of counseling and the role of nursing are identified.

Divorce has become a common rather than a rare event in Western society. According to the *Los Angeles Times*,[1] the United States divorce rate has increased 96 per cent in the last decade. Lambert and Lambert[2] state that in this nation, which leads the world in divorce, it is found that the largest proportion of divorce occurs among childless couples and that the peak period (95 per cent) is in the second year of marriage. Although there may be a greater acceptance of this growing social problem in America, there is increasing evidence of the high stress divorce causes among couples and that children are often the innocent victims of the process.

Divorce is one of the most traumatic crises a family may face . . . and nursing is long overdue in taking its share of responsibilities in recognizing the powerful impact of change that occurs within divorced families.[3]

The purpose of this chapter is to reveal to nurses more information about divorce in our society and its significant effect on the women involved. The growing role of the nurse as a counselor is addressed.

CHANGING ATTITUDES

According to Lytle,[4] the traditional marriage relationship of the past is "out" in America and a relationship of greater convenience to both parties is "in," as women begin to assert their rights and make their wishes known. The institution of marriage has long been in need of redefinition: marriages are no longer expected to endure for a lifetime; permanency in relationships is no longer a value held by society at large; men and women are groping for alternatives to marriage. Equality, freedom, flexibility, privacy, companionship, absence of dominance or submission, and, most of all, growth are used to describe the "utopian" partnership in marriage that individuals today are seeking; the marital role of the female of the past has been outgrown.[4]

"Divorces are etching a deeper mark on the social landscape of America," commented Cherlin,[5] a sociologist at Johns Hopkins University, in 1981. With his work on the changing patterns in marriage, divorce, and remarriage, he speculates that family life will never revert to previous patterns of the "traditional" marriage. Some of his respected, futuristic statistics are: One out of two recent marriages are projected to end in divorce; one out of six women will still be unmarried by age 30; one third of all adults can expect to find themselves in a remarriage following a divorce; and the majority of children alive today will probably witness the disruption of either their parents' marriage or their own marriage by divorce.

Cherlin's analysis of the marital trends of parents during the 1950s is interesting. He felt that that generation was a historic oddity; he felt that couples in the 1950s married too young, had few divorces, and had too many children. He added that these parents were shaped by the traumas of the Great Depression and World War II. On the other hand, he believes that the current generation is marrying too late, divorcing too much, and having too few children. The reasons for this, according to Cherlin, are that economic prospects for young adults today are not as good as they were for their parents and that the attitude toward divorce in recent years is becoming more positive. He believes that the main reason for current high trends for divorce is because many women are in the workforce. He states, "Widening job opportunities for women allow couples to separate who are unhappy with their marriage for other reasons." He adds that although women raising children by themselves do have a hard time, most of these women remarry, and that although divorce does cause an immediate emotional upheaval in children, Cherlin has found that long-term effects on children have not been documented. Cherlin maintains that despite all of the recent rapid change, the American family is still strong and valued.[5]

Today, there is a greater acceptance of the possibility of divorce; because of this acceptance, Aguilera and Messick[6] feel divorced persons have lost some of the feelings of failure and guilt that were formerly associated with it. The higher divorce rate may reflect new values placed on marriage. Marriage is no longer accepted as an "endurance race" that is doggedly maintained for the sake of the children. The current demands are for a "good marriage," one that meets the needs of the individuals involved. Even from the point of view of the children, who seemingly pay the highest price for marital failure, divorce may in certain circumstances create fewer psychologic problems if the children are not used as pawns by the separating parents. However, since divorce rates are so high and many marriages are centers of friction and unhappiness, something must be lacking in the preparation for marriage. No event in life of equal importance is viewed with so little realism, and marriage seems to come about with little or no preparation.[6]

It has been pointed out in an interesting article that women tend to be the "scapegoats," or victims, of divorce in American society. Brandwein and colleagues[7] state:

Related to the scarcity of studies on clients with stress of divorce is the assumption throughout the literature that the female-headed single parent family is deviant and pathological. Such families are called "broken," "disorganized," or "disintegrated," rather than recognized as widespread, viable alternative family forms . . . this is stigmatization. Stigma is ascribed to divorced and separated women for their presumed inability to keep their men. The societal myth of the "gay divorcée" out to seduce other women's husbands leads to social ostracism of the divorced woman and her family.[7]

RESEARCH STUDIES ON STRESS OF DIVORCE

Despair, hopelessness, feelings of worthlessness, difficulty in sleeping and eating, loss of energy, and thoughts of death are some of the painful symptoms of depression described by women going through the process of divorce. Bloom[8] reported that there is a growing body of evidence supporting the idea that marital disruption causes extreme stress. Without a single exception, admission rates into psychiatric facilities are the lowest among the married, intermediate among the widowed and never married adults, and highest among the divorced and separated; the divorced woman in the high-risk category is a concern for mental health professionals.[8]

Carter's descriptive research[9] (which included 13 divorced white women) found that even when women displayed assertive behavior in attempting to adjust to divorce, they felt anxiety, anger, loneliness, and depression. Carter wrote that often the woman who assumed the traditional role of dependency, which is expected of wives, was angry at herself for still allowing her ex-spouse to control their relationship as divorced people. She also found that wives need to go through a grieving process before they can accept the loss of their married role. The passive woman who has relied exclusively on her husband (for economic support, social status, living arrangements) finds she is physically and emotionally drained in trying to cope alone with these problems, often while facing the additional trauma of job-hunting. Carter learned that the assertive woman may fantasize about a carefree, single lifestyle but that, in reality, many women discover in this lifestyle a loneliness more terrible than anxiety.[9] Other problems according to Hunt[10] are that the woman's family and friends are not quite sure whether they should be sympathetic or jealous of the divorcee's freedom, while at the same time they question her failure or inadequacy. Male friends may act fatherly or seductive, whereas married female friends may be threatened by the availability she represents.[10] Perhaps the most difficult transition for the newly divorced woman is the necessary detachment from the personality and influence of the former spouse. The woman often faces a personal identity crisis and is forced to deal with issues of who she is and where she is going in life.

That the stress of divorce can be the origin of physical problems was found by Forrest[11] when she examined the relationship between adjustment to marital separation and divorce, and psychosomatic complaints. Examples given of psychosomatic disturbances that divorced women often complain of are headaches, ulcers, bronchial asthma, and high blood pressure.[11] Divorce ranks as the second most stressful life event requiring significant adjustments on the well-known instrument of Rahe and co-workers[12] and of Holmes and Masuda.[13] Divorce was preceded on the test only by the death of a spouse. In three classic studies of divorce cited by Forrest,[14] Goode reported that over 60 per cent of 425 respondents showed various kinds of personal disorganization during the divorce process (sleeping difficulties, greater feelings of loneliness, poorer health); Nager, Chiriboga, and Cutler in their study of 277 individuals in the divorce process reported disturbances in work, sleep, and health status, with increasing use of alcohol and smoking; and Chester in his study of 150 women applying for divorce reported a majority experiencing a deterioration in health. Forrest's study of 205 individuals either in the process of divorce or divorced showed that an increase in the number of psychosomatic complaints since separation was found to be significantly related to adjustment to marital separation.[14]

Hackney and Ribordy[15] studied the emotional reactions of individuals to the stress of divorce. Their research included 74 males and females in North Dakota representing couples happily married, undergoing marriage counseling, and in the process of divorce, as well as those divorced at least 6 months, but not more than 12 months. They found that the people in the divorcing group had the highest level of depression, with feelings of anxiety and hostility. During the most traumatic period of prolonged stress (counseling to actual divorce), feelings of isolation, alienation, and loneliness, boredom, self-doubt, anger, and vague bodily complaints were reported. The investigators established that by the 6- to 12-month postdivorce period, many of these feelings had diminished greatly as the individual readjusted, getting on with his or her new life.[15]

DIVORCE AND ROLE TRANSITION

Precipitating factors causing the rapid rise in divorce rates in America have been numerous. Among these are early marriages (15 to 19 years of age), mixed racial or religious marriages, dissimilar backgrounds, and unhappy parental marriages, as well as the progress of industrialism and prosperity of income that may result in the independence of marriage partners and lack of their need to rely on each other. Regardless of these reasons, there is growing concern that often couples do not understand the total legal dissolution of their marriage bonds, the complete final severance of all ties between the marital partners. That divorce poses a crisis when one goes through the initial shock, feelings of ambivalence, and disorganization, along with a period of recovery and reorganization to begin anew, is well documented. However, current research studies are focusing on the definite role transitions women need to be aware of during the tremendous changes occurring when the woman "takes over" as head of the family.

Kaseman states, "Like every other segment of our society, the family is in a state of transition. Institutional marriage over the last two decades has undergone radical changes—more and more families are headed by one parent and this single parent family is typically headed by females."[16] Most of the individuals seen by Kaseman were women of different cultural backgrounds and of moderate to low socioeconomic backgrounds, with an eleventh- to twelfth-grade educational level. They ranged in age from 19 to 35 years, and the number of children they had varied. As might be expected, most of these women found a need to be "super-mothers" or "super-women." They were particularly concerned with proving that they could "take care of everything." They felt guilty about depriving the children of their father, and wondered if divorce had been a good decision. Frequently, these mothers were so caught up with plans for the children and with the children's feelings that their own feelings were given low priority.

A common problem was that of sexual desire. Many women said that they felt guilty about their need for male companionship and sexual relationships. Some admitted feeling helpless and missing the identity associated with their husband's status. There was some ambivalence toward relationships with men. Casual sex brought on feelings of anger, depression, and low self-esteem. Many of the women gained weight and tended to be unkempt. By gaining weight and neglecting their appearance, they were able to avoid the issue of a male-female relationship.

The anger these women experienced often prevented or covered up their feelings of loss, which arose later. Most women needed additional support to "work through" their loss before they were able to discuss the implications of the divorce with the children. Many women's thoughts were unclear as to why the divorce took place and wondered whether they could have prevented it, which led to self-blame. They felt isolated and lonely and stated that their greatest need was for companionship. They felt left out of society, being neither single nor married but in transition. For many, the children were viewed as the remnants of the marriage, either positively or negatively, depending on the woman's view of the marriage.

Kohen's research,[17] involving 30 divorced or separated mothers in Boston, focused on role transition and changes reported by the women when accepting full responsibility as family head. Kohen learned that divorced mothers were not trained in the skills necessary for their new role as head of the family. In the study, 70 per cent of the participants recalled that their teenage ideas of marriage were to be married, have children, and walk hand-in-hand in love, as in the movies. Leaving marriage and becoming a divorced mother, they found, involved a major change. During the initial postdivorce period, these women defined themselves as estranged, displaced, and depersonalized. Family and friends appeared uncomfortable and unaccepting of their situation. The women were not seen as the family authority by relatives. The stereotype of the divorced woman was not flattering: they reported situations in which they were treated as irresponsible, incapable, childlike, and sexually promiscuous. Tied to the problems of social support were problems of material support; the mothers experienced a sudden drop of over one half of their income. Getting or keeping jobs consistent with their family responsibilities was a real factor in their loss of income.

The women in the study had endless problems getting housing, credit, repair service, and so forth. They reported that they felt inadequate, tended to isolate themselves, and

questioned their ability to head the family. It became clear to them that heading a family requires mastery, control, and assertiveness—skills and attitudes that were neither consciously taught nor valued for women, before or after the divorce.[17]

Two factors became apparent in the study that seemed to make a difference regarding these women's ability to handle this new "head of family" situation. One was the degree to which they could maintain their previous life—that is, to bring with them and "build on" aspects of responsibility of their former married life. The other was whether they wanted to leave the marriage or had been forced out of it (for example, by a violent or alcoholic husband).

Three factors appeared to be the index of stability in these female-headed families: (1) occupational security; could the woman depend on continuing her employment or staying home as the full-time housekeeper? (2) financial regularity; could she rely on her current source of income? and (3) absence of additional chronic family difficulties such as health problems, demands from ex-husbands, family, or manipulation (for example, in return for a loan, a parent may feel free to interfere or to run the life of a divorced daughter).

In summary, current research does report an apparent increase in symptoms of depression in the divorced woman and evidence of high, continuous growth of nontraditional female-headed families in this era of serious economic problems. It is apparent that this family in extreme role transition will be in great need of understanding and support by all health professionals.

RESEARCH STUDIES ON WOMEN'S REACTIONS TO DIVORCE

The emotional isolation felt by the woman in divorce implies the trauma of loneliness. Divorce counselors Wabrek and associates[18] in 1980 found that often the problem of loneliness is the first one that the woman will want to discuss. Her feeling of being "alone" is also one of grief. Her anger toward her spouse for the hurt and pain she has endured must be dissipated before she can move on to a more positive relationship. Her denial of her loss and her continued need for love, affection, and sexual involvement need to be recognized. Lambert and Lambert felt that the divorced elderly person may show the highest rate of loneliness with depression.[19] Frieda Fromm-

Reichmann, psychoanalyst, believed the most common problem shared by distressed people was loneliness. In her sensitivity and gentleness in describing the depressed, she states "Loneliness is almost unbearable . . . for that reason few can tolerate recalling periods of their lives when they were very lonely."[19a] H. S. Sullivan, the distinguished sociologist, agreed, writing that the "toneless quality of loneliness can in itself be more terrible than anxiety . . . and few people can empathize with people who are lonely because it is so threatening a state to be in."[20]

Guilt is another reaction women have felt as a result of still-prevailing societal attitudes that divorce is a wrongful act and the expectation that women should maintain marriage at all costs. Peterson's research of 170 people recently granted divorces investigated the relationship between guilt and resolution of the divorce crisis.[21] That religiosity and the act of initiating the divorce were significant related to guilt was not surprising; however, a most important result of the study was the conclusion that the level of guilt is not as crucial in resolving the divorce crisis as the person's ability to respond and take action in one's own behalf.

The preponderance of depression among women compared to that among men (2:1) was documented by Weissman and Klerman in 1977.[22] At every age in every country, women are more likely than men to experience depression, yet we know little about the stresses in women's lives and the impact of stress on women's health. Stress research has been dominated by studies of men, and the findings and theories developed from such studies have been improperly generalized to women. It is evident that men and women respond differently to the same stressful events. Furthermore, stress research has ignored social changes, such as those in women's roles, while much marital therapy has been designed to help women adjust to existing social roles and demands. Feminist therapy (which attributes women's pathology primarily to social and external rather than personal sources) can be a force for changing social roles—to the extent that depression is a disease of women's powerlessness and hopelessness. Guttentag and colleagues[23] in 1980 wrote that political efforts to broaden women's options and their ability to control their own lives should aid the cause of women's mental health.

The relationship of depression to two life events, divorce and bereavement, was studied by Briscoe and Smith.[24] These investigators' study of 128 individuals included three groups of depressed persons: (1) hospitalized patients with no history of stress, (2) recent widows and widowers, and (3) recently divorced men and women. Matching age and sex, the divorced depressed group significantly more often reported somatic complaints (45 per cent versus 10 per cent), self-pity (45 per cent versus 8 per cent), blaming others (65 per cent versus 29 per cent), and death wishes (58 per cent versus 7 per cent) than did the hospitalized depressed group. The divorced individuals were a younger population than the widows and widowers. This was probably due to the fact that divorce is a phenomenon of the young, whereas death of spouse occurs more frequently in the older segment of the population. However, it was found that even though they were younger, they had had significantly more episodes of depression (47 per cent versus 5 per cent) than had the bereaved depressed persons.[24] Although evidence is far from conclusive, it appeared that among divorced depressed persons there was a high incidence of chronic depression and alcoholism in their families. The study points out the need for awareness that the death of a spouse very likely causes the depressive syndrome of bereavement, whereas divorce could either cause *or* result from depression.

An earlier study by these two investigators[25] revealed that divorce may well play a role as a precipitating factor in depression. They found that of the 45 divorced depressed persons in their study (female to male ratio, 2:1), 96 per cent had had an episode of depression of more than a month's duration at the time of their divorce, and 47 per cent of these people had suffered depression prior to their marital disruption. The women most frequently had episodes of depression associated with their separation, whereas men were more frequently depressed at the time of their divorce.

Maggie Scarf[26] identifies clearly the difference between depression in women and depression in men. She writes that the depressed woman is someone who has lost someone significant and who has feelings of hopelessness and worthlessness. *Attachments* are the critical variable to nonworking, working, and highly professional women; what matters most to them is their highly invested and important loving attachments. Women are supposed to be warmer, more expressive, and more eager to relate on a personal level; to have failed in those relationships is equated with failing in everything. It is around "attachment issues," more than any other issues, that depressive episodes in women tend to emerge. Men do not usually become depressed over the rupture of emotional bonds; their depression has more to do with work issues, their status and success difficulties, with "making it out there" in the world at large. Although career issues may be important to women, these issues do not set the stage for severe depression. For men, in contrast, depression has much to do with their perceived failure to live up to self-expectations in their life work.

Women continue to be diagnosed at a very high rate as mentally ill, especially psychoneurotic. McGrory[27] writes that as a nurse she believes these statements to be true. Focusing on the "sexist trap" women may be in, caused by traditional sex role stereotypes, McGrory writes: "Both men and women are conditioned from childhood to develop attitudes and behave in a manner befitting their sex. For women this is particularly destructive in that for a woman locked into the feminine stereotype of passivity, dependence and non-achieving, a feeling of low self-esteem develops and ultimately has its effect on her mental health."[27] McGrory cites sociologists Gove and Tudor on why women who do not work outside the home may become mentally ill: (1) Women in contrast to men have only one major source of societal gratification—their families—whereas men have both work and family. If a woman is unhappy in the family situation, she has no other source of fulfillment. (2) Women often find housework and raising children frustrating, as some of the tasks do not require a great deal of skill and are given low prestige. (3) The housewife role is unstructured, invisible, and sometimes boring. (4) Married women in the job market often suffer from fatigue. They hold jobs below their educational preparation and abilities, and they carry a triple load of responsibility of their children, their housework, and their jobs. (5) The high expectations of women (to be fulfilled wives, "super" mothers, and achieving employees) create problems.

Studies have found that sex role stereotyping is pervasive in our society in general and occurs within the mental health professional community as well. One study of this issue has found sex role stereotyping to be a more serious problem with male therapists who have described the female patient as dependent, submissive, highly emotional, and less able to make important decisions than men.[28] This researcher also found that frequently the goal of therapy is to retain women's compliance with the expected feminine role. Female therapists tend to have more understanding attitudes toward female patients.[29] Consistent with the findings of Kjervik and Palta,[30] psychiatric nurses were identified as the professional group adhering to the fewest traditional sex role stereotypic attitudes. Repeatedly, traditional treatment approaches reinforce the passivity and negative self-image of women, thus only perpetuating the problem, rather than resolving the depression.[31]

McGrory's[32] supportive suggestions are that women be encouraged to learn more about their bodies, be more assertive against media advertising, and be more vocal about their needs; and that psychotherapists be more sensitive to what it means to be a woman in a male-dominated society, be more active as agents of social change by supporting legislature, and encourage training of more female therapists. McGrory writes: "Today mental health care of women needs much improvement. Women can and should make a difference in the care they receive."[32]

Divorce and the Impoverished Woman

One of the most alarming findings in the four-year Stress and Families Project at Harvard[33] was the high rate of use of mental health facilities by impoverished women who headed families without spouses. These formerly married, poorly educated women and their children appeared to be at particular risk for mental illness. Interviews conducted in the Boston area revealed that the worsening economic situation, the social isolation, and impairment of their maternal role functioning in the difficult life circumstances appeared to result in depression. Neither the women's ex-husbands nor their boyfriends were a sure protection against depression. Half of the women in the study who shared a household with a man experienced about as much depression as the women living alone with their children. Although some women lived with men who provided financial and emotional support, others reported little support from their partners, and several reported severe beatings.

A most relevant article has been written by Ehrenreich and Stallard entitled "The Nouveau Poor" (new poor). These single women, middle class by birth, are now raising their children alone through a tenuous combination of welfare, child support, and native ingenuity in many American cities. These authors report that the fastest-growing segment of the female poor are single women (divorced or never married) raising children on their own. Between 1978 and 1980, the number of these women moving into poverty rose to 150,000 per year. All in all, the number of women heading families with children increased by 81 per cent during the 1970s. Most women are making a valiant effort to support themselves before turning to welfare. Their former husbands cannot be depended on. Departed fathers (40 per cent) contribute nothing to their children's support, and the average payment provided by the 60 per cent who do contribute is less than $2000 a year.

For women, jobs are no sure antidote to poverty. The majority of employed American women work in poor-paying "service" jobs (clerical, waitresses, nurses aides, sales). The reality is that whether through divorce, desertion, or death, an estimated 85 per cent of American women can expect to have to support themselves and their children at some time in their lives. These deep-seated injustices in a white male–dominated society crucially need a feminist vision for a just and economically viable reality is long overdue.[34]

Divorce and the Middle-Aged Woman

An unusual and extremely interesting paper has been written by Ruth Moulton,[35] a psychoanalyst in New York, about five lonely professional women, aged 35 to 45, who decided to divorce because their husbands seemed to become too dependent on them, holding them back from the freedom found in their careers. Studied also were five divorced men, ages 40 to 55, patients of Dr. Moulton's husband, who courted and had affairs with women but who were reluctant to remarry. Moulton's research is enlightening as well as relevant. She begins her article explaining that the causes of divorce in both middle adulthood and early adulthood are considerably different. Midlife is defined as a time when one realizes the finiteness of one's own time, the waning of physical powers, and the certainty of one's death. It is a time of loss, as in the maturation and departure of children; the deaths of parents, friends, and spouses; and the sense of a decrease in future opportunities unless action

is taken immediately while there is still time. The person is apt to reappraise life in terms of success in parenting, in finding sexual satisfaction, and in professional attainment. As people re-evaluate their lives and fail to find satisfaction and fulfillment, they often try to avoid disappointment and depression by making changes in job, marital status, or lifestyle. This may result in turmoil and sudden shifts, as occur in divorce.

Until the last decade, being married and having children was assumed by most people to be the most desirable, normal lifestyle. Marriage has always been considered the best solution for loneliness as well as the most practical way to raise and protect the next generation. Women felt a strong need for marriage as their main source of security, both financially and socially. Divorce was formerly seen as a disgrace and a failure for the wife.[35]

Moulton believes the greatest change in America has been the increase in women working in their middle years. In the midlife period, when family demands decrease and women are prone to depression, it is useful for them to have human contact and satisfactions outside the home. Moulton became aware of a new aspect of the problems these working women had as she studied in detail five women who were born in the 1920s and 1930s.[35] These women did not grow up with the goals of female autonomy and self-sufficiency. They were molded in the traditional pattern when girls were raised to be sweet, compliant, nurturing, supportive figures for men's pleasure. However, as older married professional women became more financially independent, they saw divorce as an emancipation from domesticity; they could earn their own way and wanted a new chance for autonomy. They also expected to find new and more exciting men. Those seen in therapy by Moulton reported disappointment in their new hope. They found men who were sexually exciting but who withdrew from any real intimacy, leaving these women feeling used, unloved, and abandoned. The divorced women discovered to their surprise that they missed the feminine role, that sex alone was not enough, and that they needed male admiration and affection to feel successful as whole women. Without this feedback, they felt isolated, lonely, and dissatisfied that their professional success was not enough for total happiness. They had wished for more autonomy than they could manage. The men they dated seemed to have all the charm and vitality that their husbands lacked, but these men had no interest in remarriage; and when the women discovered this they became more clinging and desperate, thus precipitating the men's withdrawal. The thought of never being caressed by a man again was unbearable; even a reliable lover was not enough. They could not believe they were lovable unless men were present. Since they could run their own businesses without male assistance, they could not understand why they needed the personal affirmation of a man to feel valued. In summary, although women were just as realistically independent as men, they still wanted more commitment, predictability, and finally marriage, whereas men did not.

Moulton states that divorced men and women in middle age both suffer from a social isolation; that many of them are ashamed of their loneliness, avoiding phone calls and contacts; and that many are simply pretending to be self-sufficient. Regarding treatment, Moulton reveals that the patients described in her research were in unusual distress, partly because they lacked proper preparation for divorce. Skilled therapists also play an important role in evaluating the need for divorce, in making an effort to avoid divorce, or in preparing middle-aged persons for the turmoil of separation. Because the concept of marriage is changing (many no longer expect it to last a lifetime) and the rate of divorce is increasing, Moulton says that therapists may be called on more and more to help facilitate decisions about marriage and divorce, as well as to alleviate the suffering of separation and readjustment.[35]

Catron, Chiriboga, and Krystal[36] investigated divorce at midlife, while exploring the concept of liminality: the "betwixt and between" state seems most often to occur with middle-aged persons in the process of divorce. The condition is lack of a clear-cut separation from one's former mate. These individuals tend to remain connected, unable to break the bond and once and for all to end the relationship, free themselves of each other, and move ahead to re-establish themselves in a world of their own choosing. This condition appears to be more prevalent among the middle-aged and may also be fostered by the number and complexity of issues they face. Their disposition of extensive property, protesting children and grandchildren, and the long and well-entrenched history of shared life emerge as problems.

Seventeen patients, aged 40 to 64, were involved in the study in the San Francisco Bay area.[36] These individuals all entered therapy within eight months of their separation with complaints of depression, anxiety, loneliness, hopelessness, restlessness, and feelings of fear and inadequacy concerning social relations. Underlying these complaints were indications of the stage of liminality: they could not seem to "cut off" from their divorced spouse. They tended to isolate themselves to the point of becoming "hermits," refusing to call old friends or to answer the phone. The use of ritual to treat their problems was initiated as a treatment approach.

The therapy consisted of three phases. The first phase included teaching the patients how to achieve a state of deep relaxation. They were then instructed in the performance of visualization to achieve psychologic separation. The patients were then asked to use this meditation technique at least once but preferably several times a day, for no less than two weeks. This first encourages patients to "confront their partners," to be angry, sad, resentful, and so on. Written lists describing mutual dependencies, as well as their partner's positive and negative characteristics were required. These lists provided material for discussion in therapy sessions, and they facilitated the mourning process.

In the second phase of the ritual, patients were asked to visualize "cords" that connected them to their partners, during the deep relaxation state that accompanied their daily meditations. The patients almost always could "see" some connections, describe the cord's shape, size, color, and so on. The patient was then asked to remove and destroy the cord. After the cords had been destroyed, a bath in a stream, lake, or ocean was followed by a process of thanking, apologizing to, and forgiving the partner.

The final phase of the ritual involved the writing of an unsent letter to the separated partner, expressing all positive and negative feelings, affirming freedom, independence, and farewells. The letter was "destroyed" through a rite of the patient's own choosing, usually involving actual burning or burial.

During the postritual period, patients reported changes in their outlook and behavior. Most found it possible to at last forgive their partner or themselves. In the weeks that followed, they experienced more energy, felt more positive, more independent, and less angry—they felt themselves to be free. Patients consider the ritual, especially that of the unsent letter, as signifying the end of their attachment to something old and the beginning of a new life. This divorce ritual is designed for an individual, rather than a group.

Women Existing in a "Loveless Marriage"

"More puzzling than divorce—and ultimately more painful . . . is the loveless marriage, where discord, misery and hopelessness become a way of life, and the two partners little more than prisoners, chained together by fear instead of united by love," states Koslow,[37] who writes of the surprising staying power growing in a number of empty marriages across America. Her article includes the three general marriage classifications of noted family therapist Sonya Rhodes: (1) the rare, unusual, durable marriage that retains an element of passionate romance or recaptures it from time to time; (2) the more common, less-passionate marriage that is endowed with compatibility and friendship and (3) the "loveless" marriage, which is comprised of couples who stay together despite little emotional bonds and no companionship. London, a psychiatrist at New York University, states that "there are an awful lot of married people who realize they don't like each other . . . often this troubled couple hasn't grown together or their expectation of marriage hasn't been realistic." He finds that the majority of these couples do not care to work on improving their marriage. Their resentments have become entrenched, communications have shut down, and the relationship has taken on a rigid quality.[37] Koslow goes on to point out that "loveless" marriages are not new and that to marry for love alone is only a contemporary notion. She reveals that as recently as during our mothers' era, many women sentenced themselves to lifelong unhappiness rather than contemplate divorce, which was even then still considered taboo or at least disreputable. In the interesting and relevant article, this author explains why, in the decade of the 1980s, when divorce is prevalent, loveless marriages persist.[37]

Women today stay in such vacant marriages as these for emotional as well as practical reasons. *Fear of the unknown* is the one pervasive anxiety that lies at the root of all the emotional explanations for tolerating a loveless marriage. London states, "In spite of the liberating influence of the woman's movement, there is still a vast cadre of women—young, old, middle-aged—who cling to the title of "Mrs. So and So." He maintains that they have painfully discovered that unless one is a superwoman, doing a man's job, one still needs a husband to avoid second-class citizenship. Hammer, a psychoanalyst in New York, found that *fear of lost status* is further aggravated if a woman plays a visible role in her community by virtue of being "Mrs. John Important." The more distinguished her husband (congressman, judge, professor of surgery), the more prestige she stands to lose. Hammer found that this woman holds talents and capabilities herself but chooses not to assert them for fear of appearing exceptional; instead, she elects to identify with her husband's success. The researcher finds, among other worries common to wives in loveless marriages, is *fear of sexuality*. According to Hammer, being in a bad marriage gives people an excuse not to have sex.[37] Existing quite apart from sexual anxiety is the adjacent *fear of intimacy*, fear of being emotionally close and vulnerable to a partner. "Intimacy is stressful," writes Zeisel, a psychotherapist New York City: "Some people stay in a marriage where intimacy is minimal because they are afraid of what might happen if they feel more."[37]

Fear of criticism is another panic haunting the unhappily married woman. "She may have been a good little girl," suggests Hammer, "and in order to please her parents she stays married to someone who quite likely was originally their choice." Finally, writes Koslow,[37] *fear that all marriages are unloving* is a significant concern of women in loveless marriages. Thinking all marriages are as cold, remote, and often as hostile as theirs keeps many women from ending an emotionally drained relationship. Pinto, a psychiatrist also in New York City, says, "Many women in unfulfilling relationships lack a well-developed sense of what defines a loving marriage . . . they seem to think that mutual trust, love and reciprocity are unattainable dreams." Women in disappointing marriages tend to see the obstacles to happiness as insurmountable and themselves as relatively helpless. A woman like this allows herself to be psychologically abused by her husband, the object of harsh and unwarranted criticism, cruel put-downs and browbeating. Pinto adds that this woman suffers from low self-esteem, lacks confidence, and typically tends to think that there is something wrong with her rather than with her abuser.[37]

Pragmatically, women today are growing more aware of the difficulty in living with the nation's tightening economy. Koslow states:[37]

Many women in unsatisfying marriages are simply and unsentimentally aware that divorce is a luxury that they cannot afford . . . they don't feel they could survive economically if they split up. Whether a woman is a homemaker with limited education or employed and making a decent salary, economic stress is a powerful reason for staying married."

Financial help from the ex-husband, once the Rock of Gibraltar for the newly divorced woman, adds Koslow, is no longer a forgone conclusion. Suan Prescott, editor and counselor, writes: "Except for marriages of long standing, most women don't get alimony at all . . . if an ex-wife receives anything, it's only a temporary maintenance payment."[37] When a woman has children, the issue becomes further complicated; the refusal of ex-husbands to contribute their share of child support is fast becoming a national disaster. Prescott estimates that nearly 95 per cent of divorced mothers become custodial parents. In sum, the many financial hardships awaiting the newly single woman are reason enough to stop short of divorce.

Dr. London finds that, monetary worries aside, the mere presence of children keeps many women married. He maintains that especially when young children are involved, the classic reason to sustain a marriage—staying together "for the kids' sake"—is as operative today as it ever was. Also, mothers are staying in dissatisfying marriages because they may be justifiably terrified of trying to rear their children alone. Koslow describes a case in which the woman explained that her husband was cold and a philanderer but that he was very good at reading bedtime stories and pushing swings.[37]

Responsibility and effort by both husband and wife toward a more loving marriage is seen as important to these mental health professionals. The question of the fairness of "settling" for a bland, flawed, hostile relationship without exerting some work to make it richer and more rewarding was asked. Dr. Rhodes concluded that "married people, like everyone else, have to grow personally as they travel through life and they have the added responsibility of seeing that their own marriage continues to develop."[37]

Divorce and the Woman in Violence

Carmen Warner's book[38] on conflict intervention in social and domestic violence proposes that divorce may be the most humanizing option for physically and psychologically damaged married women. She quotes Clinebell, a counselor in Philadelphia, who looks at factors important to assess while making the decision: "Divorce counseling is not the same as marriage counseling. Divorce counseling is based on the assumption that it may be better for some couples to separate, rather than on the traditional attitudes of the church that a marriage must be saved if possible and that divorce is always a tragedy. Divorce counseling is a kind of counseling and consciousness raising that affirms singleness as an option for human wholeness."[38] Warner suggests lists of issues and questions that will help women to understand more clearly the problems and alternatives for discussion in therapy. These questions can be used to help any woman making her decision of divorce. Five leading questions are: (1) Are you willing to risk living alone? (2) Are you willing to have custody of the children? (3) Are you willing to risk supporting yourself? (4) Are you willing to risk relocating? and (5) Are you willing to risk facing the unknown? Warner's pragmatic questions include realistic "pros and cons" of each of these situations that would be most beneficial for women to reflect on before making divorce decisions that might lead to disillusionment and a sense of failure.

APPLYING CONCEPTS OF NURSING CARE

Divorce is a difficult and complex crisis that denotes loss. Loss and separation are painful. It is crucial that nurses be aware of the feelings of patients experiencing divorce and lend interpersonal support to help them adjust and move through stages of trauma to a more secure, fulfilling lifestyle. To this end, nurses must be informed and must understand the stress of divorce. They need to care enough to get involved and to risk using a more direct approach to learn "where the patient is." Nurses might well expect the divorced woman (who has felt rejection from husband or relatives or friends) to have a hesitant, guarded, mistrusting attitude toward them. The divorced woman will probably wait for clues from the nurse indicating a sincere interest in her and a willingness to listen.

That the woman in the hospital is in a divorce crisis might be detected in the initial interview. Examples of verbal clues are such statements as "No, my husband won't be visiting" and "My husband isn't with me; we feel we both need time to think about our marriage." Sarcastic remarks about men in general are easy to pick up, and clarifying them might give information. A woman who does not speak to her husband or mention him phoning her; whose husband does not visit her or send gifts or flowers; or who appears depressed, is seen crying, isolates herself, and eats poorly is giving nonverbal clues about her situation.

Perhaps the best opportunity to become aware of the deep loneliness the divorced woman feels would be open to the night nurse. Nights are long and lonely for most patients; however, this time is acknowledged by the divorced (especially the newly divorced) woman to be utterly desolate. She misses her husband to talk to and to touch; she misses knowing someone is in the room who can comfort her and hold her. This is the time for the nurse to stop by her bed, to sit down, and to listen—and to use touching for reassurance. These nurses should know and accept that perhaps the patient cannot express her feelings, and they need to reinforce that they care enough to be with the patient.

It is essential for the nurse to really listen, to given total attention to the patient by good eye contact, by sitting near the patient, and by conveying the attitude that "no one is more important right now to me than you and your problems." These nurses must think deeply about what the woman is telling them by observing her nonverbal communication. The patient needs to know that she can weep, shout with anger, or tremble with anxiety. She needs to know that these discharges will release her tension and her inner, stored-up feelings, and that by doing this she will be able to think clearly again, evaluate her situation with the nurse's support, and take better charge of herself.

That the stages the divorced patient goes through are similar to those most people go through in any crisis may be easy to acknowledge, but to identify which stage the patient is in requires more perceptiveness. Women move back and forth through stages, often confused and with real fears of insanity. At various times they will confide that they are unable to sleep without thoughts of "losing their mind," "going crazy," or "going out of control." These women need reassurance; often, inquiring about and discussing their fears provide relief.

People in the denial stage are frightened; they need to talk about their insecurity. The nurse must help the patient by listening and by presenting reality with perceptiveness. For example, the nurse may ask the patient who, with father absent, would be a good role model for her sons. This is one way of bringing the issue out in the open. Although the patient may deny that her husband is not coming back, she will be aware of that possibility and that meanwhile her sons need men to communicate with. The nurse needs to interpret the patient's needs accurately by again attemping to clarify what she is saying, without irritating her.

The anger stage can be uncomfortable for both patient and nurse. It is important that the nurse listen with understanding, no matter how the anger is expressed. The feeling of disappointment and the frightening concrete (finances, housing, and automobile) and abstract (relatives, neighbors, friends, and social outlets) issues that this woman is facing alone need to be talked about. The thought of helping her children readjust to life without a father can be overwhelming to the mother who is undergoing additional physical problems. Cline[39] believes that the nurse must and can help the mother become aware that the parents' bitterness and anger toward each other affect the children far more negatively than does any other factor. The mother needs to know that it is normal for children to try to manipulate their divorced parents. Children usually have a secret wish for their parents to reunite and will often do all they can to manipulate the situation so that parents will talk to each other. Parents need to talk about how they also tend to manipulate their children by sending messages to each other through them and by gaining affection from them unfairly. Cline adds that "children almost always feel guilty and partially responsible for the divorce." Nurses also need to help children express such feelings. Kaseman believes strongly that *both* parents need to know how each child comprehends the absence of one of the parents and how the total picture is perceived.[40]

COUNSELING

"Marital therapy is often one of the most rewarding but also most frustrating areas of involvement with people," state Holdsworth and Daines.[41] The role of the therapist is to help the couple discover what they really want and to enable them to carry this through. Counselors tend to focus on the couple's lack of communication and on the risk of a therapist who "takes sides." These authors advise the need for two therapists in trying to disentangle the web of communication problems in complex situations. They write of their frustrations in finding misunderstandings and resentments established over years so resistant to change. However, despite the recent rise in the divorce rate, these authors find that many people still take marriage very seriously and are often prepared to put up with a great deal of disharmony and suffering rather than see their marriages fall apart.

The goal of a therapist's intervention with the woman in the process of divorce is to help her recognize and cope with her feelings of ambivalence and guilt.[42] Unrecognized feelings about the marriage and impending divorce should be explored, with direct questioning and reflection of verbal and nonverbal clues. Assessment would include identifying the woman's realistic perception of the event, her support system, and her coping mechanisms. With the support of the therapist, she should be able to explore what she wants and expects from a marriage in the future.[42]

Wabrek, Wabrek, and Burchell,[43] divorce counselors helping women cope with termination of their marriage, state that grief is commonly experienced by the divorced woman. They advocate helping the woman understand her needs for love, affection, and sexual involvement. Often, if the marriage has been of long standing, woman are unprepared for the tremendous shift in sexual mores that have occurred in this country. This transitional period can cause a women to feel very insecure. As old friendships are disrupted, new relationships will need to be formed. Usually the problem of loneliness is the first one to be discussed. The love of a child, family member, or very close friend may be truly wonderful when one is grieving. These counselors suggest pragmatic ideas in order to help the woman be aware of and cope with her stressful changes (such as moving from her old house, which provided security but also afforded painful memories). They add that the postponement of unnecessary change during this transition period makes good common sense.

Women in the process of divorce may also be dealing with the conflict of an unwanted pregnancy. Rosenthal and Young state, in a poignant article on abortion counseling:

As women achieve the right to determine their destiny, nurses and other health professionals must reexamine their own beliefs in relation to their participation as care providers . . . the goal of counseling is to help each woman make a decision that is right for her. Ventilating her feelings prior to any

procedures with some time to consider the alternatives gives her a chance to lessen her anxiety, conflict and guilt . . . one of the most important responsibilities for only nursing care for abortion patients is that of contraceptive counseling. The nurse should be well versed in all methods of contraception and be able to help the woman select a method that is most appropriate for her. Emphasis needs to be on future planning as opposed to past failure to either use a method or fail to use it successfully.[44]

To refer individuals to marriage counselors at family service centers in the area is perhaps the most important help that nurses can give, as these counselors are experts in the field. Clubs, churches, and community organizations also provide healthy and realistic ongoing support systems (for example, the group called Parents Without Partners). While the woman is still in the hospital, other resources may include having her talk to other hospitalized divorced women of the same age or to other hospitalized women with similar medical/surgical problems. After discharge, referral to a women's support group (for example, an outreach group) may help.

PREVENTION

In the area of preventing the stress on women that accompanies divorce, nurses might do well to plan and become involved in the teaching of high school students in community classes about the psychologic aspects and responsibilities of marriage and good parenting. If nurses are unprepared to do this, then they should support such courses in their community. Since divorce rates are so high and since many marriages are centers of friction and unhappiness, it would seem that marriage comes about with little or no preparation. Women's support groups may also be helpful in preparing young women for the realities of marriage.

In summary, with today's increasing divorce rate, nurses need to be aware of and also to recognize the need for intervention and the need for improvement of methods of total patient care that help women survive this crisis.

References

1. Aguilera, D. C., and Messick, J. M. *Crisis Intervention: Theory and Methodology.* St. Louis: C.V. Mosby, 1982, pp. 109.
2. Lambert, Clinton E. and Lambert, V. A. Divorce: A psychodynamic development involving grief. *Journal of Psychiatric Nursing and Mental Health Services,* vol. 15, January 1977, pp. 37–42.

3. Herman, Sonya J. Divorce: A grief process. *Perspectives in Psychiatric Care,* vol. 12, 1974, pp. 108–112.

4. Lytle, Nancy A. *Nursing of Women in the Age of Liberation.* Dubuque, IA: William C. Brown Co., 1977, pp. 20–21.

5. Cherlin, Andrew J. *Marriage, Divorce, Remarriage.* Harvard University Press, 1981.

6. Aguilera and Messick, op. cit.

7. Brandwein, Ruth A., Brown, Carol A., and Fox, Elizabeth Maury. Women and children lost: Divorced mothers and their families. *Nursing Digest,* January-February 1976, p. 39.

8. Bloom, B. L. *Community Mental Health.* Monterey, CA: Brooks/Cole Publishing Co., 1977.

9. Carter, Judy W. Assertiveness and post-divorce adjustment in women. *Issues in Mental Health Nursing,* vol. 3, 1981, pp. 365–379.

10. Hunt, M. M. *The World of the Formerly Married.* New York: McGraw-Hill, 1966.

11. Forrest, Deborah A. Marital adjustment and psychosomatic complaints. *Issues in Mental Health Nursing,* vol. 2, December 1979, pp. 21–37.

12. Rahe, R. H., Meyer, M., Kjaer, M., Holmes, G., and Holmes, T. Social stress and illness onset. *Journal of Psychosomatic Research,* vol. 8, 1964, pp. 35–44.

13. Holmes, T., and Masuda, M. Life change and illness susceptibility. Chicago: Annual Meeting of the American Association for the Advancement of Science, December 1970.

14. Forrest, D. A. Marital adjustment and psychosomatic complaints. *Issues in Mental Health Nursing,* vol. 2, December 1979, pp. 21–37.

15. Hackney, Gary R. and Ribordy, Sheila. An empirical investigation of emotional reactions to divorce. *Journal of Clinical Psychology,* vol. 36, January 1980, pp. 105–110.

16. Kaseman, Charlotte M. The single-parent family. *Perspectives in Psychiatric Care,* vol. 3, 1974, pp. 113–118.

17. Kohen, Janet A. From wife to family head: Transitions in self-identity. *Psychiatry,* vol. 44, August 1981, pp. 230–240.

18. Wabrek, Alan J., Wabrek, C. J., Burchell, R. C. Divorce counseling: Helping the woman cope. *Connecticut Medicine,* vol. 44, May 1980, pp. 295–298.

19. Lambert and Lambert, op. cit., p. 40.

19a. Fromm-Reichmann, F. *Principles of Intensive Psychotherapy.* Chicago, University of Chicago Press, 1967.

20. Scarf, Maggie. *Unfinished Business: Pressure Points in the Lives of Women.* New York: Ballantine Books, 1980, pp. 94, 95, 373, 374.

21. Peterson, Linda C. Guilt, attribution of responsibility and resolution of the divorce crisis. *Image,* vol. 10, June 1978, p. 57.

22. Weissman, Myrna M. and Klerman, G. L. Sex differences and the epidemiology of depression. *Archives of General Psychiatry,* vol. 34, 1977, pp. 98–111.

23. Guttentag, Marcia, Salasin, Susan, and Belle, Deborah. *The Mental Health of Women.* New York: Academic press, 1980, pp. 155–157.

24. Briscoe, C. W., and Smith, J. B. Depression in bereavement and divorce. *Archives General Psychiatry,* vol. 32, April 1975, pp. 439–443.

25. Briscoe, C. W., and Smith, J. B. Depression and marital turmoil. *Archives General Psychiatry,* vol. 29, December 1973, pp. 811–817.

26. Scarf, op. cit., pp. 94–95.

27. McGrory, Arlene. Women and mental illness: A sexist trap? *Journal of Psychiatric Nursing and Mental Health Services,* October 1980, pp. 16–21.

28. Broverman, I. K., Broverman, D., Clarkson, F. E., et al. Sex Role stereotypes and clinical judgments of mental health. *Journal of Counseling and Clinical Psychology,* vol. 34, 1970, pp. 1–7.

29. Brown, C. R., and Hellinger, M. L. Therapists' attitudes toward women. *Social Work,* 1975, pp. 266–270.

30. Kjervik D. K., and Palta, M. Sex role stereotyping in assessments of mental health. *Nursing Research,* vol. 27, 1978, pp. 166–171.

31. Weissman and Klerman, op. cit., pp. 98–111.

32. McGrory, op. cit., pp. 16–21.

33. Belle, Deborah, Marshall, N., Kline, P., and Tsang, L. Fighting stress and depression: Exemplary programs for low income mothers. *The Stress and Families Project,* Harvard University, 1980.

34. Ehrenreich, Barbara, and Stallard, K. The Nouveau Poor. *Ms.,* Special Report, August 1982, pp. 217–224.

35. Moulton, Ruth. Divorce in the middle years: The lonely woman and the reluctant man. *Journal of the American Academy of psychoanalysis,* vol. 8, 1980, pp. 235–250.

36. Catron, Linda, Chiriboga, David, and Krystal, Sheila. Divorce at midlife: Psychic dangers of the liminal period. *Maturitas,* vol. 2, 1980, pp. 131–139.

37. Koslow, Sally P. The surprising staying power of loveless marriages. *Ladies Home Journal,* No. 3, March 1982, pp. 42–45.

38. Warner, Carmen G. *Conflict Intervention in Social and Domestic Violence.* Bowie, MD: Robert J. Brady Co., 1981, pp. 208–214.

39. Cline, Foster W. Generalities concerning children and divorce. *Nurse Practitioner,* March-April 1977, pp. 29–30.

40. Kaseman, op. cit., pp. 113–118.

41. Holdsworth, Vanessa, and Daines, B. Marital therapy, a risky business. *Nursing Mirror,* July 10, 1980, pp. 18–20.

42. Aguilera and Messick, op. cit., p. 113.

43. Wabrek, Wabrek, and Burchell, op. cit., p. 295.

44. Rosenthal, Miriam, and Young, F. R. Voluntary interruption of pregnancy. *In* Lytle, Nancy. *Nursing Women in the Age of Liberation.* Dubuque, IA: William C. Brown Co., 1977, pp. 147–150.

22

THE EXPERIENCE OF WIDOWHOOD

MARIE ALBRECHT

Marie Albrecht's chapter on the experience of widowhood starts by identifying the cultural, sociologic, and psychologic factors affecting a woman who has lost a spouse through death. The process of bereavement from initial impact to recovery is included. Nursing intervention is based on a crisis model, and the importance of the perception of reality and support is stressed.

Loss is a part of life. Life consists of giving up old behaviors and learning new ones, of having and losing, of holding onto and letting go. Life is a cycle of beginnings, endings, and new beginnings. Human life is temporary, but this fact is resisted and often denied. Consequently, when a loved one dies, the impact may be overwhelming.

The loss of a spouse through death is viewed as the life event that results in the highest level of stress.[1] Although it appears that the state of widowhood increases general vulnerability[2] and that the stress level may be high, a newly widowed woman may experience little tolerance of her grief by those around her.[3] It is a serious problem with such profound overtones that few people are prepared either emotionally or socially to cope with death or to come to the assistance of those touched by death.[4]

Many cultural, sociologic, and psychologic factors affect a widow and the manner in which she grieves. These factors, the grieving process, and an approach to stress and crisis intervention are addressed here.

FACTORS AFFECTING NORMAL GRIEVING AND ADAPTATION TO LOSS

Cultural Factors

An individual's bereavement is conditioned by his or her early reaction to loss, as well as by the institutionalized ways that a culture deals with loss.[5] Our culture is death denying; so, with denial of death, there is denial of free expression of grief. This creates problems for the bereaved. Overt expression of grief is thus treated as though it were a weakness instead of a psychologic necessity. The period of shock is given recognition, but tradition generally denies mourning following the funeral.[6]

With such denial, death then is often not viewed as a natural part of life. Death, if it happens, is perceived as something that happens to others—at least not to oneself or to one's family. Denial leads to avoidance and discomfort.[7]

In this setting, when death does occur, it is traumatic. Our culture sends out messages to the bereaved that say, "Thou shalt not fall apart."[8] Stoicism is expected; feelings need not be expressed. Messages are given that children should be protected from death, that grief is time limited, is limited to loss by death, and should be concealed.[7] Furthermore, it is thought that feelings can be cut off by thinking only of pleasant thoughts, by avoiding reminders of the dead, and by idealizing the dead. The myth of a geographic cure may lead one to travel from place to place seeking that cure.[9]

Feifel adds further insight: "With increasing fragmentation of the family, decline in kinship and neighborhood groups, the growing impersonality of a culture dominated by technology, and the waning of providential faith, death signals . . . man's loneliness and a threat to his pursuit of happiness."[10]

Sociologic Factors

Societies develop ways of containing death's impact, because mortality tends to disrupt the ongoing life of relationships and social groups. A social vacuum is created when a member of society dies. This disruption is more evident for a person in the middle years. Thus, in modern society, in which death is more frequent among the old, society rarely interrupts its business. Death may simply remind the survivors of the social and psychologic debts they owe, so the funeral and memorial may become attempts to compensate for this. Even funerals have become relatively unimportant. Often only family members and a few other individuals are affected, so bereavement and adjustment become a private responsibility. This can cause serious problems in adjustment; that is, at a time when death becomes less disruptive in society, its consequences can be more serious for the bereaved individual, who experiences grief less frequently but more intensely.[11]

Our youthful orientation, receptivity to innovation, and dynamic social change increase the distance between the dead and the living. The aged become disengaged in present and future status and are left more powerless, anonymous, and ignored. As traditional values of the aged and dead lose significance, there is less sense of identity and belonging with kinship and community. When the threat of death is present but for many does not fit into a religious or philosophic context, our society experiences a crisis.[11]

The social changes wrought by death are far more significant than those attending birth, puberty, or marriage. A mourner may need to depend on his or her own resoures, with little help in finding a comfortable social status. If the mourner has few intimate relationships, bereavement is personally more significant and anxiety producing.[5] Along with this, the nuclear family orientation provides fewer opportunities for people to be bereaved; therefore, there is little if any past experience for guidance.[12]

"Differing mortality rates and the tendency of men to marry women younger than themselves, especially in second and third marriages, leave older women widowed. The result is that eighty-five per cent of surviving spouses are female. The average age of widowhood is 56, which leaves one third of a life-span to go."[13] The increased life expectancy makes it unlikely that one will experience death while young; thus, the loss of a spouse may be the first experience with death in a family. This heightens the effect of the loss of a spouse, which is probably the loss of an intimate, very meaningful relationship. The problems of bereavement following loss of a spouse may be intensified by the expectation that the marriage relationship had compensated for less meaningful relationships elsewhere in society.[14]

Also, the typical American family fails to utilize its opportunities to educate its children in preparation for facing death. Social distance is unnecessarily created when adults do not practice their professed beliefs or share with their children their actual beliefs regarding death. There is a need for blending the realism and directness in confronting death with new patterns of socialization of children. Personal experience could be melded with contemporary understandings and a renewed sensitivity to people.[15] This could enhance the emotional adjustment to loss.

Psychologic Factors

A glaring exception to humanity's ability to solve most problems confronting it is its powerlessness to conquer death. Thus, there is the paradox of people today who believe in science and use the scientific method but who resort to magic and irrationality in handling the anxiety of death. The study of death and the defenses against it is extremely important, for it is the consistent experience of psychiatry that "any defense which enables us to persistently escape the perception of any fundamental internal or external reality is psychologically costly."[16]

Death needs to be put in proper perspective. The person who can accept the thought that one day he or she will die can spend time unfettered by fear. Energies bound up by fear can then be released for the constructive aspects of living.[16]

GRIEF

The Grieving Process

Grief is a normal adaptive process that enables a bereaved person to deal with the psychologic disequilibrium caused by the loss of a significant other. Grief is the emotional reaction to loss. To adapt successfully to loss, the grieving person needs to accomplish four major tasks; that is referred to as the work of grieving. These tasks are (1) to make psychologically real an external event that is not desired (that is, to accept the reality of the loss); (2) to emancipate oneself from the strong emotional bondage to the deceased, to allow oneself to experience the painful emotions; (3) to readjust to the environment from which the deceased is missing; and (4) to form new relationships and patterns of behavior.[12, 17]

There seems to be agreement that there are phases of grief. These phases or stages are referred to by the use of various terms. I prefer the terminology suggested by Tyhurst (cited in Rapaport); namely, that of impact, recoil, and recovery.[18]

Each phase of grief has certain characteristics. The line between impact (with its shock) and recoil (with its awareness) is more distinct than that between recoil and recovery. I agree with Bowlby in quoting Shand that the nature of "sorrow is so complex, its effects in different characters so various, that it is rare, if not impossible, for any writer to show an insight into all of them."[19]

Phases

Impact. With impact, there is numbness, shock. The numbness may be preceded by great distress. Pollock states that the first reaction may be panic, accompanied by shrieking, wailing, and moaning, or perhaps by complete collapse, with paralysis and motor retardation. The response may vary according to the suddenness of the death and the degree of preparation preceding the death.[20] The bereaved finds herself in disequilibrium, is bewildered, cannot believe what has happened, has a tendency to act as though the lost partner is still present, and may weep or express anger, be accusing or express ingratitude.[19]

Lindemann provides a picture of the physical symptoms, the striking features being a marked tendency toward sighing respiration, lack of strength and exhaustion, digestive symptoms of anorexia, and a feeling of hollowness.[21]

This initial period of shock and disbelief may be followed by a stunned, numbed feeling in which the grief-stricken person does not permit herself any thoughts acknowledging reality. The loss may be accepted intellectually, but the painful character of the loss is denied or muted.[22] This denial may be a defense mechanism, a means to deal with painful feelings.

This period of impact is described by Phyllis Silverman as a time when people restrict their time orientation to the immediate present.[23] It is a time when there is a sense of being lost, of not knowing what to do, of being suspended in life. One is unable to concentrate, is indifferent to needs, and does not believe the deceased is gone. The feeling that life can never again be worth living hinders the ability to plan for ongoing needs.[24]

Recoil. The second phase of grief is one of awareness, when there is emergence from the protective fog of numbness. This is a painful period not cushioned by shock. Bowlby[19] describes the period as a state of mental helplessness when the bereaved has conflicting, ambivalent reactions; for example, there is intensified conflict between the desire for reunion with the deceased and hatred of the deceased and the desire for detachment. The bereaved cries for help, yet may reject those who respond. This is a time when there is restlessness, an inability to sit still, a continuous searching for something to do, an inability to initiate and maintain organized patterns of behavior, a feeling of emptiness of self and world, loss of self-esteem, lack of interchange with others, and loss of a significant goal. That changes in the external world are experienced as changes in the internal world of feeling is not only painful but also alarming.[19]

Psychologic loss is felt most acutely at this time; so the bereaved experiences acute loneliness. Silverman's research has shown that loneliness and depression are most difficult six months to a year following the husband's death. Superficially, the widow may appear to carry on, but underneath she is lonely.[25]

A woman I interviewed described her loneliness as that of being on an island surrounded by people who could not touch her, nor could she touch them. She felt alone, completely alone.[26]

The loneliness of widows is very complex. Lopata found in studying widows that a widow missed *that* man, her love object; she missed being the love object, being important to somebody; she missed not having someone who thought what she said was important enough to argue over, her companion, her escort, someone with whom to organize time, someone with whom to work, someone living in the house.[27]

Bornstein and co-workers, in a research study of the depression experienced by widows, concluded that "grief is grief," that there is a normal depression of widowhood that is different from that of clinical affective illness.[28]

During the recoil phase, there is also a loss

of interest in sources of gratification, and the world is viewed as insecure and hostile. The denial continues. There is a marked increase in affect, and insomnia is common. The intense pining, expressed through crying, restlessness, anger, and searching, creates a strong urge to recover the lost person. There is preoccupation with thoughts of the deceased, and attention is directed to the places and objects in the environment associated with him. There may be a sense that the loved one is present.[17]

Intense psychic pain may be compounded by feelings of guilt. With guilt, the widow may resent having exposed herself to the experience of loss and may also resent the dead person for having taken with him certain parts of her inner self. This loss of parts of oneself leads to mourning and loss of identity.[29]

Loss of a widow's identity affects her self-concept, which is the most important factor affecting behavior. Self-concept relates to all the aspects of one's perceptual field. It is the organization of ideas that is more important to its owner than the body in which it exists. The extension of self is observable with respect to other persons or groups; this is the feeling of oneness with those who have special value. This experience is a feeling of identification, which makes us human. In essence, one's self-concept is who one is; its very existence determines what is perceived. Self-concept corroborates the already-existing beliefs about oneself and so tends to maintain and reinforce its own existence. Significant others affect self-concept; the feeling that one is loved by someone who matters is positively reinforcing. Without that reinforcement, self worth is questioned.[30]

It is no wonder that a widow has difficulty accepting the fact that she is a widow, a single person. To lose identity while experiencing painful emotions leading to fear, anxiety, disruption, despair, and detachment can be overwhelming.

Recovery. There is no clear-cut transition from the recoil period to that of recovery, but some form of more or less stable organization does begin to develop, if the widow has been able to accept the reality of the loss and allow herself to experience the painful emotions. Behavior oriented to the lost one changes. Recovery is not painless, but the depressed periods become less intense and less frequent. Because of trigger events and the ebb-and-tide cyclic nature of grief, painful emotions are still experienced, sometimes at the least expected times. The widow continues to miss her husband, but she learns to assume new roles and to adjust to the environment without her spouse. She functions more effectively in the present, can give up the past, and is able to plan for the future. Gerald Caplan states that this period provides the "opportunity for many widows to gain a maturity, to develop psychologically, to be tempered by the fire."[31] Thus, growth is a part of recovery.

Time Required for Grief Work

There is disagreement over the length of time it takes to pass through the phases of grief. This is not a quick process, for there are many associations with the lost person, and for each association the tie must be dissolved. The breaking of ties and mourning are not only for the lost person but also for intangibles like missed experiences and relinquished hopes.[23]

Vachon does not believe that people move through their grief work within a specified time period. She suggests that the length of time it takes to "get over a death" takes "longer than one expects."[33] Probably each person has his or her own inner time needs for grieving.

APPROACH TO STRESS AND CRISIS INTERVENTION

Crisis

In a crisis, there is an upset in a steady state, or disequilibrium. A person is faced with a need to resolve a problem, but the normal repertoire of coping skills does not provide the answer. Where there was equilibrium, there is now disequilibrium and a need to again seek equilibrium. When this happens, there is tension followed by discomfort and a rise in tension.[34] This tension may motivate an individual to either perceive the situation as a challenge and thus initiate action toward solution or perceive the situation as a threat too great to be tackled.[18]

Model of Intervention

When working with a widow who feels a need to restore equilibrium where there is an imbalance, a nurse can find it helpful to use a stress and crisis model as a tool for assessing needs, planning interventions and evaluative criteria with the widow, and then intervening in the areas of need. One such model that seems to be appropriate for persons who are grieving following a significant loss is the "paradigm" of intervention. This model concerns three balancing factors, the presence or absence of which may determine whether a person who feels a need to restore equilibrium does or does not regain that equilibrium. These three vital balancing factors that may tip the scale one way or the other are identified as perception of the event, situational support, and coping mechanisms. If the perception is realistic, the situational support and the coping mechanisms are adequate, and the problem is resolved, with equilibrium regained. However, if one or more of these balancing factors are weak or missing, the problem remains unresolved, disequilibrium continues, and the stressful event becomes a crisis situation.[35]

Relationship Between Balancing Factors and Tasks of Grieving

The balancing factors will be viewed in relationship to the tasks of grieving: accepting the reality of the loss, experiencing the painful emotions of the loss, developing new patterns of behavior to adjust to the environment without the lost person, and forming new meaningful relationships.

Perception of Reality. Before a widow can adequately see and accept herself as a widow, she needs to recognize her loss not only intellectually but psychologically as well. This takes time. The cushioning effect of shock may initially be a merciful balm, but as the numbness subsides, the full blast of realization of the loss may hit. The blow is so severe that the widow wants to recoil; hence, the appropriateness of the term for this painful second phase of mourning. Because of the degree of anxiety at this time, there is a narrowing of perception, which also makes it more difficult to perceive the situation realistically.

Vachon reports that the period of acute grief following a sudden death is different from that following a lingering illness. When loss is sudden and the resulting death unexpected, denial is common; the shock progresses to alternating times of denial and beginning acceptance. However, for the relative of someone experiencing a long-term life-threatening illness, there may be several periods of acute grief. These may occur at the time of diagnosis, when the relative learns death is inevitable, or possibly at the time of death if the relative has previously used denial as a predominant manner of coping.[36]

Painful grief reactions may be delayed by persistent denial of the reality of the loss.[37] Davidson says that yearning and searching for the presence of the loved one is a way of testing reality; then, as the griever shifts from testing reality to awareness of the reality, painful disorganization occurs.[38] Slagle also says that searching is a means of making the loss real, for when one searches and does not find what is missing, then one becomes conscious of the fact that loss has truly occurred, that it is real.[7]

Nadeau (cited in Morphew), in sharing some findings of the St. John's Hospital Bereavement Study, says of the bereaved, "Immediately they know intellectually that their loved one is dead. But after a year, they know emotionally that their loved one will never come back."[39]

To recognize the reality of loss, Gorer thinks that there is a growing awareness of the need for a bereaved person to see the loved one dead and that this is indeed a necessary prerequisite for carrying out successful grief work.[6] Also, talking about the circumstances of the death and the relationship with the deceased, and doing so over and over, helps the mourner acknowledge the reality of the loss. The widow should be encouraged to talk about circumstances surrounding her husband's death, to recall memories, and to verbalize her feelings.[37] Early opportunities for this are provided when relatives and friends of the dead person gather for a wake, funeral, or other event of mourning.

Vachon suggests that the use of heavy tranquilizers is usually inappropriate at this time;[36] sedation impedes the ability to perceive reality. A funeral director reported that one widow was so tranquilized at the time of her husband's death and funeral that for six months thereafter she refused to believe her husband was dead. Only after the body was exhumed and she saw her husband's corpse while she was not tranquilized did she accept the reality of his death.

Recognizing the reality of loss is necessary not only for a widow to see herself as a widow but also to accept herself as such; to accept herself as a separate individual with an identity, not as a wife, but as a widow and a single person. This acceptance of a change in identity and self-concept takes time, a fact that in itself may be difficult to recognize and accept.

Besides realistically perceiving and accepting herself as a widow, the bereaved woman needs to recognize that grief has ebbs and tides, to perceive grieving as not only normal but indeed as necessary, and to recognize and accept her feelings.

The balancing factors of perception of reality are indeed pertinent to the determination of whether a widow can progress from recognition to acceptance of the reality of her husband's death and to the self-allowance of feeling her emotional pain.

Support. Gerald Caplan and others have felt that supportive intervention at a time of crisis is more readily accepted than at other times and can be preventative. Preventive intervention during bereavement could tip the balance between high- or low-level wellness.[31]

More and more, the results of research studies are demonstrating the value of a strong support system, both external and internal, in helping widows do their work of grieving. Lopata discovered, while studying widows in the Chicago area, that these women are often left alone to do their grief work; but she says that widows cannot do their grief work alone—they need to do it with others.[27]

Grief must be released. Although there is a need for a widow to release her feelings privately, there also is a strong need for her to express her thoughts and feelings publicly. Gorer believes that the mourner is at this time in need of social support and assistance more than at any time since early childhood.[6]

Research by Maddison indicates that some widows at high risk for unsatisfactory outcome can be identified shortly after bereavement. One factor of outstanding importance appears to be the widow's perception that the persons in her environment are failing to meet her needs or are actively blocking her expression of affect and her review of her past relationship with her husband.[40] It is therefore important to determine a widow's perception of her support system.

Vachon and colleagues, in their study of 162 widows to determine variables that were related to "high distress" after bereavement, found that the most important variable associated with high distress at one month was the woman's perception that she was seeing old friends less than before her husband's death.[41]

A two-year study of conjugal bereavement by Vachon et al. indicated that deficits in social support correlated with the enduring high distress of 26 of the 99 subjects. Most of these women, even after two years of bereavement, viewed themselves as relatively isolated with respect to some aspects of their social network.[42]

This study also indicated that the presence of certain core personality factors seemed to play a protective role in the widows who experienced enduring "low distress." These factors were emotional stability, conscientiousness, regard for social reputation, and tolerance of traditional difficulties.[42] Although

core personality factors, beliefs, values, and a sense of meaning and purpose may not be viewed as situational supports in the crisis paradigm, I view these internal factors as supportive.

The key conclusion in the St. John's Hospital Bereavement Study is that it is important to get the families of bereaved individuals involved as much as possible, for the people in this study who were making the best adjustment were those who had active relationships with their families.[43]

In a study to observe the effects of sudden death versus those of chronic illness death on bereavement outcome, Sanders produced results that extended beyond this. These results indicated that bereaved individuals need support to help them rejoin the social environment best suited for meeting their needs. It also appears that this support is needed over a much longer period of time than was previously viewed appropriate.[44]

Roy and Sumpter determined, on the basis of experience with more than 200 mourners, that professional help in a bereavement group can assist mourners through their work of grieving. Group discussions revolved around five major themes: time perspective, emotional states of members, family problems and support, significance of social roles, and a changing sense of identity.[45]

New widows in the "widow-to-widow" program in Boston reacted positively to the supportive intervention of aides who were themselves widowed and who understood what the new widow was experiencing. Empathetic support was needed, appreciated, and beneficial. It was found also that such support, at least the availability of it, was usually welcomed until the widow was on her way to recovery, especially during the period of recoil.[46]

Matz has summarized the support needs of a bereaved person: acceptance and warm understanding; an opportunity to express feelings and to share them with others; and friends who are willing to stay and listen, who understand, who can help the bereaved to know that expressions of sorrow are a sign of strength and dignity that eventually will enable her to face the harshness of reality, to recall the life that was lived with its meaning and limitations as well as its blessings, and to create a framework of meaning for memories so that an enduring image can emerge.[47] Support that helps a widow to accept reality and experience feelings will also help her adjust to an environment without her husband.

Coping. Because the loss of her husband

may be the first time that a woman has had to deal with the death of a significant other, she may have no repertoire of coping skills with which to adjust to the loss. Hence, accomplishing all the tasks of grieving may be crucial.

Although the relationship between support and coping is significant, that among physiologic, psychologic, and social functioning is significant as well. Vachon and associates have shown that poor adjustment of widows to bereavement is consistent with their self-ratings indicating that their health was less than good; that tranquilizers, sedatives, or antidepressants were used; that they perceived widowhood as very stressful; and that instead of freely expressing feelings, they felt a need to maintain a facade.[42]

A recent study of 15 widowers after the death of their spouses concluded that suppressed immunity may be related to the increased morbidity and mortality associated with bereavement.[48] As exemplified by this study's conclusion, it seems that only a dent has been made in determining how grief may affect a mourner's coping ability. Fortunately, a widow in stressful situations may be more amenable to receiving assistance in coping and in learning how to cope more effectively.

Widows need permissive support to carry out the work of grieving.[40] The person who is supportive in accepting the widow, in allowing her to talk about her reaction to her loss and about her relationship to her husband, and in providing the opportunity for the widow to express and share her thoughts and feelings may be giving the widow the chance to express and explore feelings that help her to perceive her situation more clearly and arrive at her own solution to her problems.

Sometimes a grieving person's ability to cope may be underestimated. Therefore, it is important to ask the widow what she thinks needs to be done, for it is she who needs to grieve in her own unique manner.

If a widow can successfully accept the reality of her loss and can experience the painful emotions of grief, she will be more capable of adjusting to the challenging role changes necessitated by becoming a "single" person and perhaps also a single parent. Although she may need assistance, she may be reluctant to ask for it, or she may welcome assistance when and if it is offered. Needs for coping include facing reality, expressing emotions, identifying most pressing concerns, learning problem-solving skills, examining values and beliefs, determining goals and setting priorities, learning new skills, and recognizing and building on the strengths and positive coping skills that she already possesses. Maddison thinks that it is not necessary to direct all approaches at the widow herself, "for in some instances it may be considered that she has the resources to work through her own problems . . . provided certain aspects of the environment can be modified so as to reduce the amount of interference with her . . . coping techniques."[40]

As a widow adjusts to her environment without her husband, she may find that she needs a looser, more flexible social network to allow her to receive support from persons who have had similar experiences or who can meet her changing emotional needs as she frees herself from the ties associated with her lost spouse.[3] As the energy once invested in grieving is released, she has more energy to invest in new, satisfying relationships—to accomplish the last task of grieving.

CONCLUSION

I firmly believe that, although many cultural, social, and psychologic factors may negatively influence grieving, a widow may successfully work through grief and accomplish the tasks of grieving if the balancing factors of reality perception, support, and repertoire of successful coping skills are present. Indeed, progression through the grieving process can be a freeing, growing experience. Alla Bozarth-Campbell expresses this beautifully: "Grief is a passion to endure. People can be stricken with it, victims of it, stuck in it. Or they can meet it, get through it and become quiet victors through the active, honest, and courageous process of grieving."[8]

References

1. Holmes, T. H., and Rahe, R. H. The social adjustment rating scale. *Journal of Psychosomatic Research*, vol. 11, 1967, pp. 213–218.
2. Helsing, K. J., and Szklo, M. Mortality after bereavement. *American Journal of Epidemiology*, vol. 114, 1981, pp. 41–52.
3. Walker, K. N., MacBride, A., and Vachon, M. L. S. Social support networks and the crisis of bereavements. *Social Science and Medicine*, vol. 11, 1977, pp. 35–41.
4. Fulton, R. Widow in America: Some sociological observations. Boston: Harvard Medical School of Laboratory and Community Psychiatry, *Proceedings of Workshop for Widows and Widowers*, April-May 1971, p. 8.
5. Krupp, G. R., and Kligfeld, B. The bereavement reaction to a cross-cultural evaluation. *Journal of Religion and Health*, vol. 1, 1962, pp. 222–246.
6. Gorer, G. *Death, Grief and Mourning: A Study of Contemporary Society*. New York: Anchor Books, 1965.

7. Slagle, K. W. *Live with Loss*. Englewood Cliffs, NJ: Prentice-Hall, 1982.
8. Bozarth-Campbell, A. *Life is Goodbye Life is Hello*. Minnesota: CampCare Publications, 1982.
9. Worden, J. W. *Grief Counseling and Grief Therapy: A Handbook for the Mental Health Practitioner*. New York: Springer Publishing Company, 1982.
10. Feifel, H. The meaning of death in American society. *In* Green, B., and Irish, D. (eds.) *Death Education: Preparation for Living*. Cambridge, MA: Schenkman Publishing Company, 1971, p. 405.
11. Blauner, R. Death and social structure. *Psychiatry*, vol. 29, 1966, pp. 379–394.
12. Gerber, I. Bereavement and acceptance of professional services. *Community Mental Health Journal*, vol. 5, 1969, pp. 487–491.
13. The White House Conference on Aging. Report of the mini-conference on older women. DHHS Publication No. MCR-19. Washington, DC: U.S. Government Printing Office, 1981.
14. Reiss, P. J. Bereavement and the American family. *In* Kutscher, A. H. (ed.) *Death and Bereavement*. Springfield, IL: Charles C Thomas, 1969, pp. 219–221.
15. Irish, D. Death education: preparation for living. *In* Green, B., and Irish, D. (eds.) *Death Education: Preparation for Living*. Cambridge, MA: Schenkman, 1971, pp. 45–67.
16. Brantner, J. P. Death and the self. *In* Green, B., and Irish, D. (eds.) *Death Education: Preparation for Living*. Cambridge, MA: Schenkman, 1971, pp. 17–24.
17. Parkes, C. M. The first year of bereavement. *Psychiatry*, vol. 33, 1970, pp. 444–467.
18. Rapaport, L. The state of crisis: Some theoretical considerations. *In* Parad, H. J. (ed.) *Crisis Intervention: Selected Readings*. New York: Family Service Association of America, 1965, pp. 22–31.
19. Bowlby, J. Process of mourning. *International Journal of Psychoanalysis*, vol. 42, 1961, pp. 319–338.
20. Pollock, G. H. Mourning and adaptation. *International Journal of Psychoanalysis*, vol. 42, 1961, pp. 323–355.
21. Lindemann, E. Symptomatology and management of acute grief. *American Journal of Psychiatry*, vol. 101, 1944, pp. 141–147.
22. Engel, G. L. Grief and grieving. *American Journal of Nursing*, vol. 60, 1964, pp. 94–96.
23. Silverman, P. Services for the widowed during period of bereavement. *In* Social Work Practice Proceedings: Conference on Social Welfare, 93rd Annual Meeting, New York City: Columbia University Press, 1966.
24. Silverman, P. Services to the widowed: First steps in a program of preventive intervention. *Community Mental Health Journal*, vol. 3, 1967, pp. 38–43.
25. Silverman, P. The widow-to-widow program: An experiment in preventive intervention. *Mental Health*, vol. 53, 1969, pp. 225–336.
26. Accola, K. M., and Albrecht, M. *In* Snyder, M. (ed.) *A Guide to Neurological and Neurosurgical Nursing*. New York City: John Wiley & Sons, 1983, pp. 307–320.
27. Lopata, H. Social change and older women's roles. Paper presented at the Minnesota Gerontological Society Spring Conference, Brooklyn Park, MI, April 1983.
28. Bornstein, P. E., Clayton, P. J., Halikas, J. A., et al. The depression of widowhood after thirteen months. *British Journal of Psychiatry*, vol. 122, 1973, pp. 561–566.
29. Grinberg, L. Two kinds of guilt: Their relations with normal and pathological aspects of mourning. *International Journal of Psychoanalysis*, vol. 35, 1964, pp. 367–368.
30. Combs, A. W., Avila, D. L., and Purkey, W. W, *Helping Relationships: Basic Concepts for Helping Relationships*. Boston: Allyn and Bacon, 1971.
31. Caplan, G. Foreword. Proceedings of Workshop for Widows and Widowers. Boston: Harvard Medical School of Laboratory and Community Psychiatry, April-May 1971.
32. Grayson, H. Grief reactions to the relinquishing of unfulfilled wishes. *American Journal of Psychotherapy*, vol. 24, 1970, pp. 287–296.
33. Vachon, M. L. S. Grief and bereavement: The family's experience before and after death. *In* Gentles, I. (ed.) *Care for the Dying and the Bereaved*. Toronto: Anglican Book Centre, 1982, pp. 62–74.
34. Caplan, G. *Principles of Preventive Psychiatry*. New York City: Basic Books, 1964.
35. Aguilera, D. C., and Messick, J. M. Problem-solving approach to crisis intervention. *In Crisis Intervention Theory and Methodology*, Rev. Ed. St. Louis: C. V. Mosby, 1982, pp. 59–72.
36. Vachon, M. L. S. Type of death as a determinant in acute grief. *In* Margolis, O. S. (ed.) *Acute Grief: Counseling the Bereaved*. New York City: Columbia University Press, 1981, pp. 14–22.
37. Brown, J. T., and Stoudemire, A. Normal and pathological grief. *American Journal of Medicine*, vol. 250, 1983, pp. 378–382.
38. Davidson, G. Problems the hospice is designed to correct. *In* Wass, H. (ed.) *Dying; Facing the Facts*. New York: Hemisphere Publishing Corporation, 1979, pp. 169–181.
39. Morphew, C. Coping with grief: When need is greatest, church often fails. St. Paul, MN: Pioneer Press, January 1984.
40. Maddison, D. The relevance of conjugal bereavement for preventive psychiatry. *British Journal of Medical Psychology*, vol. 40, 1968, pp. 224–231.
41. Vachon, M. L. S., Robers, R. N., Lyall, W. A., et al. Predictors and correlates of adaptation to conjugal bereavement. *American Journal of Psychiatry*, vol. 139, 1982, pp. 998–1002.
42. Vachon, M. L. S., Sheldon, A. R., Lancee, W. J., et al. Correlates of enduring distress patterns following bereavement: Social network, life situation and personality. *Psychological Medicine*, vol. 12, 1982, pp. 783–788.
43. Hoval, G. Widows idealize husbands, study indicates. *Minneapolis Star and Tribune*, January 20, 1984, pp. 1B, 4B.
44. Sanders, C. M. Effects of sudden vs. chronic illness death on bereavement outcome. *Omega*, vol. 13, 1982–1983, pp. 227–241.
45. Roy, P. F., and Sumpter, H. Group support for the recently bereaved. *Health and Social Work*, vol. 8, 1983, pp. 230–232.
46. Silverman, P. Widow-to-widow program. Paper presented at the Widow-to-Widow Workshop, Boston, June 1971.
47. Matz, M. Judaism and bereavement. *Journal of Religion and Health*, vol. 3, 1968, pp. 350–351.
48. Schleifer, S. J., Keller, S. E., Camerino, M., et al. Suppression of lymphocyte stimulation following bereavement. *Journal of American Medical Association*, vol. 250, 1983, pp. 374–377.

23

LOSS OF THE CHILD: TWO CASE STUDIES

IDA MARTINSON

This chapter by Ida Martinson about death of a child is introduced by a brief review of the literature. Two case studies from the mother's perspective provide the chapter's main material, and it concludes with the challenge of nursing to support these mothers during the end stage of their child's life.

One of the most emotionally painful situations encountered by a mother is the death of her child. When the death follows a long illness, sometimes years in the case of childhood cancer, the mother not only faces the stress of losing her child but also must cope with the accumulated effects of the ups and downs of treatment, the uncertainty of prognosis, overwhelming physical demands, and often isolation from other family members and friends. During this time of stress a mother must maintain herself and her family throughout the traumatic experience. "A crisis experience may thus be seen as a transitional period, a turning point."[1] Health professionals should try to make the experience as positive as possible.

SEPARATION OF CHILD AND MOTHER

In our society, it is usually the mother who has the most consistent and intimate contact with her child. When a situation arises in a family in which a child is dying, the mother most frequently will have the greatest involvement in the case of that child. Health professionals need to know how best they can help a mother who is in the process of caring for a child whose death is imminent. One way this knowledge might be gained is by understanding what a mother experiences during this extended period of stress.

A literature review shows that the child's need for the mother increases during serious illness; hospitalization significantly reduces the child's access to her.[2] Because of the reduced access, the child can reject the parent for not stopping the painful procedures and long hospitalizations. Dependence on hospital staff for relief bypasses the parents and strips them of responsibility and the chance to care for the child.[3] Therefore, parents need the opportunity to participate in this care. A study done at the City of Hope Hospital showed that there was a better adjustment and alleviation of many problems for both parents and child when they could be in constant contact.[4-7]

A great deal of literature has been written on the effects of hospitalization on children.[8-11] For children up to age five, the worst fear is separation from the mother. Involved in this separation is separation from family, home and belongings. Add to this the introduction to new people, new places, and new routines, many of them painful. Hospitalization can be traumatic no matter what the diagnosis is. The child over age five is confronted with the same losses and also fears procedures and mutilation. Questions of the dying child about death usually express concern for three things:[12, 13]

1. Am I safe?
2. Will there be a trusted person to keep me from feeling helpless and alone and to overcome pain?
3. Will you make me feel all right?

There has been a gradual development of the concept of home care as one segment in the continuum of progressive patient care. The professional health team, hospitals, and consumer have shown a growing interest in developing home care services in which a patient and family can receive adequate care at an affordable cost.

HOME CARE AND THE DYING CHILD

For over 10 years, I have been studying the home as an alternate institution to the hospital for nursing care. One aspect of this research is a study of the feasibility and desirability of home care for the dying child.* Since 1972, 84 families who have had a child die from cancer participated in these studies. Over three fourths, or 60, of the children died at home with one or both parents having the role of primary caregiver to the dying child. Whatever technical procedures that were necessary for the care of the dying child were provided by the parents. The lone exception was the insertion of a Foley catheter. There was sufficient time prior to the death of the child to teach procedures to the parents. A home care nurse was also available for help if the parents felt this was needed.

The educational level of the parents in these 84 families ranged from eighth grade to college postgraduate degree. Economic status ranged from a single parent receiving welfare assistance to a family in the upper middle–income level. Family size ranged from zero to nine siblings. Several were single-parent families. Some had large extended families or community resources they were able to use. Other families had very few outside resources to call on for emotional, financial, or physical support. All of the families had the support of a home care nurse they could call at any time, 24 hours a day, 7 days a week. The option of the child's returning to the hospital was always available.

A result of this nursing research study appears to be that the two most important factors necessary for home care for a child dying of cancer are (1) the child's desires to be at home, and (2) the primary caregiver's perception of an ability to care for the child at home.

Two case studies are included that describe situations in which a mother has cared for her child at home until death occurred. The two

mothers are the first and last of the 84 families I personally provided with nursing support. One mother had no professional nursing experience and the other was a registered nurse.

CASE 1*

Emily Kulenkamp is the mother of Eric, who died in November 1972 at the age of 10. He had been diagnosed with acute lymphocytic leukemia 27 months prior to his death.

A few months ago I was asked, "What has been your greatest achievement in life?"
"Surviving the illness and death of my son," I replied.
"And your geatest disappointment?"
"Losing Eric."
I did not have to ponder my answer to either question but I had never before thought of how ironic it was that my greatest achievement and disappointment were closely tied together.

It had been a beautiful July day in the summer of 1970, the kind of day that compensates for long Minnesota winters. "The kids," as we usually referred to them—Eric, 7, and Betsy, 4—had been tucked into bed. Del, my husband, and I may not have counted our blessings that evening, but we had many times. After having slept peacefully for several hours, were awakened by a cry. "I hurt all over," Eric said, as I came to his bedside. Seeming particularly distressed, as we tried to soothe him he asked, "Mommy, am I going to die?" We took him to bed with us.

The next morning, Eric told us, "It felt like a giant worm crawled through my body."

Our pediatrician was not available, so Del carried Eric to another doctor's office without even attempting to make an appointment. The doctor examined Eric, took Del aside, and said, "He must be faking; he doesn't hurt in the right places."

The seed of doubt kept lurking in the background, with denial in the foreground, over the next four weeks, as we continued our search for an answer to Eric's ailments. Eric was finally admitted to the hospital for tests. It was suspected that he had either rheumatic fever or rheumatoid arthritis. I was very upset with the doctor's speculations but Del was somewhat relieved. "Thank God," he said, "I thought it was leukemia."

Acute lymphocytic leukemia. The diagnosis was made the next day. I had heard the word, knew it was some awful disease, but that was all that came to my mind. I can remember blasting at my sister, "Of all the rotten, stinking people in the world, why Eric?" And I thought, "Why me? How can I possibly survive without Eric?"

*Supported in part by funds from DHEW, National Cancer Institute, CA 19490.

At a conference following diagnosis, the disease was explained and we were told, upon asking, that Eric would probably live 2 to 2½ years. I could remember very little of what was said other than Eric would most likely die and some comments about our lives to come.

As I recall, the physician said, "You have two children, one that is going to live and one that is going to die. The one that is going to live is the most important." His words sounded simple enough at the time, reasonable, good advice to follow. But over the next years of illness, frustration, sometimes despair, we found it was not always an easy task treating our children equally, much less "the one that is going to live" as the most important. Our youngest, in those so vulnerable years, did not always get the love and attention that she so dearly needed and deserved. Our world began to revolve around Eric as hard as we tried not to make it seem that way. Part or all of one out of four days—over 200 in all—were spent with Eric either being hospitalized or at the outpatient clinic. At gatherings, Eric would be the center of attention and was showered with gifts, some from people we hardly knew. Betsy often seemed relegated to only being Eric's sister, hardly an entity on her own. She loved, admired, and depended on her older brother, but life was very confusing for her at times.

The doctor also said to make the most of the time we had—live life a day at a time. Some parents told him those last years were the best of their lives. Living a day at a time is a good way to live, and we did have some good times, but I am more thankful for the years previous to Eric's illness, as those last ones always had a cloud hovering over. I couldn't forget that our son had been given a death sentence. I grieved—anticipatory grief—and had nightmares of his funeral.

I had been thrown into a situation where the responsibility for my son's health was beyond that customary for a mother. The routines of caring for an ill child had taken a different overtone; the drugs I dispensed were much more potent than anything I had previously dealt with. There were side effects to watch for, symptoms to be aware of, all of which had to be related to the doctor in meaningful context. There were too many times when I didn't know whether physical disturbances were a natural or unnatural part of the disease process or a drug reaction. I found that telling a doctor my son's breathing was "short and fast" was much less impressive to him than when I related his respiration was in the 90s.

Six months before Eric died, the leukemia infiltrated the central nervous system for the third time in his illness, leaving him with hemiparesis. He improved some, for a while, and went on another series of chemotherapy, but then he began to go downhill again with more loss of function involving both sides.

Aggressive therapy was discontinued. Eric became bedridden, but we kept him at home.

No matter how many people are around, living with a dying child is in many ways a very lonely life. There are few who can accept the intensity of feelings that a parent goes through or who will acknowledge the fact that a loved one, especially a child, is dying.

When Ida Martinson became part of our life, we were constantly reassured that the care we gave Eric at home was comparable, if not better, than what he would receive in the hospital, and I desperately needed that encouragement. The thought of having Eric die at home wasn't the prime consideration at that point, and it would not have even been given any deliberation had she not gently brought up the possibility.

There were some difficult times, times when we really wondered whether what we were doing was right—keeping Eric at home—but it was what he wanted and we wanted and that made it right in itself.

Eric died November 21, 1972. Del and I had been with him, alternately, through the night. I was sitting on his bed, holding his hand, when Eric found peace.

Eric will always have a special place in my heart, but I have found that I can survive without my beloved son. It hasn't been easy, and there have been times when I really didn't care whether I survived or not. I am very proud to have been his mother, as I am of Betsy, a 12-year-strawberry blonde, and the light of my life.

CASE 2

Joyce Lindgren, a mother who is also a registered nurse, is from a small city, Olivia, in western Minnesota. Her husband is a Lutheran pastor. Her 18-year-old daughter, Brenda, died in June 1978 as a result of astrocytoma, which had been diagnosed 16 months prior to her death. There are nine other children in the family ranging in age from 19 to 4 years. The six youngest children have been adopted by the family. Three of the children are legally blind.

Joyce responds to a statement made in the manual on implementation of home care services that "occupation, education or religious belief, number of children in the home, marital status, etc., need not be a factor for implementation of home care services."[14]

I think one of the things that annoys me most is when I hear somebody putting labels on others and saying, "She's so busy she can't do that," or "This would never work for them because . . ." or "The reason it worked so well for her is because she was a registered nurse," or

"How could they possibly take care of her with all the kids they have?" I really believe that "a desire to have the child home and the perceived ability to care for the child are the two major criteria."[15]

My daughter had a very unrealistic faith in her mother because I am a registered nurse. She placed great emphasis on a lot of the mothering type things that I did at home for her. She felt it was because I am an R.N. that I was "doing it so good." I was quite aware of the fact that the majority of the things I did any mother could do. There really were very few things that I did for Brenda that any mother couldn't do; in fact there weren't any, because mothers can certainly be taught to give shots, too.

I looked at the home care nurse as a professional consultant. I wanted to be the one to make the decisions about my daughter and to give my daughter her shots. I wanted to be the one to talk to the doctors, unless I specifically asked the nurse to make a phone call. A couple of times on a weekend more medications were needed and the clinic doctors, who were familiar with the family and Brenda, were out of town. I did not feel emotionally up to dealing with a doctor that I didn't know very well. I called the nurse and said, "Look, I only have enough meperidine for one shot. Do you think you could get more for me?" And she got it for me.

We bought an intercom because Brenda wanted to stay in her bedroom which was down in the basement. She shared the room with her sister. I would have been in worse shape if it hadn't been for that intercom because I wouldn't have been getting enough sleep. I knew I could call her and she could call me. There were some nights when I had her keep the intercom open so that I could hear her when she turned around and moved. That really eased my mind a lot at night. The last two weeks of her life, I moved her up into the dining room. Her sister was on a canoeing trip, and I didn't want her alone. Brenda was not eager to make the move because she loved that bedroom. We made the dining room into a bedroom. There was a queen-sized hide-a-bed there. Brenda used the dining room table for all the stuff that she was working on. The piano and stereo were in there, and she got so she really enjoyed the room. She did not spend too much time in bed although she began to sleep more and more toward the last.

It was very comforting to me to be able to be the primary caregiver for my daughter; to give her her shots, to rub her back and to love her up. I slept with her on the hide-a-bed after she went into the coma. One of the intercoms was then plugged in by me and the other by my husband so that I could call him. This worked out effectively for us.

During this time, I didn't want a lot of people in the house. We live in a parsonage and people are used to coming in. Yet at this point I couldn't bear to share her with anybody. She was ours, and I didn't want people coming in and looking at her. I didn't think Brenda would want that either—I know Brenda would not have wanted that. I stopped at the doctor's office and said, "In the hospital sometimes you put notes up on doors 'No visitors, check at desk' or something. Could you do something like that on our front door?" He said, "I don't see any reason why not." So he wrote a note requesting that nobody come into the house without checking with one of the two doctors or the home care nurse and he put his home phone number on it. We were not bothered with numerous visitors after that. Our neighbor across the street said that many people came up, read the note, turned away and left. This was hard for some people to accept I think, but I felt we had a right to do that. This was our family and we were a family unit. We just locked our front door and used the side door so that we weren't seen going in and out.

The day after Brenda's death was an entirely different thing. I needed support then. There was nothing more that I could do for Brenda and that kind of support was helpful to me.

People were very supportive. They brought in meals for almost a month when she wasn't really all that sick and I could have done it. Actually it was me that was collapsing, not Brenda. It seemed, somehow, that I couldn't muster the energy to make the meals. This help was so appreciated.

One of the heavy burdens for me was the feeling of such major responsibility for meeting the emotional needs of the other children. Having Brenda at home helped immensely because they were able to verbalize with her as well as with me. She was adult enough to handle this. Having her at home seemed to reassure them a lot and seemed to make death a much less frightening thing and heaven more real to them.

We certainly realize that we're really only at the beginning stages of the grieving process. Even though we rejoice with Brenda in her new life, our grief is great. I'm sure there will be many times ahead which will be very rough.

CONCLUSION

As the case studies illustrate, mothers undergoing the difficulties of a child dying of cancer have demonstrated ability to care for their child at home.

It is important for those who work with mothers of dying children to recognize the strengths women have and to help these mothers build on these strengths and to support the decisions they make.

References

1. Moos, R. H., and Tsu, V. D. *The Crisis of Physical Illness: An Overview*. Stanford University Medical Center and Veterans' Administration Hospital, Palo Alto, CA, 1978, p. 7.
2. Knudson, A. G., and Matterson, J. M. Participation of parents in the hospital care of their fatally ill children. *Pediatrics*, vol. 26, 1970, p. 482.
3. Larson, André D. The family and the dying child. *Medical Times*, vol. 97, May 1969.
4. Binger, C. M., et al. Childhood leukemia: Emotional impact on patient and family. *New England Journal of Medicine*, vol. 280, February 1969, pp. 414–418.
5. Friedman, S. B., et al. Behavioral observation on parents anticipating the death of a child. *Pediatrics*, vol. 32, 1963, pp. 610–625.
6. Friedman, S. Care of the family of the child with cancer. *In* Green, M., and Haggerty, R. (eds.) *Ambulatory Pediatrics*. Philadelphia: W. B. Saunders Co., 1977.
7. Goldfogel, L. Working with the parent of a dying child. *American Journal of Nursing*, vol. 70, August 1970, pp. 1675–1679.
8. Bloom, G. E. The reactions of hospitalized children to illness. *Pediatrics* vol. 22, 1938, pp. 509–599.
9. Freund, Anna. The role of bodily illness in the mental life of children. *In* Eissler, R. S., et al. (eds.) *The Psychoanalysis Study of the Child*. New York: International University Press, 1952, pp. 69–81.
10. Pearson, G. H. L. Effect of operative procedures on the emotional life of the child. *American Journal Diseases of Children*, vol. 62, 1941, pp. 716–729.
11. Prugh, D. G. Investigations dealing with the reactions of children and families to hospitalization and illness. *In* Caplon, G. (ed.) *Emotional Problems of Early Childhood*. Basic Books, 1955, pp. 307–311.
12. Green, Morris. Care of the dying child. *Pediatrics*, vol. 40, September 1967.
13. Waechter, Eugenia H. Children's awareness of fatal illness. *American Journal of Nursing*, vol. 71, June 1971, pp. 1168–1172.
14. Martinson, I. M., et al. *Home Care: A Manual for Implementation of Home Care For Children Dying of Cancer*. School of Nursing, University of Minnesota, 1978, p. 6.
15. Ibid.

INDEX

Note: Page numbers in *italics* refer to illustrations. Page numbers followed by (t) refer to tables.